Pathophysiologic Principles of Urology

Pathophysiologic Principles of Urology

Grannum R. Sant, MD
Professor and Vice-Chairman
Department of Urology
Tufts University School of Medicine
Associate Urologist-in-Chief
New England Medical Center Hospitals
Boston, Massachusetts

BOSTON

Blackwell Scientific Publications
Oxford London Edinburgh Melbourne Paris Berlin Vienna

Blackwell Scientific Publications
EDITORIAL OFFICES:
238 Main Street, Cambridge, Massachusetts 02142, USA
Osney Mead, Oxford OX2 0EL, England
25 John Street, London WC1N 2BL, England
23 Ainslie Place, Edinburgh EH3 6AJ, Scotland
54 University Street, Carlton, Victoria 3053, Australia
Arnette SA, 1 rue de Lille, 75007 Paris, France
Blackwell-Wissenschaft, Düsseldorfer Str. 38, D-10707 Berlin, Germany
Blackwell MZV, Feldgasse 13, A-1238 Vienna, Austria

DISTRIBUTORS:
USA
Blackwell Scientific Publications
238 Main Street
Cambridge, Massachusetts 02142
(Telephone orders: 800-759-6102
or 617-876-7000)
Canada
Times Mirror Professional Publishing
130 Flaska Drive
Markham, Ontario L6G 1B8
(Telephone orders: 800-268-4178
or 416-470-6739)
Australia
Blackwell Scientific Publications (Australia)
Pty Ltd
54 University Street
Carlton, Victoria 3053
(Telephone orders: 03-347-5552)
Outside North America and Australia
Blackwell Scientific Publications, Ltd.
c/o Marston Book Services, Ltd.
P.O. Box 87
Oxford OX2 0DT
England
(Telephone orders: 44-865-791155)

Typeset by The Type Shoppe, Inc.
Printed and bound by BookCrafters

Printed in the United States of America
94 95 96 97 5 4 3 2 1

Library of Congress Cataloging-in-Publication Data

Pathophysiologic principles of urology / [edited by] Grannum R. Sant.
p. cm.
Includes bibliographical references and index.
ISBN 0-86542-221-4
1.. Urinary organs—Pathophysiology. I. Sant, Grannum R.
[DNLM: 1. Urologic Diseases—physiopathology. 2. Urogenital System—physiology. . WJ 100 P297 1994]
RC800.8.P38 1994
616.6'07—dc20
DNLM/DLC 83-42937
For Library of Congress CIP

Dedication

To my wife Kathleen
and children, Justin and Sinead,
for their enduring love and support
of my quest for continuous learning.

To my parents and teachers
who instilled into an early generation
of the Trinidadian diaspora
the study ethic of. . .

"The heights by great men,
reached and kept,
were not attained by sudden flight;
But they, while their companions slept,
were toiling upwards in the night. . ."
(H. W. Longfellow)

Contents

Contributors

Paul Abrams, M.D., FRCS, Consultant Urological Surgeon, Southmead General Hospital, Bristol, England

Anthony A. Caldamone, M.D., Professor of Surgery, Brown University Medical Center; Director of Pediatric Urology, Rhode Island Hospital, Providence, Rhode Island

Marc Cendron, M.D., Assistant Professor of Urology, Tufts University School of Medicine and Pediatric Urologist, Boston Floating Hospital for Infants and Children, Boston, Massachusetts

Christopher T. Coughlin, M.D., Professor of Medicine, Dartmouth Medical School; Radiation Oncologist, Dartmouth-Hitchcock Medical Center, Hanover, New Hampshire

Colin P. N. Dinney, M.D., Assistant Professor of Urology, University of Texas—M.D. Anderson Cancer Center, Houston, Texas

John M. Fitzpatrick, MCh, FRCSI, Professor of Surgery, University College, Dublin, Ireland; Consultant Urologist, Mater Misericordiae Hospital, Dublin, Ireland

Stuart M. Flechner, M.D., Staff Urologist, Department of Urology, Section of Renal Transplantation, Cleveland Clinic Foundation, Cleveland, Ohio

Simon C. W. Harrison, MA, MChir, FRCS, Consultant Urologist, Pinderfields Hospital, West Yorkshire, England

Joseph M. Hayes, M.D., Medical Director for the Carilion Transplant Center, Roanoake Memorial Hospital, Roanoake, Virginia

John A. Heaney, MB, FRCSI, FACS, Professor of Surgery (Urology), Dartmouth Medical School; Chief, Section of Urology, Dartmouth-Hitchcock Medical Center, Hanover, New Hampshire

Paul G. Horgan, MCh., FRCS, FRCSI, Lecturer in General Surgery, University College Dublin; Senior Registrar in Surgery, St. Vincent's Hospital, Dublin, Ireland

Prahalad Jajodia, M.D., Research Fellow, Department of Veteran Affairs Medical Center of San Francisco, San Francisco, California

George T. Klauber, M.D., Professor of Urology and Pediatrics, Tufts University School of Medicine and Chief of Pediatric Urology, Boston Floating Hospital for Infants and Children, Boston, Massachusetts

Michael O. Koch, M.D., Associate Professor of Urology, Vanderbilt University School of Medicine; Chief of Urology, National Veteran Affairs Hospital, Nashville, Tennessee

Badrinath Konety, M.D., Research Fellow, Department of Veteran Affairs Medical Center of San Francisco, San Francisco, California

Mary Lee, Pharm.D., Associate Professor of Pharmacy, University of Illinois at Chicago College of Pharmacy; Associate Professor of Surgery, University of Illinois at Chicago College of Medicine; Pharmacotherapist, University of Illinois Hospital; Clinical Pharmacist, West Side Veteran's Administration Hospital, Chicago, Illinois

John P. Long, M.D., Assistant Professor of Urology, Tufts University School of Medicine; Director of Urologic Oncology, New England Medical Center Hospitals, Boston, Massachusetts

Kevin R. Loughlin, M.D., Associate Professor of Surgery, Harvard Medical School; Urologic Surgeon, Brigham and Women's Hospital, Boston, Massachusetts

Tom F. Lue, M.D., Professor of Urology, University of California and Attending Urologist, University of California at San Francisco, San Francisco, California

Edwin M. Meares, Jr., M.D., Charles M. Whitney Professor and Chairman, Department of Urology, Tufts University School of Medicine; Urologist-in-Chief, New England Medical Center Hospitals, Boston, Massachusetts

Mani Menon, M.D., Professor of Surgery and Physiology, University of Massachusetts School of Medicine; Chairman, Department of Urology and Transplant Surgery, University of Massachusetts Medical Center, Worcester, Massachusetts

Perinchery Narayan, M.D., Associate Professor of Urology and Oncology, Co-Director, Section of Urology/Oncology, University of California at San Francisco; Chief of Urology, Department of Veteran Affairs Medical Center, San Francisco, California

Andrew C. Novick, M.D., Chairman, Department of Urology, Cleveland Clinic Foundation, Cleveland, Ohio

Michael P. O'Leary, M.D., M.P.H., Assistant Professor of Surgery, Division of Urological Surgery, Brigham and Women's Hospital and Harvard Medical School, Boston, Massachusetts

Howard M. Price, M.D., Assistant Professor of Urology, University of Massachusetts School of Medicine, University of Massachusetts Medical Center, Worcester, Massachusetts

John P. Pryor, MS, FRCS, Consultant Uroandrologist, King's College and St. Peter's Hospital, London, England

Jerome P. Richie, M.D., Elliott Carr Cutler Professor of Surgery and Chairman, Harvard Program in Urology, Harvard Medical School; Chief of Urology, Brigham and Women's Hospital, Boston, Massachusetts

Grannum R. Sant, M.D., FRCS (Ed), Professor and Vice-Chairman, Department of Urology, Tufts University School of Medicine; Associate Urologist-in-Chief, New England Medical Center Hospitals, Boston, Massachusetts

Roohollah Sharifi, M.D., Professor of Surgery/Urology, University of Illinois at Chicago Medical Center; Chief, Service of Urology, West Side Veteran's Administration Medical Center, Chicago, Illinois

R. Ernest Sosa, M.D., Associate Professor of Surgery, Department of Urology, New York Hospital-Cornell Medical Center, New York, New York

Robert A. Stephenson, M.D., Associate Professor of Surgery, Division of Urology, University of Utah, Salt Lake City, Utah

Notice

The indications and dosages of all drugs in this book have been recommended in the medical literature and conform to the practices of the general medical community. The medications described do not necessarily have specific approval by the Food and Drug Administration for use in the diseases and dosages for which they are recommended. The package insert for each drug should be consulted for use and dosage as approved by the FDA. Because standards of usage change, it is advisable to keep abreast of revised recommendations, particularly those concerning new drugs.

Preface

As a specialty, urology originated as a craft but current urologic practice is increasingly based on scientific principles. New developments in technology, therapeutics, diagnosis and treatment rely heavily on an understanding of the pathophysiology of urologic disease. Regrettably, much of the information relative to urologic pathophysiology is scattered throughout the literature.

This book is meant to complement rather than compete with the larger textbooks of urology. It emphasizes pathophysiologic concepts, correlates diagnostic testing with pathophysiology and documents the scientific basis for the treatment of the common diseases of the genitourinary tract. *Pathophysiologic Principles of Urology* bridges the gap between basic science and the clinical practice of urology by filling the existing void between large, standard texts and urologic journals.

It is my hope that urology residents and postgraduate trainees will find this book stimulating, informative and up-to-date. It should have primary appeal to individuals preparing for certification by the American Board of Urology, the Royal Colleges of Surgeons and other certifying bodies. Practicing urologists and medical students should also benefit from its emphasis on pathophysiologic concepts and treatment. As a concise reference to urologic disease, obstetricians, gynecologists, nephrologists and general surgeons should find it readable.

I would like to thank the contributors for the painstaking preparation of their manuscripts, their willingness to emphasize pathophysiologic principles and their acquiescence to my strict editing to ensure uniformity of the text.

With humility, I also thank my urologic mentors on both sides of the Atlantic: J. Dermot O'Flynn, M.D., FRCS, who initially kindled my interest in urology while I was a medical student, and Edwin M. Meares, Jr., M.D. who nurtured and facilitated my clinical training and academic career.

The need for this book grew out of many stimulating and challenging interactions with medical students, surgical residents and urology residents over the last ten years. Hopefully, this book is a testament to those who believe in its underlying premise—a concise, easily readable text dealing with urologic pathophysiology. My editors at Blackwell Scientific Publications, Mike Snider and Patricia Tyler, maintained their enthusiasm and vision for the book from its gestation to its final form. My loyal secretary, Susan Mayo, was a constant source of support throughout the genesis, editing and final word-processing phases of its preparation. My wife, Kathleen, was a bedrock of inspiration and the "wind beneath my wings" from inception to completion of this writing project.

Finally, I wish to acknowledge the lessons learned from my patients and teachers over the years. Through them, I have come to a better understanding of disease pathophysiology. It is my hope that the readers of this book will do likewise.

Grannum R. Sant

Pathophysiologic Principles of Urology

CHAPTER 1

Embryology

Anthony A. Caldamone

The embryologic development of the genitourinary tract is a complex yet integrated sequence of events. An understanding of embryology provides a clear understanding of many clinical problems encountered in urology. This understanding explains the associated disorders within the genitourinary tract and in related organ systems and provides the necessary background for a meaningful approach to diagnosis and management of congenital genitourinary disorders.

This chapter discusses the embryology of the various components of the genitourinary tract. Within each section, embryologic disorders are addressed in the hope of integrating embryologic events with clinical disorders.

SEXUAL DIFFERENTIATION

Normal and abnormal sexual differentiation are superb examples of how an understanding of embryology is absolutely necessary to approach and manage a group of complex and intriguing clinical disorders. Normal sexual differentiation is the result of an integrated sequence of events. When one or more of these steps are interrupted or interfered with, disorders of sexual differentiation result.

Sexual differentiation is a sequential process that can be divided into three stages. Jost established the sequence as follows: chromosomal sex is determined at fertilization and dictates the differentiation of the gonad (gonadal sex), which in turn dictates the phenotypic sex (differentiation of the internal ductal system and external genitalia) (Figure 1.1). The gonadal blastoma is undifferentiated until the sixth week of gestation, at which time differentiation occurs based on the chromosomal complement. The differentiated gonad, ovary or testis, directs the development of the internal ductal system and external genitalia, which is mediated by hormonal secretions.

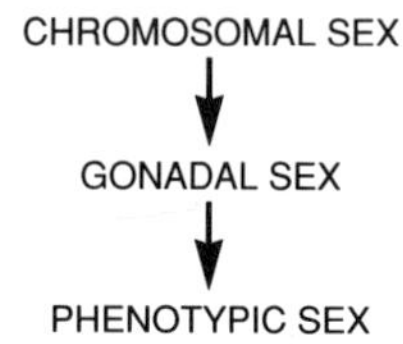

Figure 1.1: Sequential sexual differentiation

New genetic and biochemical technologies have advanced our understanding of the mechanisms responsible for sexual differentiation. Chromosomal sex is determined at the moment of conception by the sex chromosome complement of the fertilizing sperm. If this sperm carries an X chromosome, a 46XX complement results (normal female); if the sex chromosome is Y, a 46XY, or normal male genotype, results (Figure 1.2). While early experimental evidence pointed to the X chromosome as the sex-determining chromosome, later evidence indicated that the genetic information necessary for male sexual differentiation was located on the Y chromosome. The critical gene or genes, located close to the centromere on the short arm of the Y chromosome, express the H-Y (histocompatibility) antigen: a male-specific antigen located on the cell membrane of virtually all male tissues which is thought responsible for testicular differentiation from an undifferentiated gonad. Testicular differentiating factor (TDF), also produced by a gene on the short arm of chromosome Y, attaches to the surface of gonadal primordia to induce development into testes.

However, it is evident that in some clinical situations phenotypic female patients with 45X gonadal dysgenesis are H-Y antigen positive. In addition, there has been a report of an H-Y antigen negative patient with 45XO/46XY mixed gonadal dysgenesis and bilateral intra-abdominal testes. These factors have cast some doubt on the role of the H-Y antigen in sexual differentiation. More recent work by Page and his associates has identified a sequence of genes located on the distal portion of

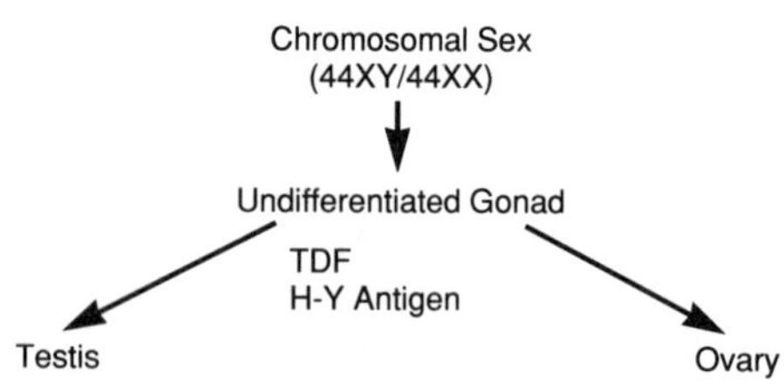

Figure 1.2: Sexual genotypic differentiation

the short arm of the Y chromosome. These genes encode a protein, testicular differentiating factor (TDF), which is thought to be the main determinant of testicular differentiation.

The gonad develops from both somatic and germ cells. The somatic cells are located at the ventral region of the mesonephros and arise from the mesonephric cells and the coelomic epithelium. Somatic cells become the Sertoli cells of the testis and granulosa cells of the ovary. The germ cells migrate from a more inferior position on the yolk sac to the genital ridge. Once the germ cells reach the gonadal ridge, they become surrounded by the somatic cells, which seem to regulate germ cell differentiation.

Prior to the seventh week of gestation, the gonad remains histologically undifferentiated. However, submicroscopic differentiation occurs. The predetermined testis grows at an accelerated rate compared to the predetermined ovary due to an increased number of cell divisions. Therefore, although there are no histological differences apparent until the seventh week of gestation, the growth rate of the fetal testis is more rapid than that of the fetal ovary. In contrast, ovarian histologic differentiation occurs later in gestation, usually about the twentieth week. The initial event is that of meiotic prophase, which is thought to be under the influence of elevated gonadotropins, somatic cell influences, or as yet undetermined factors. Most of these primordial germ cells are lost, because of the absence of a surrounding protective layer of follicular cells and stroma. The development of this protective layer is under the control of ovarian determining genes.

The gonadal sex is established by the seventh week of gestation. Differentiation of the internal ductal system and the external genitalia is based on the gonadal sex. At this stage the fetus contains two internal ductal systems (wolffian and müllerian), and an undifferentiated external genital primordia recognized as protuberances anterolateral to the cloacal membrane. Both internal ductal systems are derived from the mesonephric system. The wolffian, or mesonephric, duct is a tubular structure that connects the capillary network of the mesonephros to the urogenital sinus. Evagination of the coelomic epithelium leads to formation of a second tubular structure adjacent to the mesonephric duct, the paramesonephric, or müllerian, duct. The distal ends of these two ducts are joined. In some way, the wolffian duct is essential for müllerian duct development. That portion of the urogenital sinus distal to the termination of these ducts contributes to external genital development, whereas the proximal portion develops into the bladder, trigone, and posterior urethra.

Phenotypic sexual differentiation is predicated on establishment of gonadal sex. If an ovary develops, the wolffian duct involutes and only its terminal portion persists as Gartner's duct. Some of the mesonephric excretory tubules and a portion of the wolffian duct form the epoöphoron in the mesovarium. The müllerian ducts develop into the proximal vagina, uterus, and fallopian tubes (Figure 1.3).

The cephalic portion of the müllerian ducts form the fallopian tubes, while the caudal ends fuse to form the uterus. The union of the fused caudal ends of the müllerian ducts and urogenital sinus forms the vagina. The proximal two-thirds of the vagina is of müllerian-duct origin and the distal one-third of urogenital-sinus origin. The exact role that ovarian development and secretion play in female phenotypic differentiation is uncertain. Because ovarian development lags somewhat behind genital development and female phenotypic development occurs in cases of gonadal agenesis regardless of the chromosomal complement, the ovaries may not play the critical determining role in early female differentiation. It is possible that this process occurs under the influence of the high estrogen milieu from the placenta and maternal circulation. However, estrogen and progestin secretion by the ovary is more active in the development of the secondary sexual structures later in fetal development.

The vagina develops from the müllerian duct, wolffian duct, and urogenital sinus. A protuberance (urethrovaginal plate) between the distal terminations of the müllerian ducts into the urogenital sinus is apparent at the 9-week stage. Proliferation of this urethrovaginal plate occurs, causing the uterus and urogenital sinus to separate; by 20 weeks canalization of the vagina is complete. The lateral genital swellings enlarge to form the

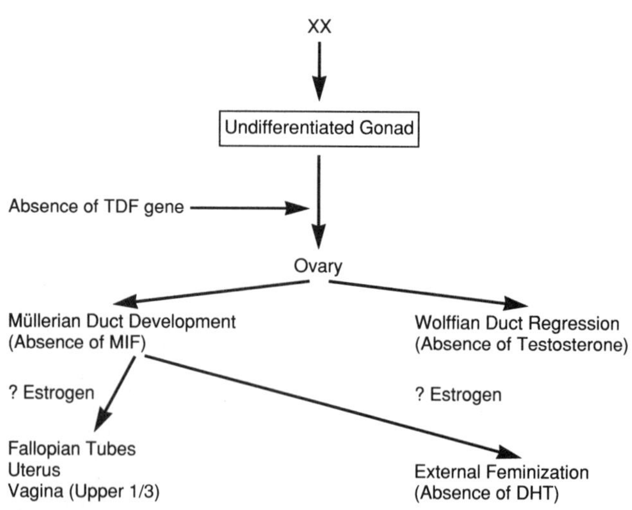

Figure 1.3: Female ductal system development

labia majora and fuse inferiorly, forming the posterior forchette; the genital fold remains separate and becomes the labia minora.

Male phenotypic differentiation is the result of the elaboration of two distinct testicular hormones, testosterone and müllerian inhibiting factor (MIF) (Figure 1.4). These are produced and secreted by the 8-week stage of development, and are essential for normal male differentiation. Involution of the müllerian ducts is caused by MIF, which is secreted by the fetal Sertoli cells. The remnants of the müllerian ducts persist caudally as the prostatic utricle and cephalically as the appendix testis. The absence of MIF results in a disorder (hernia uterus inguinali) in which a phenotypic and chromosomal male also has a uterus and fallopian tube. MIF exerts its action unilaterally and locally rather than bilaterally via the circulation.

Immediately after müllerian duct regression, the wolffian ducts develop under the influence of testosterone secreted by the fetal Leydig cells. This occurs at 9 to 10 weeks of gestation. The wolffian ducts evolve into the epididymis, vas deferens, and seminal vesicles. This process occurs as a direct action of testosterone on the ductal structures. By the twelfth week of gestation, virilization relies on the ability of the tissues involved to convert testosterone into a more potent androgen, dihydrotestosterone. The cytoplasm of the target cells possesses the enzyme 5-alpha-reductase, which is necessary for this conversion. Dihydrotestos-

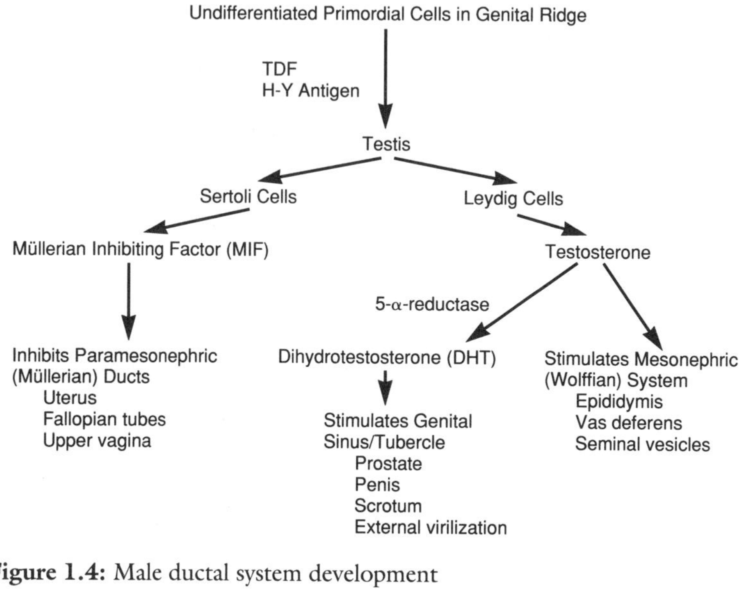

Figure 1.4: Male ductal system development

terone binds to a cytoplasmic receptor and is transported to the cell nucleus, where it acts on deoxyribonucleic acid to direct the formation of various proteins necessary for virilization of the external genitalia. It is unclear whether testosterone synthesis from the fetal testis is dependent on gonadotropins or whether it is an intrinsic function of the fetal testis. The ductal remnants (müllerian and wolffian) seen in both sexes are listed in Figure 1.5. A summary of the various mechanisms involved in sexual differentiation is provided in Table 1.1.

Disorders of Sexual Differentiation

Intersexuality results from overandrogenization of the female or underandrogenization of the male. These processes result from events occurring at the chromosomal, gonadal, or phenotypic stages of development. Not all intersex states lead to ambiguous genitalia. Intersex conditions in which chromosomal, gonadal, or internal phenotypic disorders do not affect external phenotypic expression may be accompanied by normal-appearing external genitalia. In some disorders with normal external genitalia, the internal ductal system is either poorly developed or develops along lines inconsistent with external genital and sexual differentiation. Such patients may have infertility, delayed puberty, primary amenorrhea, inguinal hernia with müllerian contents in a phenotypic male, or inguinal hernia with a gonad in a phenotypic female.

Disorders of chromosomal sex occur when either the number or structure of each of the sex chromosomes is abnormal. These include Klinefelter's syndrome, 46XX male (sex reversal syndrome), gonadal dysgenesis (Turner's syndrome), mixed gonadal dysgenesis, and true her-

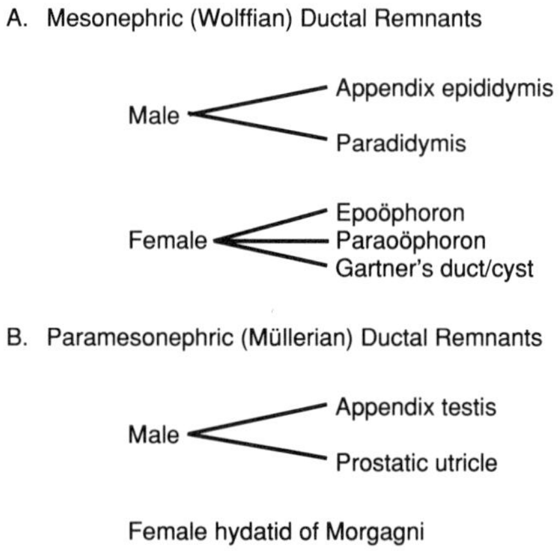

Figure 1.5: Ductal remnants

Table 1.1: Sexual Differentiation: A Summary

Embryonic gonad has inherent tendency to become an ovary, in absence of testicular differentiating factor (TDF)

Embryonic testis imposes masculinity, represses femininity

Mesonephric (wolffian) ductal system
- Male reproductive system
- Mostly disappears in female

Paramesonephric (müllerian) ductal system
- Female reproductive system
- Few vestigial remnants in male
- Inhibited by müllerian inhibiting factor from testis

Testicular differentiation
- Testicular differentiating factor (TDF) from gene on short arm of chromosome Y
- H-Y (histocompatibility) antigen on chromosome Y

maphroditism. The common denominator in disorders of chromosomal sex is an abnormality of the structure or number of sex chromosomes or of the autosomal chromosome that is responsible for differentiation of the gonad into an ovary or testis. For example, in the 46XX male syndrome a defect in production of antigens is responsible for testis differentiation. Gonadal dysgenesis (45XO), mixed gonadal dysgenesis (46XY/45XO), and Klinefelter's syndrome (47XXY) are all characterized by an abnormality in the sex chromosome number. The exact mechanism responsible for gonadal development in true hermaphroditism is poorly understood, because many genetic patterns have been described, including 46XX (most common), 46XY, and various mosaicisms. It is thought that testis development in true hermaphroditism in which no Y chromosome is present is probably derived from translocated genetic material from a Y chromosome. Alternatively, differential growth rates of the undifferentiated gonad may lead to development of a testis on one side and an ovary on the other. The gonad with accelerated growth forms a testis despite the presence or absence of testis-determining antigens.

Disorders of gonadal sex are caused by abnormalities of gonadal development in which the chromosomal sex does not correlate with the gonadal or phenotypic sex. These disorders include pure gonadal dysgenesis, either 46XY or 46XX, and gonadal agenesis (testicular regression). Pure gonadal dysgenesis occurs in phenotypic females with streak gonads who lack the somatic features of gonadal dysgenesis (Turner's syndrome) and who may have either a 46XX or 46XY complement. Regardless of the chromosomal complement, a female phenotype develops with a rudimentary internal müllerian ductal system as a result of failure of gonadal development.

Absent testis syndrome, or gonadal agenesis, is a disorder in which variable amounts of MIF and testosterone are produced for variable periods during fetal development. At one end of the spectrum is the 46XY phenotypic male with bilateral anorchia, absence of müllerian structures, and external virilization. In contrast, there are patients in whom very little testosterone is produced, resulting in the 46XY phenotypic female with absent gonads and absence of müllerian and wolffian derivatives. Such a defect occurs at the time between the development of Sertoli cells and Leydig cells because MIF, but not testosterone, is synthesized.

Disorders of phenotypic sex are those syndromes in which a normal chromosomal complement and appropriate gonadal development are seen; however, the phenotypic expression is either incomplete or in contradistinction to the chromosomal and phenotypic sex. These syndromes are categorized into female and male pseudohermaphroditism.

Female pseudohermaphroditism, or virilization of a 46XX patient with ovaries, is caused by one of two conditions: endogenous androgen production (congenital adrenal hyperplasia, maternal virilizing tumor) or exogenous androgen administration. Congenital adrenal hyperplasia is an inherited disorder in which one of five enzymes responsible for the production of cortisol from cholesterol is deficient (Figure 1.6). Androgen synthesis shares the initial three steps of this pathway. A deficiency of the two enzymes responsible for glucocorticoid synthesis (21-hydroxylase and 11-beta-hydroxylase) affects only hydrocortisol production. Lack of hydrocortisol induces increased production of adrenocorticotropin hormone, which in turn forces the steroid pathway toward increased production of adrenal androgens. Deficiencies of the proximal three enzymes in the pathway (20,22-desmolase, 3-beta-hydroxysteroid dehydrogenase, 17-hydroxylase) affect both glucocorticoid and androgen production, leading to congenital adrenal hyperplasia and undervirilization of the male. In the female, therefore, normal ovaries, müllerian structures, and varying degrees of external virilization are found, depending on the severity of the enzyme deficiency.

Other causes of female pseudohermaphroditism are rare in comparison to congenital adrenal hyperplasia. Maternal ingestion of certain progestins used to maintain pregnancy may cause external virilization; however, it is usually not seen to the same degree as occurs in congenital adrenal hyperplasia. This is also true for maternal virilizing tumors, for example, arrhenoblastomas or luteomas.

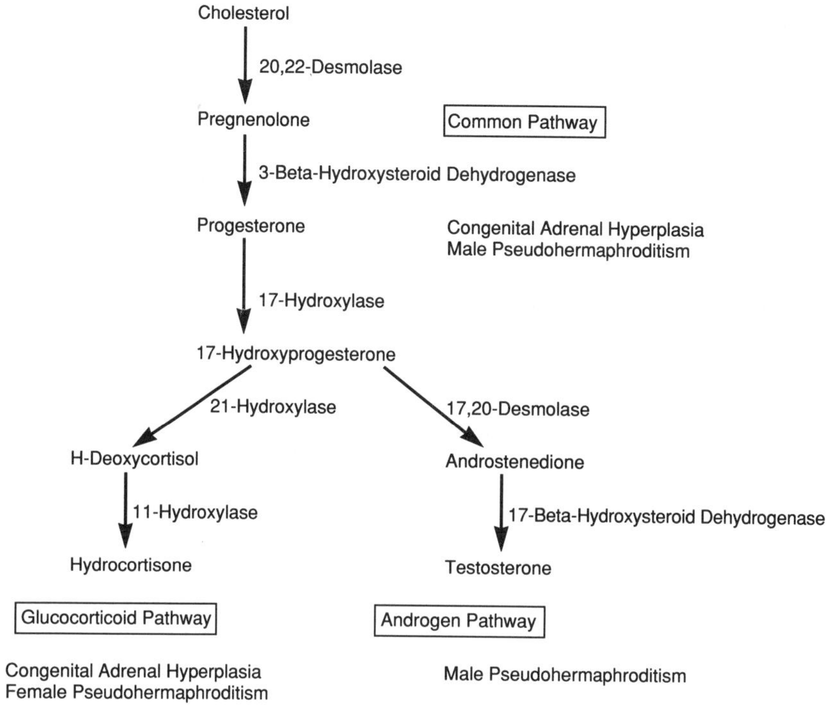

Figure 1.6: Intersex disorders and steroid synthesis

Male pseudohermaphroditism, or inadequate virilization of the 46XY male with normal testes, is the result of one of the following: (1) deficient MIF (hernia uteri inguinali), (2) defective androgen synthesis (five enzymatic steps), (3) defective androgen action, or (4) deficiency of 5-alpha-reductase (pseudovaginal perineoscrotal hypospadias).

Deficiency of MIF leads to persistent müllerian duct syndrome. These 46XY males are fully virilized because testosterone is produced normally; however, they have either unilateral or bilateral fallopian tubes, a uterus, and the upper third of the vagina. This is thought to occur because of deficient MIF production by the fetal testis or inability of the müllerian ducts to respond to MIF.

A defect in one of five enzymatic steps in the synthesis of testosterone from cholesterol leads to deficient androgen production. As noted, the initial three enzymatic steps are common to adrenal glucocorticoid synthesis as well; therefore, a deficiency in one of these initial enzymes results in congenital adrenal hyperplasia in an undervirilized male.

Androgen insensitivity of defective androgen action is a result of a deficiency of the cytoplasmic receptor protein needed to transport dihydrotestosterone into the cell nucleus to mediate virilization. The same, or a similar, protein is necessary to transport testosterone into the nucleus to stimulate spermatogenesis. The result is an undervirilized male with normal testes. The degree of undervirilization depends on the degree of deficiency of the androgen-binding protein. When severe deficiency is present, the external genitalia are completely feminized with a short vagina, no internal müllerian structures, and intra-abdominal testes (complete testicular feminization). These patients present with either a palpable inguinal testis in a hernia sac or primary amenorrhea. Incomplete forms of testicular feminization are also seen, although they are much less frequent. Incomplete forms may be seen as mild virilization of what appears to be female genitalia (Lubs syndrome) or infertility because of azoospermia (infertile male syndrome).

Lack of 5-alpha-reductase in target cells results in a failure of conversion of testosterone to dihydrotestosterone, which causes undervirilization of the external genitalia. The wolffian ductal system, because of adequate testosterone production and action, develops normally. The syndrome is sometimes referred to descriptively as pseudovaginal perineoscrotal hypospadias. Such children appear feminized with a mild degree of clitoral hypertrophy. Most are assigned a female gender and may not be seen by a physician unless a testis is palpable inguinally or masculinization occurs at puberty because of increased testosterone production.

DEVELOPMENT OF THE URETHRA

Posterior Urethra

The urorectal septum grows caudally to reach the cloacal membrane and, in so doing, divides the cloaca into anterior urogenital and posterior hindgut portions. During this process the wolffian ducts, which entered the primitive cloaca, become incorporated into the ventral wall of the urorectal septum, forming Müller's tubercle. The portion of the urogenital sinus that is proximal to Müller's tubercle forms the entire urethra in the female and the prostatic urethra in the male. The more proximal portion of the urogenital sinus just distal to the tubercle develops longitudinal striations in its lateral walls extending from the tubercle to the site of origin of Cowper's glands in the male and Bartholin's gland in the female. In the male, these folds persist as the plicae colliculi in the posterolateral urethral wall.

The embryologic basis for the four types of posterior urethral valves is variable. Type I valves consist of posterior mucosal leaflets that originate distal to the verumontanum and fuse anteriorly to a variable degree, thereby creating an elliptical opening that is widest proximally. Tolmatschen proposed that these valves are an exaggeration of the normal urethrovaginal folds. Stephens believes that an abnormal junction of the wolffian duct and the urogenital sinus results in persistence of the distal portion of the wolffian duct and type I valves.

Type II valves are urethral folds originating at the verumontanum and diverging toward the bladder neck. These are commonly seen in association with type I valves and are not considered obstructive. Type III valves represent either a severe form of type I valves with extensive anterior and posterior fusion or a congenital urethral membrane. They occur in either the membranous or proximal bulbous urethra and may appear as a diaphragm with a central lumen, or as a redundant membrane that prolapses into the bulbous urethra ("windsock"). Type III valves may be caused by a persistence of urogenital membrane, the anterior portion of the cloacal membrane. Thickening of the urogenital membrane, because of an abnormal amount of mesoderm between the epithelial layers, would impede dissolution and result in type III valves.

Stephens described a type IV urethral valve, characterized by a deep infold of the anterior and anterolateral urethral walls, that overrides the lumen of the membranous urethra. These folds are noted on voiding cystourethrography in some children with prune-belly syndrome.

Anterior Urethra

During the fourth week of gestation, paired swellings appear anterolateral to the cloacal membrane; they later fuse in the midline to form the genital tubercle. The phallic portion of the urogenital sinus (the anterior portion of the cloaca) remains undifferentiated between the fifth and tenth weeks of gestation. The urethral and genital folds are formed from the posterolateral anal tubercles and the lateral mesoderm. The mesodermal components convert testosterone to dihydrotestosterone and allow external virilization. The phallic portion (bulbar and penile) of the urogenital sinus near the urogenital membrane and the proximal portion near the bladder become the posterior urethra. The primary urethral groove forms from elongation of the urogenital sinus outward onto the ventral phallic surface. The anterior walls of the urogenital sinus converge to form an endodermal urethral plate. The urogenital sinus then disintegrates, to expose the urethral groove. Under the influence of testosterone and dihydrotestosterone, the genital tubercle enlarges, causing elongation of the phallus and extension of the urethral groove to the level of the corona. The penile urethra is tubularized by fusion of the endodermal edges of the urethral groove. The ectodermal edges fuse to create the median raphe. External genital virilization is under the influence of dihydrotestosterone.

The glandular urethra appears during the fourth month of gestation. The exact mechanism of its development remains controversial. It is thought by some that the glandular urethra forms in the same manner as the bulbous and penile urethra. Others believe that the glandular ectoderm forms a solid core of tissue that joins the penile urethra formed by closure of the urethral groove. It has been proposed that canalization of this core by epithelial ingrowth forms the distal urethra. The point at which the penile and glandular portions of the urethra meet is the fossa navicularis. The coalescence of mesenchyme dorsal to the urethra forms the corporal bodies and neurovascular channels. The mesenchyme is also responsible for the development of Buck's fascia, dartos fascia, and the corpus spongiosum. The labioscrotal swellings migrate medially and fuse at the base of the penis, to form the scrotum.

Hypospadias mechanically results from failure of fusion of the endodermal edges of the urethral groove (urethral folds) at variable levels between the perineum and distal penile shaft. Distal shaft, coronal, and glandular hypospadias may be caused by anomalous canalization of the glans penis. Formation of the glandular urethra is a relatively late embryologic event compared to renal development, and this accounts for the infrequent association of upper tract anomalies with distal hypospadias. Biochemically, any defect that results in inadequate androgen synthesis (testosterone or dihydrotestosterone) or defective androgen action (androgen receptor deficiency) may lead to hypospadias. This need not be a continuous deficiency; rather, the deficiency must be manifest at the appropriate gestational time corresponding to genital differentiation. Attempts have been made to determine androgen receptor and 5-alpha-reductase levels in penile tissue obtained from hypospadiac patients, but the results have been conflicting. Progesterone administration during pregnancy can be associated with hypospadias.

DEVELOPMENT OF THE BLADDER

The body of the bladder is derived principally from the anterior portion of the cloaca following separation of the cloaca into anterior and posterior sections by the urorectal septum. The base of the bladder and trigone are derived from the distal ends of the wolffian duct: the common excretory duct. The cloaca is a pouch having a short extension to the caudal portion of the embryo, the tail gut; it receives in its cephalad portion the allantoic duct and the hindgut. The cloacal membrane regresses as the mesoderm migrates from medial and caudal directions, leaving only the lower two-thirds of the cloaca covered anteriorly by the cloacal membrane. Mesodermal migration proceeds to form the anterior abdominal wall. Impediment to this migration results in lateral displacement of the musculoskeletal elements of the abdominal wall.

This mesenchymal plate migrates between the endodermal and ectodermal layers of the cloaca. These lateral ridges proliferate and fuse to form the genital tubercle. Enlargement of the genital tubercle is accompanied by outward migration of the cloacal membrane, which forms the floor of the phallus and later becomes the urethral groove (see section on development of the urethra). As this process occurs, the cloaca becomes divided by the urorectal septum, which migrates in a cephalad to caudad direction. The anterior portion of the cloaca forms the bladder and the posterior portion the hindgut. The residual communication between the anterior and posterior portions of the cloaca is a narrow channel called the cloacal duct of Reichel. Persistence of this duct, as occurs in imperforate anus, results in a urethrorectal or vesicorectal fistula. The urinary tract becomes separated from the hindgut when the advancing urorectal septum reaches the cloacal membrane. The anterior cloacal membrane, or urogenital membrane, perforates to establish the urogenital orifice. In the female, the urogenital canal shortens, allowing for separate urethral and müllerian duct openings. In the male, the urogenital sinus progressively lengthens.

The urachus is derived from the allantoic duct and bladder. The bladder retains its connection to the umbilicus through its communication with the allantoic duct. This duct undergoes complete obliteration during development of the bladder. Except for the portion closest to the umbilicus, the urachus is felt to be derived primarily from the apex of the bladder.

The wolffian ducts enter the posterolateral wall of the cloaca. The ureter arises as a bud off the wolffian ducts at a specified point just cranial to the cloaca. The segment of the wolffian duct between the urogenital sinus and the ureteric bud is termed the common excretory duct. The ostia of the wolffian ducts migrate caudally to take position at the müllerian tubercle of the urogenital sinus, absorbing the common excretory duct, and the ureteric bud migrates cephalad, forming the trigone.

Agenesis of the Bladder

Agenesis of the bladder is one of the rarest anomalies of the urinary tract. Only 37 patients have been reported in the literature, 29 of whom were stillborn; 7 of the 8 survivors were female. The exact embryogenesis is not clear. If other associated anorectal malformations are present, persistence of the cloaca and failure of urogenital sinus development result in the ureteric orifices terminating in the rectum. Failure of the lower portions of the mesonephric ducts to form the trigone and proximal urethra is a likely sequence, leading to bladder agenesis. In the female, because the müllerian duct structures are likely to develop normally, the ureteric orifices end in the uterus, anterior vaginal wall, or vestibule. The ureters may remain separate or form a common channel. The upper tracts are often hydronephrotic and dysplastic.

Anomalies of Bladder Compartmentalization

Anomalies of bladder formation occur during the fifth to seventh weeks of gestation, the time corresponding to the early stages of bladder development. Various theories of embryogenesis for these rare anomalies have been proposed. A sagittally oriented urorectal septum or supernumerary urorectal septa may divide the cloaca into four parts, thereby dividing both the bladder and hindgut into two compartments each. This accounts for the association of bladder and hindgut duplications. Other theories for bladder septation include fusion of redundant mucosal folds during early intrauterine life; persistence of Chwalle's membrane in duplicated ureteric systems, resulting in a multilocular bladder; and unequal growth rates of ectodermal and mesodermal bladder components, causing the "hourglass" bladder.

Anomalies of the Urachus

As the urachus develops, it loses its attachment to the umbilicus. Differential growth rates of the urachus and anterior abdominal wall, along with bladder descent, produce four anatomic variants of urachal termination. In type I, the urachus fails to atrophy, retains its attachments to the bladder dome and umbilicus, and is separate from each umbilical artery. The remaining variants are formed when the upper portion atrophies as the urachus fails to grow commensurately with the anterior abdominal wall. In type II, the urachus merges with one or the other of the umbilical arteries and continues as a single structure to the umbilicus. In type III, a common ligament to the umbilicus is formed by the merging of the umbilical arteries and urachus. In type IV, the urachus forms an atrophied tube that terminates before fusing with the umbilical arteries to form the plexus of Luschka. If a type I variant remains patent through all or part of its length, a patent urachus, umbilicourachal sinus, or alternating sinus can result. Because of their blind umbilical termination, types II and III may result in a urachal cyst, urachal sinus, or vesicourachal diverticulum.

Exstrophy-Epispadias Complex

The embryologic basis for the development of bladder exstrophy is based on experimental work of Muecke. Exstrophy was produced in the chick embryo by inhibiting anterior cloacal membrane formation by inserting a plastic wedge above the cloacal membrane. A persisting cloaca, or an abnormally large cloaca that does not retract normally toward the perineum, accounts for bladder exstrophy and its variants. This wedge effect prevents medial mesenchymal ingrowth, causing the future abdominal wall to remain lateral. With dehiscence of the cloacal membrane in the ninth week, the posterior surface of the bladder becomes exposed to the exterior on the surface of the abdominal wall. The infraumbilical membrane is absent, causing the umbilicus to be adjacent to the bladder wall. The urogenital groove also fails to form, creating the associated epispadias. The corpora of the phallus assume a more widely divergent course proximally. The paired genital tubercles fuse inferiorly, leaving the urethral groove anterior.

If dehiscence of the cloacal membrane occurs after the urorectal septum has completed its partitioning of the cloaca, bladder exstrophy results (Figure 1.7). However, if this dehiscence occurs prior to division of the

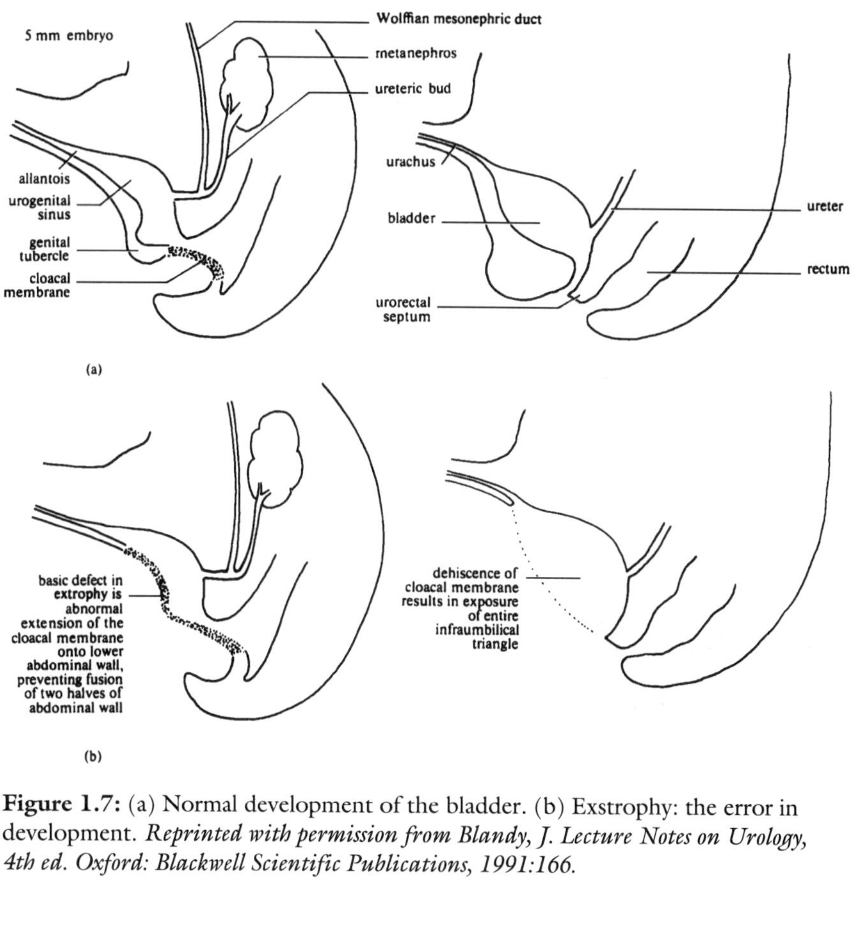

Figure 1.7: (a) Normal development of the bladder. (b) Exstrophy: the error in development. *Reprinted with permission from Blandy, J. Lecture Notes on Urology, 4th ed. Oxford: Blackwell Scientific Publications, 1991:166.*

cloaca, the hindgut becomes exposed as well, separating the bladder into two halves with the hindgut between them, leading to cloacal exstrophy. Epispadias results if the cloacal membrane persists only inferiorly, whereas a superior vesical fissure results if the persistence is superior.

Mesodermal invasion of the infraumbilical membrane may be merely delayed rather than entirely absent, so that secondary closure of the parietes occurs before formation of the exstrophy. Such development produces covered exstrophy. Rarely, sequestration includes portions of viscera not ordinarily involved in exstrophy.

DEVELOPMENT OF THE URETER AND TRIGONE

The ureteral bud appears as an outpouching from the caudal end of the mesonephric duct at the seventh week of gestation. The ureter goes through a stage between days 37 and 40 of loss of lumen throughout most of its length, with sparing of the proximal and distal ends. It then progressively recanalizes, beginning with the midsection. Rapid elongation of the ureter may be the cause of loss of patency. It is thought that hydrostatic pressure from the mesonephric secretion of urine may contribute to the recanalization process. The ureter elongates out of proportion to renal ascent, resulting in fetal folds. Postnatally, the growth rate of the infant exceeds that of ureteral lengthening, thus straightening the ureter. It is possible that persistence of these infoldings when fixed by ureteral adventitia may lead to valvelike obstruction.

The relationship between the ureteral bud and the mesonephric duct explains many of the congenital anomalies associated with the ureteral orifice. The ureteral bud originates from the mesonephric duct at a relatively fixed site. The portion of the mesonephric duct between the ureteral bud and urogenital sinus is termed the common excretory duct. This segment, a precursor of the trigone and bladder neck, contributes to its muscularization as it becomes absorbed into the urogenital sinus. The orifice of the mesonephric duct migrates caudally and the ureteral bud cranially. While this opposed migration occurs, rotation takes place. Initially, the ureteral bud is located medial and distal with respect to the mesonephric duct, which becomes the seminal vesicles, vas deferens, and epididymis. As the ureteral bud migrates cephalad and laterally, the mesonephric duct crosses over the ureter, migrating medially and caudally. The final position of these two structures is about equidistant from the bladder neck.

Vesicoureteral Reflux

Primary vesicoureteral reflux results when a ureteral bud forms from a more caudal site on the mesonephric duct (i.e., closer to the urogenital sinus) and leads to a foreshortened common excretory duct. The shorter common excretory duct is absorbed sooner, allowing the ureter to migrate more cranially and laterally, further separating it from the mesonephric duct. A wider trigone develops with deficient muscle, as there is less mesenchyme contributed by the common excretory duct. The final product is a ureteral orifice that lies more lateral and superior than normal. It is poorly fixed to the trigone, causing a shortened submucosal ureteral tunnel.

Ureteral Ectopia

If the ureteral bud forms at a more cranial position on the mesonephric duct, a longer than normal common excretory duct results. The ureter will then migrate for a longer time attached to the mesonephric duct before separating as the longer common excretory duct is completely absorbed. This leaves little or no opportunity for the ureter to migrate separately from the mesonephric duct. When the ureteral bud arises only slightly higher than normal on the mesonephric duct, the ureteral orifice assumes its final position closer to the bladder neck. In a more cephalad outpouching of the ureteral bud, it may terminate in the urethra, or in the male, it may maintain its attachment to the mesonephric duct connecting with the seminal vesicle or vas deferens. In the female the ureter may end in the urethra or in the distal remnant of the mesonephric duct, Gartner's duct, which extends from the uterine broad ligament along the lateral vagina wall down to the hymen (Figure 1.8).

With a more cephalad outpouching of the ureteral bud, separation from the mesonephric duct does not occur, resulting in a ureter that drains into the genital tract in either sex. The major difference between the two sexes is that, in the male, the sites of ectopia all lie cephalad to the level of the external sphincter; therefore, incontinence does not occur (Table 1.2). In the female, however, an ectopic ureter may terminate distal to the sphincter mechanism and result in constant urinary leakage.

With bilateral ureteral ectopia from single systems in which the ureters end distal to the bladder neck, the bladder is poorly developed and small in capacity. This is the result of two factors: (1) urine never fills the bladder, and (2) the trigone and bladder neck never develop because muscularization is dependent on mesenchyme from the common excretory duct. As a result, children tend to be incontinent when the ureters are simply reimplanted in the bladder.

Duplication Anomalies of the Ureter

Complete ureteral duplication as a result of two separate ureteral buds follows the Weigert-Meyer law (Table 1.2). This states that the bud clos-

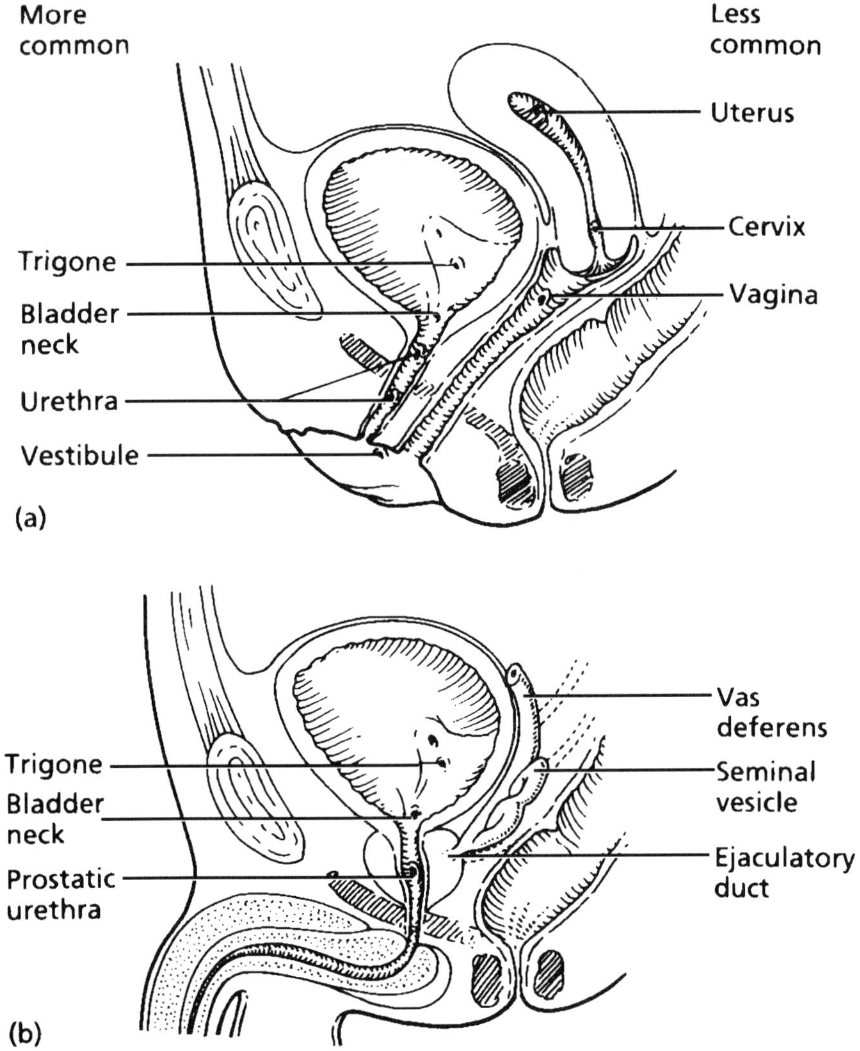

Figure 1.8: Locations in which an ectopic orifice can be, located. (a) In the female; (b) in the male. *Reproduced with permission from Webster G, Kirby K, King L, et al eds. Reconstructive Urology Vol 1. Boston: Blackwell Scientific Publications, 1993:369.*

est to the urogenital sinus, the first to migrate, is the lower pole ureter. The more cephalad bud, maintaining its contact with the mesonephric duct for a longer period of time, is the upper pole ureter. On the trigone, the lower pole orifice is more lateral and the upper more medial.

Table 1.2: Duplication, Ectopic Ureters

Weigert-Meyer law
Opening ectopic ureters outside bladder
Male
Posterior urethra
Ejaculatory duct
Seminal vesicle
Vas deferens
Female
Urethra
Vagina
Vulva

Exceptions to the Weigert-Meyer law occur if, rather than two separate buds originating from the mesonephric duct, a single bud divides immediately and leads to complete duplication. If both buds are within the normal region for outpouching on the mesonephric duct, no pathologic consequences ensue.

If one ureteral bud arises in a normal location but the other is in a more caudal position, complete duplication with reflux into the more caudal bud occurs. This bud is carried more superior and lateral on the bladder wall, accounting for reflux; because of its original position of outpouching on the ureteral bud, it corresponds to the lower pole ureter. On the other hand, if one bud is in a normal position and a second takes off cephalad to the normal zone (upper pole ureter), an ectopic ureter to the upper pole results. This accounts for the clinical observations in duplicated systems of a high incidence of reflux into the lower pole and ureteral ectopia of the upper pole.

In either complete or incomplete ureteral duplication, if one ureteral bud or a branch thereof does not reach the metanephric blastema, a blind-ending ureter results, sometimes referred to as a ureteral diverticulum.

The position of the ureteral bud on the mesonephric duct and the development off renal hypodysplasia are closely associated. Mackie and Stephens proposed that the nephrogenic ridge contains blastema with varying potential for normal renal development. The central zone, the area normally contacted by the ureteric bud, has the best potential for normal nephron induction. This potential is less in the peripheral zones. The ureteral bud that initiates from an abnormal position on the mesonephric duct may strike the blastema away from the central zone, and therefore induce abnormal renal formation. This would explain the high incidence of dysplasia found in upper pole segments of duplicated systems, and dysplasia associated with reflux from an abnormally placed lower pole ureteral orifice.

Ureterocele

The exact embryologic events leading to ureterocele formation are incompletely understood. The traditional theory involves a delayed rupture of Chwalle's membrane, a two-cell ureteric membrane that is present at the time of budding of the ureter from the mesonephric duct. Persistence of this membrane after urine excretion begins could lead to ureteral obstruction and dilatation. This obstructive theory would fit with the clinical observation that many ureteroceles have a stenotic orifice. In other ureteroceles, however, the orifice is patulous or the ureter is blind-ending: These developments are not easily explained by the Chwalle's membrane theory. An intrinsic defect in the musculature of the terminal ureter leading to dilatation of the distal segment is another plausible theory for the formation of ureteroceles.

Primary Obstructive Megaureter

A primary obstructive megaureter results from a derangement of the distal ureteral musculature that impedes the normal peristaltic wave from conveying a bolus of urine. This is often described physiologically as an adynamic segment. Early muscularization is predominantly of the circular type. Longitudinal musculature, however, is essential for proper peristalsis. A development arrest prior to formation of longitudinal musculature may lead to a nonperistaltic segment of ureter.

Infrequently, an anatomic obstruction may be the cause of obstructive megaureter. This may be explained by the persistence of fetal ureteral folds with intrinsic musculature.

DEVELOPMENT OF THE KIDNEY

Renal development proceeds through three phases: pronephros, mesonephros, and metanephros (Table 1.3). Cells from the intermediate mesoderm aggregate and differentiate into the pronephric tubules, which are evident by the third week of fetal development. These appear between the second and sixth somites. These primitive tubules are nonsecretory, and their caudal end becomes the mesonephric duct while the remainder of the pronephros involutes (Figure 1.9).

The mesonephros is formed from the descending mesonephric duct contacting mesoderm. This union induces the formation of the mesonephric nephron. By the fifth week of fetal life 40 pairs of tubules are connected to the mesonephric duct, which then drains into the urogenital sinus.

Table 1.3: Renal and Gonadal Embryogenesis

Gonads	*Kidney*
Primordial cells migrate to genital ridge (5 weeks) Undifferentiated gonad (7 weeks) Sertoli cells (16 weeks) Leydig cells (16–24 weeks)	Pronephros (0–4 weeks), then disappears Mesonephros (4–8 weeks) Disappears by 8 weeks Exception of few caudal tubules in male Mesonephric duct persists Gives uses to ureteric bud Metanephros (5–20 weeks) No metanephric duct

The final phase of renal development depends on the union of the ureteral bud and the metanephric blastema. The metanephric blastema develops from the terminal portion of the nephrogenic cord, dissociating from the cord when it contacts the ureteral bud. The blastema develops into the nephrogenic structures and supporting tissues, and the bud becomes the ureter, calices, and collecting ducts. Union of the metanephric blastema and ureteral bud occurs in the upper sacral region (fourth week). As the ureteral bud elongates and the blastema ascends (within 4 to 6 weeks) to reach the lumbar segments, nephrogenic differentiation occurs (within 6 to 34 weeks).

The ureteral bud has its origin as an outpouching off the distal portion of the mesonephric duct. The development of the ureteral bud is divided into four phases, as it undergoes a series of intricate branchings, developing into the ureter, calices, and collecting ducts.

Nephron development results from the close interaction between the ampullae of the ureteral bud and the metanephric blastema. In the absence of the ureteral bud or other inductive tissue, or if the ureteral bud does not come in close contact with the blastema, nephron development does not occur. Other tissues can be experimentally induced by the ureteral bud to form tubules (e.g., the thoracic spinal cord); however, only the metanephric blastema can form renal tubules.

Nephrogenesis begins by ureteral bud induction at about the eighth week of gestation, with function by the twelfth week. However, nephrogenesis continues until the 34th week of gestation. Beyond this time no new nephrons develop; however, tubular function continues to mature. Consequently, the timing of an insult to the development of the kidney has significant impact as to the resulting effect on renal development.

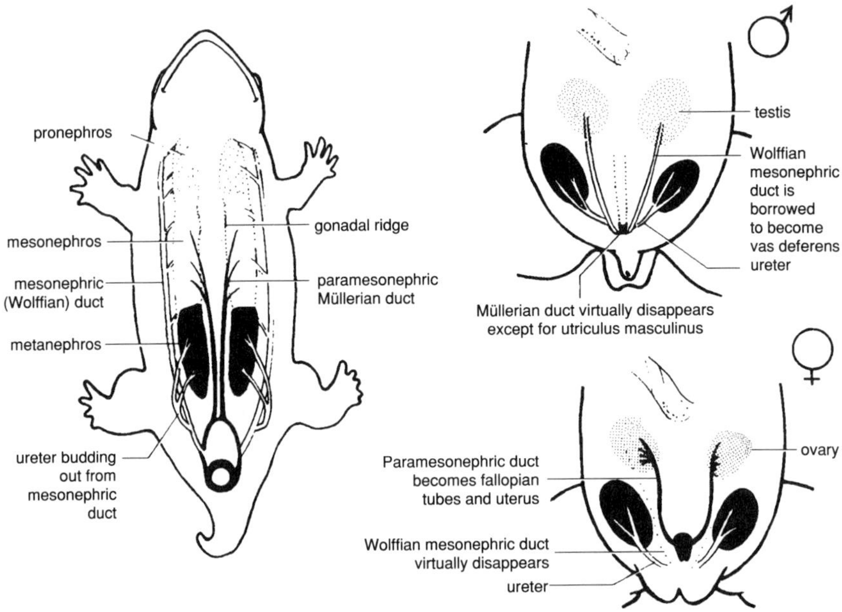

Figure 1.9: Embryologic development of the kidney. *Reproduced with permission from Blandy J. Lecture Notes on Urology, 4th ed. Oxford: Blackwell Scientific Publications, 1991:43.*

Renal Agenesis

Renal agenesis results from abnormalities of either the ureteral bud, the metanephric blastema, or their union. If the ureteral bud is absent or abnormal, or if the ureteral bud does not contact the metanephric blastema, nephron differentiation will not arise, even in the presence of a normal blastema. Alternatively, if the metanephric blastema is absent, either primarily or as the result of failure of the development of the nephrogenic cord or the metanephric precursors (pronephros, mesonephros), the kidney will not develop. In this situation, the ureter may or may not be present. Most anephric patients have a rudimentary ureter, indicating that the embryologic accident occurs after the outpouching of the ureteral bud from the mesonephric duct. In anephric patients with ureteral atresia, wolffian duct structures are normal, indicating that the insult to the ureteral bud occurs after its formation. In 10% of patients testicular agenesis is also found. This emphasizes the close association between the renal and gonadal anlage on the dorsal aspect of the coelomic cavity.

In contradistinction to bilateral renal agenesis, the embryologic insult in unilateral agenesis is most often to the ureteral bud. This theory is supported by the observation that the ipsilateral gonad is usually unaffected, and the high occurrence of abnormalities of the proximal wolffian duct structures in the male and the müllerian structures in the female.

Renal Dysplasia and Hypoplasia

Renal dysplasia is associated with obstruction (ureteral, vesical, or urethral) in up to 50% of patients and is thought by some to be the result of obstruction. Experimentally, however, simple ligation of the fetal ureter most commonly results in hydronephrosis and not dysplasia. It is likely that obstruction must be coupled with a quantitative deficiency of metanephric blastema if dysplasia is to occur. Maizels and Simpson have demonstrated that dysplasia is more likely to occur after intrauterine ureteral ligation if the ureteral buds are depleted of condensed metanephrogenic mesenchyme.

An additional factor in the development of renal dysplasia and hypoplasia (hypodysplasia) is based on the clinical observation that a ureteral orifice that is abnormal in position is more likely to be associated with renal hypodysplasia. Ureters that terminate on the trigone generally have normal renal units, whereas those that are lateral or ectopic have a higher incidence of hypodysplasia. The embryologic basis for this is that the bud of the ectopic ureter originates from an abnormal position on the mesonephric duct and therefore meets only a small amount of metanephric blastema. The dysplasia seen with urethral obstruction, that is, posterior urethral valves, is more often associated with reflux, and this suggests that an abnormal ureteral orifice position is more likely to be the cause of the dysplasia rather than the result of obstruction itself.

Multicystic Kidney

Multicystic kidney is virtually always associated with ureteral atresia or obstruction at the ureteropelvic junction. Attempts at induction of multicystic kidney by in-utero ligation of the ureter have not been universally successful. This may indicate that the obstruction causing multicystic kidney occurs at a very early stage of renal development, or that some other factor is necessary, for example, an abnormal metanephric blastema. Some investigators place multicystic kidney at the extreme end of the spectrum of hydronephrosis. This concept is further supported by clinical situations in which features of both hydronephrosis and multicystic kidney are apparent. Another theory proposes failure of union between the blastema and ureteral bud, explaining the high incidence of ureteral atresia and agenesis. Whereas multicystic kidney is most commonly unilateral, it is often associated with contralateral renal abnormalities such as ureteropelvic junction obstruction, which is seen most frequently. This is especially true for the small as opposed to the large multicystic kidney, and for the multicystic kidney with a high ureteral atresia as opposed to one with a low atresia.

Simple Renal Ectopia and Malrotation

The ureteral bud elongates to meet the metanephros in the region of the upper sacral somites at weeks 7 to 8. Factors responsible for renal ascent sequentially include: (1) caudal growth of the spine, (2) active elongation of the ureter into the metanephros, (3) elongation of the renal parenchyma with other architectural changes, and (4) further elongation of the spine when the kidney is fixed to retroperitoneal structures. The kidney adopts its blood supply from regional vessels during its ascent: the middle sacral, external and common iliac arteries, and finally the aorta. During this ascent the kidney rotates on its longitudinal axis from lateral to medial with respect to the renal pelvis. This accounts for the typical association of renal ectopia with malrotation or, rather, failure of rotation. Other factors that contribute to ascent failure include abnormalities of the ureteral bud (failure to elongate), defective metanephric blastema that fails to induce ascent, and genetic or teratogenic causes. Persistence of early vascular attachments has also been proposed as a mechanism, but it is thought that this may be effect rather than a cause.

The pelvic kidney, the most common form of renal ectopia, represents faulty ascent. The ectopic renal unit may also occur cephalad to the normal lumbar position, lying just beneath the diaphragm or in the thorax itself. It is unclear whether the kidney continues to ascend intrinsically prior to closure of the diaphragm leaflets, or if delayed closure of the leaflets allows for exaggerated renal ascent.

Crossed Renal Ectopia With and Without Fusion

Renal fusion is explained by one of two theories. The parenchyma of both nephrogenic cords may fuse along with their respective ureters, or by means of a wandering bud that crosses the midline and makes contact with the contralateral nephrogenic cord. In the former instance a horseshoe kidney develops, whereas various forms of crossed renal ectopia result in the latter. Although the exact etiology of crossover is uncertain, several theories have been proposed.

It is inferred that fusion most commonly occurs prior to or at the initial stages of renal ascent. It may also occur at later stages of ascent, explaining unusual forms of fusion, for example, the superior pole fused horseshoe kidney, or the superiorly and inferiorly fused horseshoe.

Several variations of fusion anomalies have been described, the final morphology depending on the timing and extent of fusion, degree of renal rotation, and final location of the units. Malrotation is the rule, because little if any rotation is possible once fusion takes place.

Generally, the crossed kidney lies caudal to the orthotopic unit, with fusion occurring between the superior pole of the ectopic unit and the inferior pole of the normally positioned unit. The exception, the superior ectopic kidney, is the most unusual fusion anomaly. Ninety percent of crossed ectopia involves fusion. In crossed ectopia without fusion, the orthotopic unit is in its normal position and orientation, whereas the ectopic unit is usually caudal, incompletely rotated with an anteriorly directed pelvis, and assumes a horizontal or tangential lie. Anomalies, that is, reflux, multicystic dysplasia, and ureteropelvic junction obstruction, most commonly arise in the crossed unit.

Ureteropelvic Junction Obstruction

Ureteropelvic junction obstruction is the most common congenital obstruction of the urinary tract. Its exact etiology is, however, obscure. Histologic evidence points to either a disorientation of muscle fibers (longitudinal fibers replacing the normal spiralling fibers) or excessive collagen and fibrous tissue. This effect may result from developmental arrest caused by compression of the ureter by fetal vessels or from ischemia to the ureteropelvic junction. An alternative explanation is based on work by Ruano-Gil et al., who have demonstrated that the developing ureter goes through a solid phase followed by recanalization. Ureteropelvic junction obstruction, therefore, may be caused by recanalization failure of the cephalic end of the ureter.

Other intrinsic lesions of the ureteropelvic junction include polyps, valves, and persistent ureteral folds. Congenital ureteral folds arise when the ureter lengthens out of proportion to renal ascent, providing excess ureteral length. These rarely persist beyond infancy, because postnatally the growth rate of the infant exceeds that of the ureter. Persistence of these folds containing muscle produces a valvelike obstruction at the ureteropelvic junction and at the ureterovesical junction.

Secondary causes of ureteropelvic junction obstruction are kinking and tortuosity of the ureter caused by hydronephrosis from lower tract obstruction or vesicoureteral reflux. Other urologic anomalies occur with ureteropelvic junction obstruction in up to 50% of reported series. Contralateral ureteropelvic junction obstruction is reported in 10 to 40% of patients, and this is followed in incidence by renal dysplasia, multicystic kidney, and contralateral renal agenesis (5%).

TESTICULAR DESCENT

As delineated in the section on sexual differentiation, chromosomal sex determines gonadal sex. Testicular differentiating factor (TDF), produced by genes located on the distal portion of the short arm of the Y chromosomes, attaches to the undifferentiated gonadal primordia to induce testicular development. By the sixth week of gestation the germ cells have migrated in a cephalad direction to the gonadal ridges, adjacent to the mesonephros. The gubernaculum is apparent at this stage as a mesenchymal ridge that extends from the genital swelling to the gonadal ridges. The processus vaginalis develops ventral to the gubernaculum as an outpouching of the peritoneum.

Descent of the testis is thought to occur in two phases: intra-abdominal migration and inguinal migration (Figure 1.10). By the end of the first trimester, the testis lies just proximal to the internal inguinal ring. Whether this represents true migration of the testis from the gonadal ridges or results from body growth remains unclear. Müllerian inhibiting substance may play an active role in this phase.

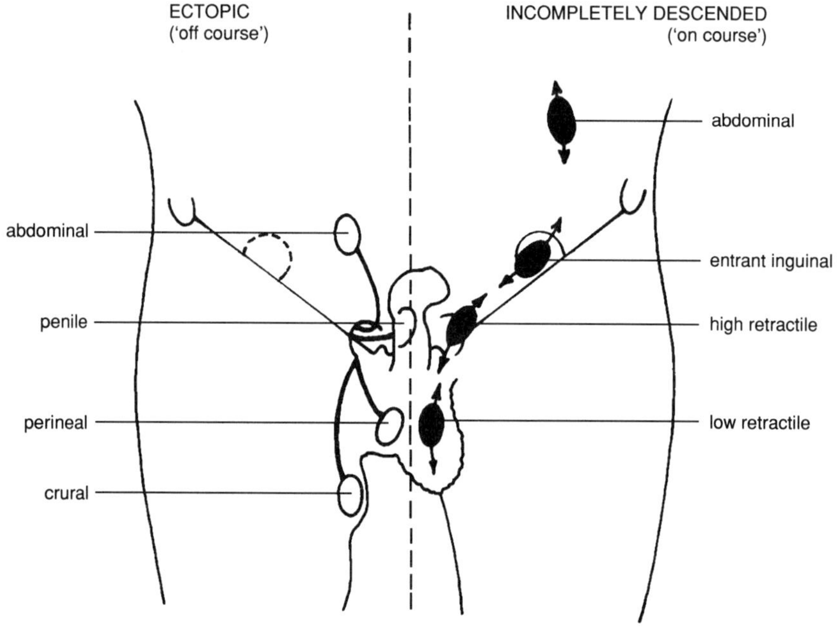

Figure 1.10: The maldescended testis may be either off course or on, i.e., ectopic (left) or incompletely descended (right). *Reproduced from Blandy J. Lecture Notes on Urology, 4th ed. Oxford: Blackwell Scientific Publications, 1991:294.*

The inguinal phase of testicular descent occurs early in the third trimester of gestation. The gubernaculum, which attaches to the epididymis, swells while the processus vaginalis extends to the scrotum. Swelling and then contraction of the gubernaculum results in descent of the epididymis, followed rapidly by the testis. Once the testis reaches the scrotum, the proximal processus vaginalis obliterates while the distal end forms the tunica vaginalis.

Various theories have been proposed regarding testicular descent (see Table 1.4). Endocrine factors, supplemented by mechanical factors, probably play the major role in testicular descent. In 1932, Engle demonstrated that premature testicular descent in monkeys could be induced by gonadotropins. Dihydrotestosterone (DHT) is thought to be the mediating agent. DHT may affect the gubernaculum either directly or through action on the genitofemoral nerve. Data indicate that cryptorchid infants have an abnormality of the hypothalmic-pituitary-gonadal axis (decreased based leutinizing hormone LH and testosterone and blunted response to gonadotrophin releasing hormone GNRH) that is not detectable before puberty.

Intra-abdominal pressure is thought to play a role in testicular descent. Evidence for this comes from experimental studies and observation of certain clinical states, such as prune-belly syndrome, abdominal wall defects, and diaphragmatic hernia, which are accompanied by an increased incidence of testicular maldescent. The traction theory proposes that the gubernaculum and/or cremasteric muscles pull the testis into the scrotum. This may be mediated by the genitofemoral nerve, which supplies the gubernaculum. The role of the cremasteric muscle has been refuted. Since the gubernaculum is thought to attach to the epididymis, abnormal development or attachment of the ductal system to the testes could also lead to testicular maldescent. The ductal system develops abnormally in approximately one-third of males with undescended testes. This incidence is higher in the case of more proximal undescended testes.

The differential growth rate theory assumes a more passive role of the testis in descent, proposing that the testis remains at an internal inguinal ring location, but rapid growth of the body wall causes the testis

Table 1.4: Theories of Testicular Descent

Theories
Endocrine
Intra-abdominal pressure
Traction
Differential growth

to find itself in the scrotum. The presence of active changes in gubernaculum development provides evidence against this theory.

CONCLUSION

This chapter reviews basic genitourinary embryology. A clear understanding of the events leading to development of the urinary tract provides insight into the management of postnatal urologic problems. These principles of embryology are even more important in today's practice, with the routine use of antenatal ultrasonography. A substantial number (approximately 30%) of prenatally detected anomalies involve the genitourinary system.

This fact has a dual effect on the practice of urology. First, more congenital anomalies are being identified earlier, requiring us to be well versed in the embryologic foundations of these lesions. Second, we will be required to observe and establish a new natural history for some of these lesions, particularly the obstructive problems. The dilemma is exemplified by the question: Does a newborn with an apparent ureteropelvic junction (UPJ) obstruction and good renal function always develop into the 5-year-old presenting with a pyohydronephrosis? Alternatively, this new postnatal natural history may in turn alter our understanding of the embryology of congenital genitourinary abnormalities.

SUGGESTED READINGS

Stephens FD. Congenital malformations of the urinary tract. New York: Payeros Publishers, 1983.

A comprehensive, detailed treatise on urinary tract embryology. Each section or congenital problem is presented with a carefully studied case or autopsy material. Masterfully written and represents a career's worth of ideas and philosophies.

Caldamone AA. Urologic applications of genitourinary embryology. Monogr Urol 1986; 7(4):89.

Discusses the embryology of the genitourinary system with particular reference to its application in clinical settings.

Diamond DA. Intersex disorders I and II. AUA Update Series 9 1990; (9 and 10):66–80.

Updated discussion of the embryology of intersex and its disorders. Presents a systematic approach to the evaluation of the newborn with ambiguous genitalia.

Stephens FD. Congenital malformations of the rectum, anus, and genitourinary tracts. London: E & S Livingstone Ltd, 1963.

A classic text on gastrointestinal and genitourinary embryology. Particularly good discussion of the relationships between the development of the lower tracts of both systems.

Bellinger MF. Embryology of the male external genitalia. Urol Clin North Am 1981; 8:375.

Excellent, concise, and understandable discussion of the embryology of the male urethra and disorders leading to hypospadias and other congenital urethral abnormalities.

Muecke EC. Exstrophy, epispadias and other congenital anomalies of the bladder. In: Walsh PC et al, eds. Campbell's urology. 5th ed. Philadelphia: WB Saunders, 1986:1856.

Discussion of the embryology of bladder exstrophy and epispadias along with cloacal exstrophy. Leads to a clear understanding of the anatomy of each condition.

Ruano-Gil D, Coca-Payeros A, Tejido-Maten A. Obstruction and normal recanalization of the ureter in the human embryo: its relation to congenital ureteric obstruction. Eur Urol 1975; 1:287.

Discusses the theory of ureteral development involving recanalization, along with events leading to obstruction based on this theory.

Tanagho EA. Embryologic basic for lower ureteral anomalies: a hypothesis. Urology 1976; 7:451.

Classic article on embryology of the ureteral bud and mesonephric duct. Discusses in detail how abnormalities of the bud lead to problems such as ureteral ectopia and reflux.

Mackie CG, Stephens FD. Duplex kidneys: a correlation of renal dysplasia with position of the ureteral orifice. J Urol 1975; 114:274.

Proposed the theory of relationship between ureteral bud position from the mesonephric duct and quality of renal parenchyma that is induced.

Maizels M. Normal development of the urinary tract. In: Walsh PC et al, eds. Campbell's urology. 6th ed. Philadelphia: WB Saunders, 1992: 1543.

Excellent discussion of genitourinary embryology, particularly the embryology of the upper tract.

Rajfer J. Congenital anomalies of the testis. In: Walsh PC et al, eds. Campbell's urology. 5th ed. Philadelphia: WB Saunders 1986:1638.

Presents a clear and thorough discussion of the embryology of testicular development and descent. Other congenital abnormalities of the testis such as torsion, hernia, and hydrocele also discussed.

CHAPTER 2

Renal Physiology

Paul G. Horgan
John M. Fitzpatrick

The kidney plays a central role in the regulation of the physiochemical status of the extracellular fluid bathing the cells of the body. The processes of glomerular filtration, selective tubular absorption, and tubular secretion maintain fluid and electrolyte homeostasis. In addition, the kidney has important endocrine activity and functions prominently in intermediate metabolism. This chapter reviews the fundamentals of the physiological functions of the kidney and examines alterations resulting from urinary tract obstruction, drug therapy, and prolonged hypotension.

BASICS

The kidneys are paired organs that lie on the posterior abdominal wall, on either side of the vertebral column. On the medial border of each kidney is the hilum, through which pass the renal vessels, nerves, and the funnel-like dilatation of the upper ureter, the renal pelvis. Bisection of the kidney reveals two macroscopically distinct regions, the outer cortex, which has a granular appearance, and the inner medulla. The medulla is made up of a number of renal pyramids whose apices project into the calyces (major and minor), which in turn empty into the renal pelvis. The pelvis plays no role in urine formation and is considered the first functional section of the ureter.

The nephron is the basic unit of renal function. Urine begins formation with filtration at the glomerulus and is altered by tubular reabsorption and secretion as it passes through the proximal convoluted tubule, the loop of Henle, and the distal convoluted tubule and into the collecting system. Each kidney contains approximately one million nephrons, and three distinct nephron populations are described based on the cortical location of their glomeruli. Superficial nephrons have glomeruli located within

1 mm of the capsular surface of the kidney. Midcortical nephrons are found more deeply, and juxtamedullary nephrons are located just above the corticomedullary junction. The major distinction between each type is the length of the loop of Henle; superficial nephrons have short loops extending to the outer medulla, whereas juxtamedullary nephrons have long loops that often reach the tips of the renal papillae.

The renal artery divides into progressively smaller branches termed interlobar, arcuate, and interlobular arteries. Ultimately, as the interlobular vessels run toward the cortical surface, afferent arterioles are given off at right angles to supply the nephron. An efferent arteriole leaves the glomerulus and subdivides into peritubular capillaries, which enmesh the tubules of a neighboring nephron. These vessels rejoin to form venous channels by which blood leaves the kidney.

GLOMERULAR FILTRATION

The renal glomerulus is a complex microvascular structure composed of endothelial, epithelial, and mesangial elements. The unit consists of a vascular tuft of capillaries embedded into the concavity of the first part of the nephron, Bowman's capsule. Within this capsule is Bowman's space. The process of filtration occurs across the barrier between vascular lumen and Bowman's space.This barrier consists of three layers: capillary endothelium, basement membrane, and a single-celled layer of epithelial cells (Fig. 2.1). The vascular endothelial layer is fenestrated with large apertures, and the basement membrane is a homogenous acellular network of mucopolysaccharides and glycoproteins. On the basement membrane is found the visceral epithelial layer of podocytes, cells distinct from the remainder of Bowman's capsule. Endothelial and mesangial cells make up the bulk of the glomerulus. The endothelial cells, which line the glomerular capillaries, play an important role in passage of macromolecules across the capillary layer. Both the endothelial and epithelial cells play a role in synthesis of the glomerular basement membrane. Podocytes possess interdigitating foot processes with intervening filtration slits, through which the ultrafiltrate passes into Bowman's space. The foot processes are coated with a thick layer of glycosialoproteins, which affects free filtrate flow. This flow is further impeded by the presence of thin diaphragms that bridge the slits at the level of the basement membrane. Mesangial cells are predominantly located at the glomerular stalk and have contractile properties.

The forces controlling the filtration of fluid from the capillary lumen to the capsular space are the same as those described by Starling in 1899 for fluid movements in other capillaries. The barrier is freely permeable to crystalloids but not to colloids. Inulin (molecular weight less

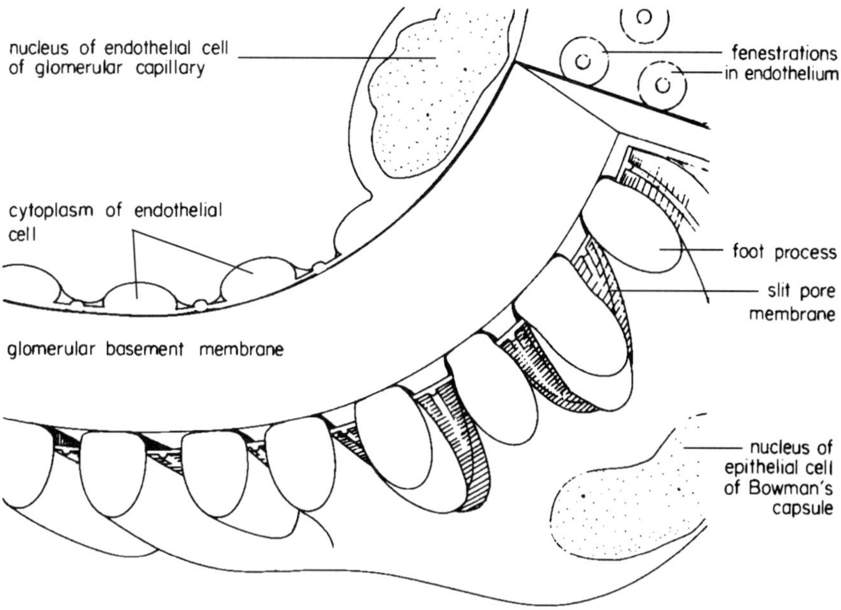

Figure 2.1: Structure of glomerular filter. *Reproduced with permission from Blandy J. Lecture Notes on Urology 4th ed. Oxford: Blackwell Scientific Publications, 1991:37.*

than 6 Kd) moves freely into the nephron, but albumin, a relatively small, anionic molecule (7 Kd), is nearly totally excluded. The electrolyte concentration of Bowman's space fluid is virtually identical to that of plasma, but does contain small quantities (50 mg/l or less) of albumin at a concentration approximately 100 times less than that in plasma. There is no hindrance to passage of molecules smaller than 7 Kd, but there is a sieving process for larger macromolecules by the endothelial fenestrae initially, then in the hydrated spaces between the glycoprotein chains of the basement membrane. Macromolecules that reach the podocytes are impeded by the slit diaphragms and foot process coats.

The triad of the glomerular barrier constituents (i.e., endothelial cell, basement membrane, and epithelial cell) is composed of fixed polyanions that tend to repel permeation of negatively charged ions across the membranes. Since most proteins bear net negative charges, this electrical barrier is another limiting factor in protein diffusion. Size is also a significant factor, and the shape of the molecule plays a role in the ease of passage across the glomerular barrier. The net forces favoring ultrafiltration, the so-called net filtration pressure (NFP), depend on the difference between the transcapillary hydraulic pressure (which aids filtration) and the difference in colloid osmotic pressures (which opposes it) (Table 2.1):

$$\text{NFP} = (P_{GC} + O_{BC}) - (P_{BC} + O_{GC}),$$

where

P_{GC} is glomerular-capillary hydraulic pressure, O_{BC} is oncotic pressure of fluid in Bowman's capsule, P_{BC} is hydraulic pressure in Bowman's capsule, and O_{CG} is oncotic pressure of plasma in capillary.

The small quantity of protein in Bowman's space is insufficient to contribute any appreciable oncotic pressure. Therefore, the equation can be amended as follows:

$$\text{NFP} = P_{GC} - P_{BC} - O_{GC}.$$

Micropuncture techniques have allowed the insertion of micropipettes into the glomeruli of experimental animals. Techniques have evolved to evaluate the nanoliter samples thus obtained and to measure directly the pressures in the individual nephron. In particular, the availability of a strain of Wistar rat that possesses glomeruli on the renal cortical surface has resulted in the direct measurement of the glomerular capillary pressure, and it has been shown to be 40% lower than aortic pressure.

Because of the inherent resistance to flow along the glomerular capillary, hydraulic pressure gradually decreases from the afferent to the efferent ends of the capillary vessel. Glomerular capillary oncotic pressure increases along the capillary because the relative impermeability of the glomerular barrier to plasma proteins results in increasing concentrations of colloids as crystalloids are filtered. The combination of decreased hydraulic capillary pressure and increased oncotic pressure can therefore result in cessation of

Table 2.1: Glomerular Filtration Rate (GFR)

Average GFR in men = 125 ml/min/1.73m^2
Lower in women
Falls by 10 ml/min per decade after age 40
Increased in pregnancy
Dependent on the hydraulic pressure difference between glomerulus and tubule
Ultrafiltration forces
Hydrostatic pressure (Bowman's capsule, glomerular capillary)
Oncotic pressure (plasma, tubular fluid)
Permeability and surface area of glomerular capillaries
GFR greater in juxtamedullary than cortical nephrons

net filtration, a phenomenon known as filtration pressure equilibrium. This situation may be seen in humans when glomerular-capillary pressure is unusually low, as occurs following severe hemorrhage. In these circumstances the major determinant of the glomerular filtration rate is then renal plasma flow.

The glomerular filtration rate (GFR) is the rate of filtration from the capillary into Bowman's space. GFR is given by the renal clearance of any substance that is freely filterable at the glomerulus but not absorbed, secreted, or metabolized by the renal tubules. In health, the average man filters 180 L into Bowman's capsule each day, or 125 ml/min/1.73 m2 surface area (Table 2.1). The GFR is dependent on the net filtration pressure, the permeability of the glomerular barrier, and the surface area available for filtration. The glomerular vessels have a much higher permeability (×10 – 100) than capillaries elsewhere in the body, and the anatomical arrangement of the glomerulus results in a large surface area, which facilitates filtration.

The product of the hydraulic (water) permeability and the surface area is designated the filtration coefficient (K_f):

$$\text{GFR} = K_f \times \text{NFP}.$$

Changes in any of the parameters in this formula will have predictable effects on the glomerular filtration rate (Table 2.2). The filtration coefficient is altered by glomerular diseases that reduce the surface area available for filtration. Such diseases include acute renal failure, hypertension, glomerulonephritis, obstructive uropathy, and experimental nephrotoxicity. It has been reported that vasoactive substances can stimulate the mesangial cells of the glomerulus to reduce surface area and

Table 2.2: Summary of Influences on GFR

Parameters affecting GFR: *GFR* = $K_f \times (P_{GC} - P_{BC} - O_{GC})$		*Changes to GFR*
K_f	Increase	Increase
	Decrease	Decrease
P_{GC}	Afferent constriction Efferent dilatation	Decrease
	Afferent dilatation Efferent constriction	Increase
P_{BC}	Tubular/distal obstruction	Decrease
O_{GC}	Increase sytemic oncotic Decrease/pressure plasma flow	Decrease

thus GFR. Laboratory study has now confirmed that the K_f is insensitive to changes in renal plasma flow (Q_A) and that it remains constant even with a doubling of Q_A.

Of the variables contributing to the NFP, the glomerular-capillary hydraulic pressure (P_{GC}) is under the most sensitive physiological control. An increase in afferent arteriolar resistance tends to decrease GFR; conversely, any decrease in inflow resistance increases filtration. Constriction of the efferent arteriole increases upstream pressure and GFR. Efferent vasodilatation tends to lower GFR.

The relationship between the afferent arteriolar plasma protein concentration (afferent oncotic pressure (O_{GC})) and the GFR is predictable; that is, the GFR varies inversely with O_{GC} (as increased oncotic pressure decreases NFP). However, experimental evidence indicates the situation is far more complex. It appears that in vivo a fall in O_{GC} is accompanied by a fall in K_f. This may be due to stimulation of mesangial cells in the glomerulus by a variety of hormones, including antidiuretic hormone, angiotension II, and parathormone.

The pressure within Bowman's capsule (P_{BC}) increases when there is obstruction in the tubular system distal to the glomerulus. Such obstruction, for example, ureteric calculi, may be within the kidney or elsewhere in the urinary tract. The obstruction leads to a damming of urine, an increase in P_{BC}, and a subsequent decrease in GFR. Assessment of GFR relies on measurement of the renal clearance of various substances (Table 2.3). GFR approximates clearance if the substance is filtered at the glomerulus but neither absorbed nor secreted in the remaining nephron segments. The advantages and disadvantages of the various methods used to measure GFR are listed in Table 2.3.

TUBULAR FUNCTION

The tubular system extends from the glomerulus to the calyx and consists of a single layer of epithelial cells resting on a basement membrane. The cells are interconnected by tight junctions and have a different structure and function in each named segment of the tubular system. The proximal tubule consists of an initial pars convoluta and the straight pars recta. This continues into the loop of Henle, which leads to the short intraglomerular macula densa and then the distal tubule. The amount of a substance transported by the tubules determines the quantity lost to the body. The tubular transport of substance x (T_x) is expressed as

$$T_x = \text{GFR} \times P_x - U_x V,$$

Table 2.3: GFR Measurement and Renal Clearance

Concept of renal clearance
  Clearance = GFR if
    Substance freely filterable
    Not absorbed, secreted, metabolized, e.g., inulin
Inulin clearance
  Accurate; complex; little clinical utility
Endogenous creatinine clearance

$$C_{cr} = \frac{U_{cr} \times V}{P_{cr}}$$

    Overestimates GFR because creatinine filtered and secreted
    Drug interference, e.g., cimetidine, trimethoprim
    Overestimation greater at lower GFR levels
Radioisotope clearance
  ^{125}I-iothalamate
  Slight overestimate of GFR
Extraction factor
  Computerized calculation of decay of injected labeled DTPA
Exogenous creatinine clearance
  Creatinine clearance measured following loading dose of creatinine
  Mainly an experimental technique

where

P_x is plasma concentration of x, U_x is urinary concentration of x, and V is volume of urine per unit time.

The value of T_x is positive with net absorption and negative with net secretion. The kidneys have a maximum reabsorptive capacity for substances such as glucose and a maximum secretory capacity for substances such as para-amino hippurate (PAH).

Tubular Reabsorption

Transfer of fluid and electrolytes across the glomerular barrier occurs by hydraulic flow. There is little such transfer in the tubule because of the lack of any effective hydraulic pressure and absence of filtration pores. Tubular reabsorption occurs by a variety of processes (Table 2.4):

1. *Simple diffusion:* dependent on membrane lipid solubility and occurs along downhill electrochemical gradients. No energy is expended, and membrane carriers are not involved.

2. *Simple facilitated diffusion:* movement along downhill electrochemi-

Table 2.4: Tubular Reabsorption Transport Mechanisms

Facilitated diffusion
Diffusion
Primary active transport (ATPase dependent)
Secondary active transport (cotransport, e.g., glucose, sodium transport)
Endocytosis
Transcellular through luminal basolateral membranes
Paracellular across tight junctions

cal gradients that is facilitated by carrier proteins in the membrane. This process has specificity and saturability and is subject to competitive inhibition.

3. *Secondary active transport:* two substances bind to the same membrane carrier, and one moves in a downhill direction by simple facilitated diffusion to release energy sufficient to transport the second substance in an uphill fashion against its electrochemical gradient.

4. *Primary active transport:* the energy for this process comes from the direct splitting of adenosine triphosphate (ATP). The substance binds to a specific membrane carrier and is transported against an uphill gradient.

5. *Endocytosis:* a form of primary transport with splitting of ATP to energize the process. The plasma membrane invaginates and envelops the substance (usually macromolecules).

Except for the few substances that are transported across the intercellular tight junctions, most transport occurs through two membranes: the luminal and the basolateral. A substance may therefore use two distinct transport processes to reach the peritubular capillaries. Sodium traverses the luminal membrane by simple facilitated diffusion and is transported across the basolateral membrane by active transport via the sodium–potassium dependent ATPase pump. Finally, the sodium ions move into the peritubular capillaries from the interstitial fluid by bulk flow along with water. This is the final step in the reabsorption of all substances.

Eighty percent of sodium reabsorption occurs in the proximal tubules, 15% in the ascending loop of Henle, and the remainder in the distal tubule via coupling to potassium (Figure 2.2). The latter process is under the influence of aldosterone. The control of sodium reabsorption in the proximal tubule, a complex process, is mediated by several mechanisms including feedback control of the GFR by the macula densa, GFR variation with the state of the extracellular fluid, and the putative existence of a natriuretic hormone. Amino acids are absorbed by at least five

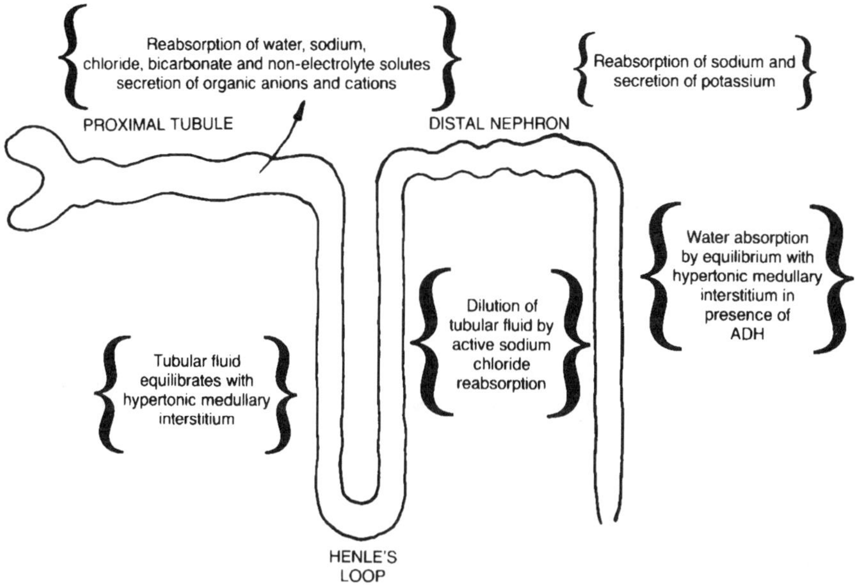

Figure 2.2: Nephron with sites of major fluid and electrolyte transport functions. *Adapted from Webster G, Kirby K, King L, et al eds. Reconstructive Urology Vol 1. Boston: Blackwell Scientific Publications, 1993:686.*

different transport systems: neutral, dibasic, dicarboxylic, iminoglycine, and beta. Phosphate reabsorption is decreased and excretion enhanced by cyclic 3'5'AMP-mediated parathormone activity. Chloride is passively reabsorbed linked with active sodium transport. Virtually all filtered potassium is reabsorbed by the proximal tubule. Low molecular proteins are reabsorbed by pinocytosis.

Tubular Secretion

Secretory processes in the tubular epithelium are categorized, like the reabsorptive mechanisms, as being active or passive. The first step for all substances is passive simple diffusion across the peritubular capillary endothelium into the interstitial fluid. Subsequent passage into the tubular lumen is effected through the tight junctions by simple diffusion or via the basolateral and luminal membranes by passive or active transport as described for reabsorption. Active carriage of substances into and out of cells leads to disruption of pre-existing electrochemical gradients and allows an element of back-diffusion.

This is termed a bidirectional transport system or a pump-leak system.

This leak renders it difficult for the transport mechanisms to shift a substance completely from one compartment to another and is more important with leaky epithelia (good crystalloid permeability) than with tight epithelia. A number of substances, for example, drugs, cations, and anions, are actively secreted in the tubules (Table 2.5). These substances are usually exogenous agents (e.g., drugs), poorly metabolized substances (e.g., para-amino hippurate), or slowly metabolized agents.

It must also be noted that along with the nephron functions of glomerular filtration, tubular reabsorption, and secretion, there is also tubular metabolism. Organic nutrients may be metabolized by the tubular cells for their own requirements. Alternatively, the metabolites may be used to alter the environment and composition of the urine or plasma, in particular via the manufacture of ammonia and bicarbonate (Figure 2.3).

RENAL BLOOD FLOW

The kidney is a unique organ with complex physiological mechanisms that optimize control of GFR and regulate the internal environment. Renal plasma flow is estimated to be 650 ml/min based on a total renal blood flow of 1100 ml/min. Twenty percent of this is filtered (125 ml/min), and the rest exits the glomerulus via the efferent arteriole (filtration fraction). The GFR is controlled by autoregulation, the sympathetic nervous system, the juxtaglomerular apparatus, and prostaglandins.

Two intrarenal mechanisms autoregulate internal blood flow: the myogenic system and tubuloglomerular feedback (Table 2.6). Increased tension on the vessel smooth muscle wall induced by afferent arteriolar blood pressure causes a reflex vasoconstriction with increased resistance to blood flow and a reduction of what would otherwise be an increased GFR. The initial increase in GFR produces an augmented flow of water and filtered solutes through the macula densa, and this triggers local release of vasoconstrictors, which increase the afferent arteriolar resistance. Angiotensin or adenosine may be responsible for these effects.

Table 2.5: Substances Secreted by Tubules

Penicillin	Creatinine
Probenecid	Cimetidine
Trimethoprim	Procaine
Chlorothiazide	Acetylcholine
Furosemide	Dopamine
Hippurates	Histamine
Prostaglandins	Serotonin

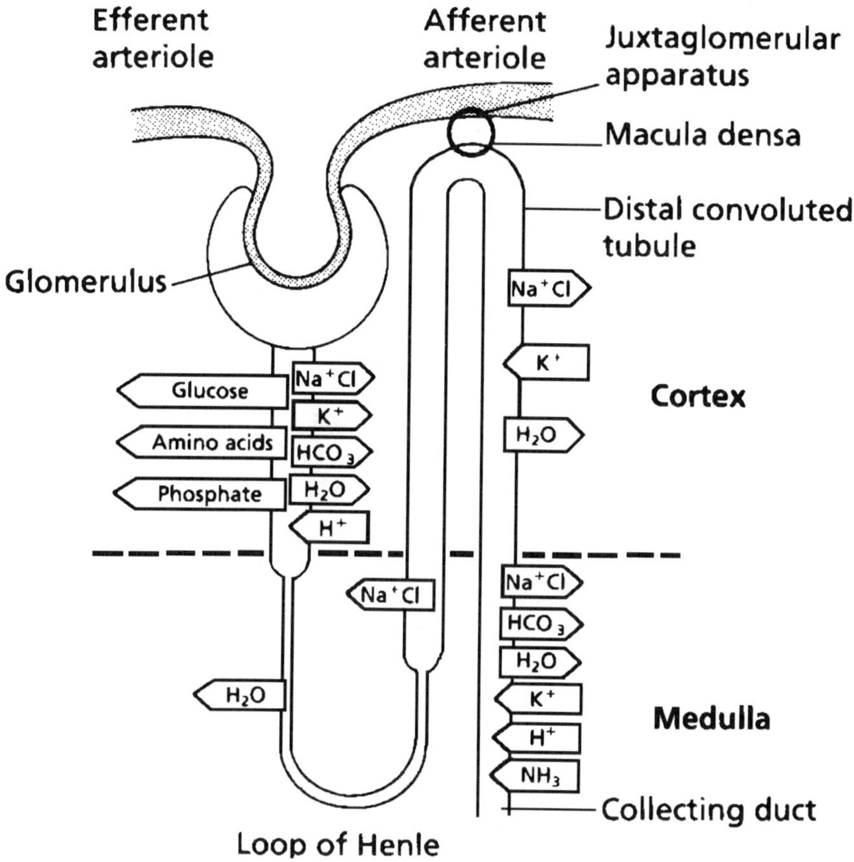

Figure 2.3: Diagrammatic representation of the main sites for removal or addition of electrolytes and solutes from or to tubular lumen. *Reproduced with permission from Webster, Kirby K, King L, et al eds. Reconstructive Urology, Vol 1. Boston: Blackwell Scientific Publications, 1991:8.*

Decreases in systemic arterial blood pressure and volume stimulate arterial and venous baroreceptors to increase sympathetic outflow. This, with the epinephrine release from the adrenals, constricts the afferent arterioles and reduces renal blood flow and GFR. However, efferent arterioles are also constricted, and this preserves GFR despite the overall drop in renal blood flow. Peripheral chemoreceptors and the higher brain centers may also be stimulated to increase sympathetic drive with the same net result. Total blood pressure recovery is aided by the increased renal peripheral resistance and by the decreased salt and water excretion resulting from a reduced GFR.

Table 2.6: Renal Autoregulation

Mechanisms
Myogenic
Tubuloglomerular feedback
Metabolic
Hormonal
Renal sympathetic innervation
Sodium/water reabsorption
Angiotensin II
Aldosterone
Atrial natriuretic factor (ANF)
28-amino-acid peptide
Produced in atria
Reduced sodium absorption
Renal sympathetic activity
Rise in activity leads to sodium retention
Renin release
Systemic baroreceptors
JG (juxtaglomerular) cells
Macula densa

Juxtaglomerular influences are also important in regulating blood flow (Table 2.6). Renin, released when renal blood flow decreases, catalyzes the conversion of angiotensinogen to angiotensin I, which is then metabolized to angiotensin II in the lungs. Renin release is achieved by (a) internal baroreceptors in the renin-secreting granular cells of the juxtaglomerular (JG) apparatus which react inversely to afferent arteriolar pressure; thus, decreased pressure induces increased renin secretion; (b) a direct stimulatory effect on renin secretion by the sympathetic nervous system and circulating epinephrine; (c) the fact that sodium and chloride concentrations in the tubule and macula densa cells have an inverse relationship with renin release by the granular cells: a low GFR and low concentration of tubular sodium chloride promotes renin secretion; and (d) the negative feedback of angiotensin II on renin release. Antidiuretic hormone (ADH), Ca^{2+}, and K^{+} all exert negative feedbacks on renin secretion. Increased sympathetic drive or angiotensin II stimulation induces synthesis and release of prostaglandins from the renal cortex. Prostaglandins E_2 and I_2 have vasodilator effects and antagonize the vasoconstrictor effects on the renal vasculature. The net effect of all these influences is to maintain a steady GFR in the face of fluctuations in total renal blood flow (Table 2.6).

RENAL HANDLING OF SODIUM, CHLORIDE, AND WATER

Sodium is transported from the tubular lumen into the cell by facilitated downhill diffusion and thence to the capillary via the sodium chloride dependent ATPase pump. Sodium moves alone, by cotransport with glucose or amino acids, and by countertransport with hydrogen ion. Water and chloride passively follow due to osmotic gradients. This process depends primarily on the permeability of membranes and tight junctions (Table 2.7).

Chloride movement occurs in three ways: (1) along the concentration gradient created secondary to flow of sodium and water, (2) along an electrochemical gradient from lumen to interstitial fluid helped by active sodium transport, and (3) by a secondary active process coupled to primary active sodium transport. The latter is the major path of chloride movement in the thick ascending loop of Henle.

Proximal Tubule

The greatest absorption of sodium and water (65% of that filtered) occurs in the proximal tubule. Sodium concentration and the fluid osmolality is the same as that of plasma at the end of this tubule segment. Sodium countertransport with H^+ drives reabsorption of filtered bicarbonate and couples with sodium reabsorption in the late tubule. The presence of osmotic diuretics—for example, mannitol or glucose in diabetics—retards sodium and water absorption.

Loop of Henle

A further 25% of filtered sodium and water is reabsorbed in the loop of

Table 2.7: Specialized Functional Segments of Nephron

Proximal tubule
Reabsorption H_2O, sodium, chloride, bicarbonate, nonelectrolyte solutes
Secretion organic anions, cations
Thin limbs of Henle's loop
Water permeable
Tubular fluid equilibration with hypertonic medulla
Thick limbs of Henle's loop
Water impermeable
Dilution tubular fluid by active sodium, chloride reabsorption
Distal nephron segments
"Fine" regulation volume, composition urine
Sodium, water reabsorption (ADH dependent)
Potassium secretion

Henle. No active sodium or chloride absorption occurs in the thin descending or ascending segments of the loops of Henle. In the thick ascending limb, primary active sodium transport results in a tubular fluid with lower sodium concentration and osmolality relative to plasma entering the distal tubule. The ascending limb is impermeable to water, a distinct contrast to the descending limb, which is highly water-permeable.

Distal Tubule

Active reabsorption of sodium chloride continues in the distal tubule, and because of low water permeability, osmolality decreases further. In the terminal segments of the distal tubule, water permeability is affected by ADH influences on the luminal membrane. Interaction of ADH with the basolateral membrane ADH receptors activates adenylate cyclase to release cyclic AMP. ADH also induces prostaglandin synthesis, which opposes adenyl cyclase activation of intracellular cyclic AMP and increases luminal membrane permeability (negative feedback).

Urine Concentration

The maximum urine concentration is 1400 mOsm/L, and the minimum obligatory water loss to excrete wastes is 0.42 L/day. Urine concentration is achieved by the countercurrent multiplier system residing in the loop of Henle. The descending limb (DLH) does not actively absorb sodium chloride but is freely permeable to water, while the opposite holds for the thick ascending limb (ALH). Thus, fluid becomes progressively concentrated in the DLH and progressively diluted in the ALH with a gradient of 200 mM/L at any horizontal level in the medulla but a variance of 300 to 700 mOsm/L from top to bottom. As tubular fluid flows along the collecting tubules it is progressively concentrated along this gradient under the influence of ADH.

Urea plays an important role in urine concentration. The distal tubule and the cortical and outer medullary sections of the collecting tubules are impermeable to urea, and luminal concentration of urea rises. The inner medullary area is permeable to urea, and thus urea diffuses out into the medullary interstitium and adds to the high osmolality and concentrating ability of the medulla. The countercurrent multiplier function of the loop is complemented by the similar looped configuration of the vasa recta, which passively protects the osmolality gradient in the medulla. The vessel loops allow sodium chloride to diffuse into and water to diffuse out of the descending limb, with opposite effects in the ascending limb. This function is termed countercurrent exchange.

RENAL CONTROL OF EXTRACELLULAR VOLUME

The most important influence on extracellular volume (ECV) is the plasma sodium concentration. Sodium excretion is the difference between filtered sodium (GFR × Plasma sodium) and the amount of sodium reabsorbed. Receptors sensitive to changes in plasma sodium are located in the adrenal cortex, kidney, and brain, but the major regulators of plasma sodium are the control factors responsible for ECV homeostasis. A fall in ECV is detected as a fall in intravascular volume and pressure, and its reflex restoration restores plasma sodium to normal. As previously described, a fall in systemic blood pressure results in a lowered GFR, which is corrected by autoregulation, sympathetic drive, and angiotensin II (Table 2.6). The net effect is a reduction in salt and water excretion and restoration of the ECV.

Aldosterone

Aldosterone is a steroid hormone secreted by the zona glomerulosa of the adrenal cortex. It promotes sodium reabsorption in the distal tubule; this is important, although 90% of filtered sodium is absorbed proximal to this site. Aldosterone binds to cell cytosolic receptors, moves into the nucleus, and stimulates protein synthesis. This results in increased luminal membrane sodium permeability and increased activity in the sodium–potassium dependent ATPase pump. Aldosterone secretion is influenced by plasma sodium and potassium concentrations, ACTH, endorphins, and dopamine, but its primary control is angiotensin II.

Natriuretic Hormone

Natriuretic hormone antagonizes the sodium–potassium dependent ATPase pump and decreases sodium reabsorption. The hormone originates in the cardiac atrium and is a 28-amino-acid peptide.

Interstitial Hydraulic Pressure

Interstitial hydraulic pressure (IHP) varies directly with peritubular capillary pressure. Elevated IHP increases back-leakage of sodium and water across tight junctions into the tubular lumen, thus reducing reabsorption. Elevated capillary oncotic pressure (induced by an increased filtration fraction) reduces IHP and favors reabsorption of sodium and water by reducing back-leakage.

There may exist two distinct nephron populations with differing abilities to reabsorb sodium. Redistribution of blood flow to either population would dramatically alter sodium excretion. Catecholamines and angiotensin II have direct effects on the proximal tubule to increase sodium reabsorptin. Cortisol, estrogen, growth hormone, and insulin also increase sodium reabsorption, while glucagon, progesterone, and parathormone all increase sodium excretion.

Antidiuretic Hormone

Antidiuretic hormone (ADH) is an octapeptide released by nerve endings in the posterior pituitary. The nerve cell bodies lie in the supra-optic and paraventricular ganglia of the hypothalamus. A fall in systemic blood pressure decreases atrial pressure and reflexly inhibits the tonic firing of baroreceptors. This leads to release of ADH with resultant increase in peripheral resistance by vasoconstriction and restoration of blood pressure. This is in addition to the sodium-sparing effects of ADH in the kidney. Angiotensin II generation also stimulates ADH release. In addition, osmoreceptors in the hypothalamus detect changes in plasma osmolality and directly influence ADH release. Secretion can be altered by pain, fear, alcohol, and the thirst center.

RENAL CONTROL OF POTASSIUM

The sodium-potassium dependent ATPase pump regulates the flow of potassium across body-cell membranes. This pump is under the influence of epinephrine, insulin, and aldosterone, all of which exert a positive effect on the movement of potassium into cells. In the kidney, potassium is freely filterable, but less than 10% is excreted. The tubules can either secrete or absorb potassium. Fifty percent of filtered potassium is reabsorbed by the proximal tubule by passive diffusion along the concentration gradient created by water absorption. Potassium is secreted along the descending loop of Henle but reabsorbed along the ascending limb.

In the distal tubules potassium is actively pumped into the tubular cells through the basolateral membrane. This raises potassium concentration and creates a chemical gradient for flow into the lumen. The luminal membrane has potassium-specific channels and a weak pump activity to reabsorb potassium into the cell. The adrenal cortex responds to elevations in plasma potassium by secreting aldosterone, which directly increases activity of the basolateral ATPase pump (and increases numbers of pumps) with net increased potassium secretion into the luminal fluid. A fall in ECV affects the renin–angiotensin system and produces the same effects via aldosterone secretion.

Acid–Base Influences on Potassium Secretion

The presence of alkalosis stimulates the basolateral entry of potassium into the tubular cell, thus increasing excretion of potassium. The opposite effects are seen with some forms of acidosis for the first 24 hours.

RENAL HANDLING OF CALCIUM

Calcium homeostasis is controlled at three sites: bone, kidney, and the gastrointestinal tract. Intestinal absorption is controlled by vitamin D, which increases uptake of dietary calcium and phosphate. Ninety-nine percent of total body calcium is sequestered in bone, and undergoes a constant flux of interchange with the extracellular fluid. Vitamin D increases reabsorption of calcium from bone and facilitates the reabsorptive effects of parathormone.

The 60% of plasma calcium unbound to protein is filtered at the glomerulus and undergoes active reabsorption throughout the nephron except in the descending loop of Henle. The majority is reabsorbed proximally and is linked closely with the reabsorption of sodium. In the distal tubules sodium and calcium absorption is under the influence of aldosterone and parathormone, respectively. The excreted calcium (1 to 2%) equals the total amount absorbed in the gastrointestinal tract. Calcium excretion is increased by the presence of metabolic acidosis.

A fall in plasma calcium releases parathormone from the parathyroid glands. Three effects ensue: increased absorption of calcium and phosphate from the intestine; tubular reabsorption of calcium is augmented and phosphate reabsorption reduced; hydroxylation of vitamin D to dihydroxycholecalciferol in the kidney increases bone and intestinal absorption of calcium and phosphate.

Calcitonin is secreted by the parafollicular cells of the thyroid gland in response to high plasma calcium concentrations (in addition to a lowering of circulating parathormone levels). This hormone decreases plasma calcium by inhibiting bone reabsorption. Cortisol depresses and growth hormone increases intestinal absorption of calcium. Growth hormone also increases urinary excretion of calcium.

ACID–BASE BALANCE

In health the pH of the circulating blood is maintained in the range of 7.36 to 7.45. The principal source of H^+ is the basic process of oxidative metabolism:

$$CO_2 + H_2O = H_2CO_3 = H^+ + HCO_3^-.$$

Formation of fixed acids such as phosphoric, sulfuric, and lactic acid and ketones also increases plasma H^+. The kidney plays an important role in acid–base balance. Extrarenally, acid–base changes are buffered by intracellular (proteins and phosphates) and extracellular (CO_2-HCO_3^- system) mechanisms. The key factors in H^+ regulation are outlined by the Henderson–Hasselbalch equation:

$$pH = 6.1 + \log HCO_3^-/0.03PaCO_2.$$

Thus renal control of bicarbonate excretion and respiratory control of plasma carbon dioxide tension are sufficient to achieve acid–base balance.

In conditions of acidosis, the kidneys reabsorb maximum quantities of filtered HCO_3 and, in addition, contribute further HCO_3 to the plasma by secreting H^+ into the tubular lumen. When alkalosis prevails, the kidneys excrete filtered HCO_3. Bicarbonate is freely filterable, and in health is reabsorbed by an active process. Passive reabsorption is negligible because the tubular luminal membranes are impermeable to HCO_3 relative to sodium chloride and water. Active HCO_3 absorption involves secretion of H^+ into the tubular fluid to join the filtered HCO_3. Formation of carbonic acid and its subsequent disassociation into CO_2 and water precedes entry into the intracellular carbonic anhydrase pathway, generating a molecule of HCO_3 to enter the plasma (Figure 2.4).

Hydrogen ion secretion occurs by countertransport with sodium (secondary active transport) and via the primary H^+ ATPase pump in the distal tubule. In acidosis, the nephron synthesizes more HCO_3 by tubular secretion of acid. In this circumstance, the H^+ binds to buffers in the lumen and is excreted; it is not reabsorbed as water as in a normal, healthy person. The important tubular buffers are phosphates (PO_4) and ammonia (NH_3). Phosphate buffering has limitations because PO_4 undergoes 75% reabsorption, with less being available for buffering. Glutamine is converted in the tubular cell by glutaminase and glutamic acid dehydrogenase to NH_3. This synthesis increases in acidosis (adaptation of ammonia synthesis). Nonionized NH_3 is lipid-soluble and passes easily along a concentration gradient into the lumen. Binding with secreted acid converts NH_3 to NH_{4+}, which is nonabsorbable and easily excreted. Buffered acid is measured in the urine as titratable acid.

Influences on Tubular Acid Secretion

The rate of tubular acid secretion is directly proportional to the GFR (by a glomerulotubular feedback system similar to that described for sodium). There is also a direct relationship to changes in plasma pCO_2 as detected by the tubular arteriole. In respiratory acidosis (e.g., pulmonary failure), there is increased pCO_2, which by mass action in the tubular cell results in tubular acid secretion, reabsorption of filtered HCO_3, and synthesis of further HCO_3 with excretion of buffered acid. The opposite holds in res-

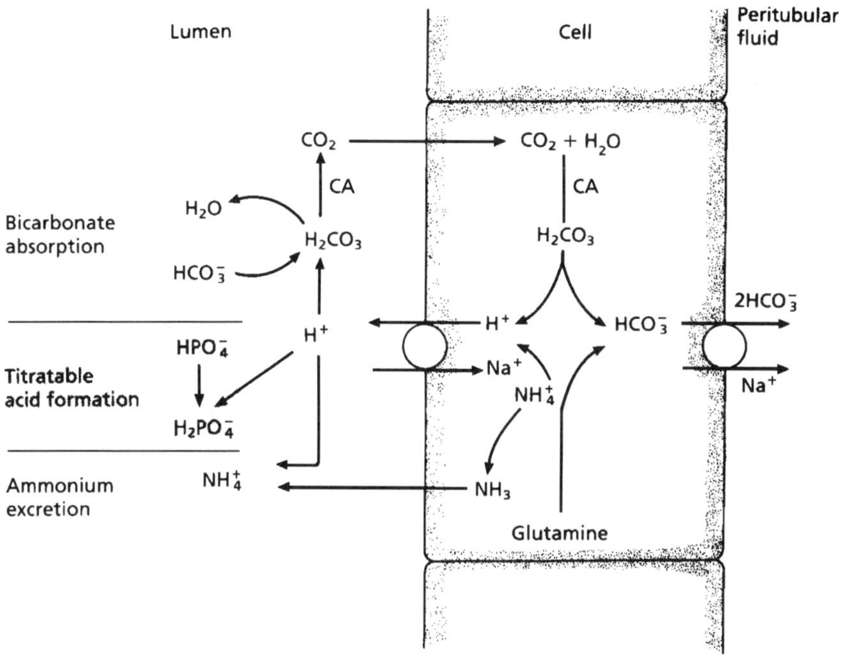

Figure 2.4: Mechanisms for the excretion of hydrogen ion. CA, carbonic anhydrase. *Reproduced with permission from Webster, Kirby K, King L, et al eds. Reconstructive Urology Vol 1. Boston: Blackwell Scientific Publications, 1991:11.*

piratory alkalosis, with net excretion of filtered HCO_3. In metabolic acidosis (e.g., increased production of fixed acids or loss of bicarbonate), the kidney compensation is the same as for respiratory acidosis but the stimulus is not an increased pCO_2. Plasma HCO_3 increases, and the tubular cell easily reabsorbs all filtered HCO_3 and secretes H^+ for luminal buffering even with an overall reduced H^+ secretion (secondary to low pCO_2). The situation in metabolic alkalosis is the opposite.

Salt depletion reduces the ability of the kidney to compensate for a metabolic alkalosis. This is due to the reflex increase in tubular reabsorption of sodium chloride, with resultant increased H^+ secretion, which then limits the excretion of HCO_3. Aldosterone has the same effects as salt depletion by stimulating sodium reabsorption and H^+ secretion. This situation is further compounded in the presence of K^+ deficiency. A fall in plasma K^+ decreases renal cell pH, stimulates H^+ secretion, and causes a worsening of the alkalotic state. In the absence of pre-existing acid–base disorders, salt depletion can induce such an alkalosis. Cortisol has mineralocorticoid effects and can cause a metabolic alkalosis by the same mechanism as aldosterone.

ACUTE RENAL FAILURE

The hallmark of acute renal failure (ARF) is a decreased glomerular filtration rate. The fall in GFR is mainly due to a decrease in renal blood flow, with diversion of flow away from the afferent glomerular arteriole. Clinically, ARF is manifest in critically ill patients by a urine output of less than 20 ml/hour (oliguria). ARF is conveniently categorized as prerenal, renal, or postrenal failure (obstructive uropathy). The urologist is most often faced with prerenal failure (often progressing to acute tubular necrosis) and obstructive uropathy (Table 2.8). ARF is also classified by etiology: vascular (major arteries, small vessels, or veins), glomerulonephritic (poststreptococcal, systemic lupus erythematosis [SLE], antibody nephritis), interstitial nephritis (infection), acute tubular necrosis (ATN), and obstructive.

Prerenal Azotemia

Prerenal azotemia, a reversible situation, occurs when either the cardiac output (e.g., in post myocardial infarction or congestive cardiac failure) or the effective extracellular volume (e.g., in hemorrhagic shock, gastrointestinal obstruction, or major burns) decreases. The ensuing reduction in renal blood flow induces three major changes in renal function.

Sodium excretion is closely dependent (direct relationship) on changes in arterial blood pressure, and the first change is a reduction in salt and water excretion. Sodium handling by the nephron is also influenced by the extrarenal hormones aldosterone and vasopressin (ADH). Secretion of these hormones is increased in hypovolemic states, resulting in further retention of sodium and water with decreased urine flow and low urinary sodium concentration (<20 mEq/l). These alterations occur even before glomerular filtration decreases.

A further effect occurring before GFR falls is the reduced clearance

Table 2.8: Biochemical Changes in Oliguria

	Prerenal	*ATN*
Plasma (*P*) urea	Rises	Rises
Plasma creatinine	Rises	Rises
Urinary (*U*) Na	<20 mM/L	>40 mM/L
U:*P* urea ratio	>10	<5
U:*P* osmolality	>1.4	<1.1

of urea. The reduction of urine flow allows maximal tubular reabsorption of urea and an increased plasma urea concentration. This may be compounded by increased formation of urea by catabolism or absorption of partially digested blood from the gastrointestinal tract. This limits the usefulness of plasma urea as an indicator of renal function. When the GFR finally falls below normal values, the deterioration in urine flow and composition is exaggerated. In prerenal failure, the urine flow is reduced and sodium, urea, and creatinine are retained.

Acute Tubular Necrosis

Acute tubular necrosis (ATN), the commonest cause of ARF, follows hypoxia, sepsis, or exposure to nephrotoxic compounds. The oliguric patient secretes an isotonic, acidic urine that contains protein and white cell and granular casts. Morphologically, extensive patchy tubular necrosis is seen with intratubular casts and leakage of tubular fluid.

Two important vascular influences on the development of ATN are (1) generation of angiotensin II, which acts as a powerful vasoconstrictor and decreases potassium filtration, and (2) prostaglandin generation, which, although usually protective via a vasodilatory effect, has a renin-releasing capability. Experimentally, infusion of the prostaglandin synthetase inhibitor indomethacin aggravates glycerol-induced ATN, and infusion of PGE_2 is protective.

Differentiating ATN from Prerenal Failure Serial measurement of the GFR is impractical in seriously ill patients, and diagnosis relies on changes in plasma and urinary osmolality and urea and creatinine levels. The urea and creatinine levels are most reliable because plasma urea is often a better indicator of catabolism than renal function. Complicated measurements of the free water clearance or fractional sodium excretion are seldom necessary. Figure 2.4 summarizes the most useful factors in differentiating prerenal failure from ATN in oliguric patients.

Postrenal Azotemia

The effects of obstruction in the urinary tract depend on whether the problem is bilateral (e.g., prostatic hyperplasia, posterior urethral valves) or unilateral (e.g., ureteric calculus). Total obstruction rapidly results in complete anuria in the affected kidney, but there may be no overall physiological changes. Partial obstruction results in a series of characteristic renal changes, which are dealt with in a later section.

DRUG-INDUCED RENAL DISEASE

Disordered renal function as a result of adverse drug reactions is common. Renal involvement may take the form of transient fluid and electrolyte abnormalities, acute renal failure due to interstitial nephritis or ATN, and chronic renal failure (Table 2.9).

Acute Interstitial Nephritis

Acute interstitial nephritis (AIN) often is first seen as acute renal failure and may be severe and oliguric. Drugs implicated as causal agents include cimetidine, beta-lactam antibiotics, diuretics, allopurinol, and non-steroidal anti-inflammatory drugs. Patients present with acute renal failure, rash, pyrexia, and joint pains. Urinary eosinophilia is pathognomonic, but hematuria, proteinuria, and pyuria are often seen. Renal biopsy is diagnostic. Gallium renal scanning shows increased uptake in nephritis but is normal in ATN.

Acute Tubular Necrosis

ATN implies direct toxicity to renal tubular epithelial cells. The aminoglycosides have a well earned reputation for nephrotoxicity. Gentamycin has the greatest potential for renal damage, followed by tobramycin, amikacin, and netilmicin. Serious damage occurs in less than 10% of patients. Brush border and lysosomal enzymes initially appear in the urine, followed by impaired tubular function and proteinuria. The aminoglycosides alter phospholipids within the lysosomes of tubular cells and cause cell necrosis. Administration of calcium supplements limits this intracellular binding and may be useful therapeutically. Renal toxicity has been reported with use of cephalosporin antibiotics, particularly cephaloridine. Synergism with aminoglycoside toxicity may occur. Amphotericin B induces a

Table 2.9: Drug-Induced Nephropathies

Renal Syndrome	*Drugs*
Acute interstitial nephritis (AIN)	Methicillin, ampicillin, diuretics, nonsteroidal anti-inflammatory drugs (NSAIDs), allopurinol, phenytoin, cimetidine, sulfonamides
Acute tubular necrosis (ATN)	Aminoglycosides, cisplatin, tetracyclines, methoxyflurane, amphotericin B, cephalosporins, contrast agents used in radiology
Chronic renal failure (CRF)	Analgesics: phenacetin, aspirin, acetaminophen, NSAIDs (especially in combination), cyclosporin

nonoliguric renal failure due to vasoconstriction, leading ultimately to concentrating defects, tubular acidosis, and potassium loss. These effects are minimized by avoidance of volume depletion during administration.

The platinum-containing anticancer agents cisplatin and carboplatin induce ATN with potassium and calcium wasting. Prehydration reduces these risks. Acetaminophen induces ATN and liver toxicity, but the latter usually dominates the clinical picture. The ionic and newer nonionic radiographic contrast compounds cause ATN in a small proportion of patients. The risk is estimated to be less than 10%. Etiological factors include volume depletion, multiple myeloma (especially with dehydration), old age, volume of contrast infused, diabetes, renal insufficiency, heart failure, and liver disease.

Chronic Renal Failure

Patients ingesting analgesics for prolonged periods are prone to develop analgesic nephropathy. This is manifested by impaired concentrating ability, sterile pyuria, and renal insufficiency. These effects are due to chronic recurrent papillary necrosis induced by toxic metabolite injury and medullary ischemia. Sloughed papillae are passed in the urine and may produce ureteral obstruction. In particular, aspirin and nonsteroidal anti-inflammatory drugs inhibit renal prostaglandin synthetase, with loss of vasodilatory prostaglandins and resultant ischemic damage. The changes can be imaged by intravenous urography (ring sign) or ultrasound examination (small kidney with thinned cortex). These patients may progress to end-stage disease and become candidates for transplantation. They are also at increased risk of developing transitional cell carcinomas of the upper tract.

OBSTRUCTIVE UROPATHY

The effects of urinary tract obstruction on renal function are diverse. Often the obstruction is gradual and reflected clinically by the development of chronic renal insufficiency. Sudden, complete bilateral obstruction causes acute renal failure accompanied by severe acidosis and hyperkalemia. The main goal of investigation and treatment is preservation of kidney function by prevention of nephron damage (particularly secondary to infection). One pathological change observed in the obstructed kidney is atrophy, which commences in the distal nephron within 7 days. Atrophy is seen in cortical regions by the fourteenth day, with eventual glomerular damage. Obstructive uropathy is associated with marked changes in renal blood flow and glomerular filtration rate. The major site of injury is the distal nephron, with inability to concentrate urine and altered hydrogen ion secretion, which leads to acidosis. Alterations in the tubular handling of electrolytes may lead to systemic electrolyte disorders and hypertension. The effects of urinary obstruction on renal function depend on its completeness, whether it is unilateral or bilateral, and its duration.

Sodium and Water Excretion

In unilateral ureteric obstruction the absolute amount of sodium excreted by the postreleased kidney is the same as that excreted by its contralateral, unobstructed mate. This is despite an overall reduction in GFR of the obstructed kidney to 10 to 20% of normal. Postobstructive diuresis does not result following relief of unilateral ureteral obstruction unless the opposite kidney is absent or severely damaged.

The situation is different following release of bilateral ureteric obstruction, which results in dramatic increases in the absolute quantity of sodium and water in the urine excreted. Increased ureteric, and hence intratubular, pressure in obstruction is associated with a fall in absolute and fractional sodium excretion due to increased tubular reabsorption of sodium and water. Thus, increased tubular pressure in itself is not natriuretic, and the postobstructive diuresis seen after chronic bilateral ureteral obstruction is due to other factors. The period of anuria before release of obstruction is important in the genesis of postobstructive diuresis.

Following release of obstruction, single-nephron GFR is reduced. In unilateral obstruction, reabsorption in superficial proximal tubules is increased, whereas it is unchanged or decreased in bilateral obstruction. Reabsorption is decreased in juxtaglomerular proximal tubules in all types of obstruction. Both unilateral and bilateral obstruction inhibit the ability of the thick ascending loop of Henle to reabsorb salt. After release of bilateral obstruction, volume of fluid delivered to the distal tubules increases, but the increase is relatively less in unilateral obstruction. The distal tubules show decreased reabsorption in bilateral obstruction and increased reabsorption in unilateral obstruction.

In obstruction, pyelolymphatic and pyelovenous pathways may also open up, allowing some reabsorption of the continuing, though reduced, volume of glomerular filtrate. Ruptures have been noted in the pelvic-papillary fornices with altered pelvicalyceal permeability and leakage of urine into the systemic circulation. There may also be leaks into the interstitial spaces and systemic absorption via renal lymphatics and damaged capillaries. The renal lymph volume approximates that of urine flow and increases with ureteral obstruction. In low-pressure obstruction pyelocanicular and pyelosinus back-flow are seen. With higher pressures, urine flows into the lymphatic and venous systems.

Renal Blood Flow

In complete ureteral obstruction (unilateral or bilateral) a transient increase in renal blood flow is seen due to changes in preglomerular vascular resistance. Renal release of vasoactive hormones contributes to these changes. This initial rise in renal blood flow (RBF) is followed by a fall to preobstruction levels within about 4 hours. The fall in blood flow continues beyond 24 hours to stabilize at a lower level, and has been estimated to be 12% of normal values at 8 weeks following complete unilateral ureteric obstruction.

Permanent focal arteriolar damage occurs following partial ureteric obstruction in the canine experimental model. These findings support the concept that postobstructive renal failure is due to a vascular injury. Following release of bilateral obstruction, renal blood flow and its intrarenal distribution return to normal. In unilateral obstruction, postrelease blood flow remains low and is shunted primarily to the outer cortex. This pattern of blood flow contributes to the increased fractional reabsorption of salt and water by the proximal and distal tubules of the outer cortical nephrons.

RBF and renin secretion effects can be reversed by cyclooxygenase-pathway inhibition, and this implies a regulatory role for prostaglandins. Adrenergic blockade has no effect on RBF. Histamine is also involved in blood-flow increases and can be abolished by H_1 receptor blockade. Following the first 4 hours of obstruction, increasing levels of thromboxane A_2 may mediate the observed vasoconstriction and reduction in flow. Atrial natriuretic peptide has also been implicated in renal blood-flow changes seen in obstruction.

Glomerular Filtration Rate

GFR falls but does not cease completely with ureteric obstruction. Decrease in renal blood flow and increases in intratubular pressure induce a fall in GFR. In addition, the ultrafiltration coefficient (K_f) decreases (perhaps by renin release), thus further reducing GFR. It is estimated that there is a four- to five-fold reduction of filtration rate in both unilateral and bilateral obstruction. Release of ureteric obstruction returns GFR to about 50% of preobstruction levels.

Postobstructive Diuresis

During partial ureteric obstruction and following release of bilateral ureteric obstruction, increased volumes of filtrate reach the distal tubules and collecting ducts. In addition, the decrease in the ability of the kidney to concentrate urine results in polyuria and an increase in urinary sodium. Following the release of chronic unilateral ureteral obstruction, the changed renal blood-flow patterns and the increased fractional reabsorption by cortical nephrons may reduce the excretion of salt and water.

Even though these changes do not occur in bilateral obstruction, there is a five-fold increase in salt and water excretion despite a reduced GFR (i.e., by 80%). It may be that accumulation of natriuretic factor(s) during anuria are contributory to the observed postrelease diuresis. Urea is a possible candidate due to its known osmotic diuretic effects. In humans, postobstructive diuresis has been observed despite normal plasma urea, and therefore other natriuretic factors must also be involved (Table 2.10).

Studies have shown that the longer the period of obstruction, the greater is the deterioration in function and the longer the period of recovery. The higher the osmotic load from retained fluids and solutes, and the higher the GFR, the greater the potential for a postrelease diuresis.

Polyuria can be prolonged with replacement therapy, which prevents the return to normal fluid and electrolyte balance. Large volumes of water and electrolytes, particularly sodium, are lost during the recovery period. The patient may, in extreme cases, become hypotensive. Defects in urine acidification and potassium excretion may induce systemic acidosis or hyperkalemia. Magnesium loss leading to hypomagnesemia has also been reported.

Recovery of Renal Function

The ability of the kidneys to recover function following release of both unilateral and bilateral ureteric obstruction depends on two factors: the severity of the renal injury and the presence or absence of infection. Supervening infection accelerates renal deterioration. Infection warrants immediate intervention by the urologist to effect renal drainage and institute aggressive antimicrobial therapy.

Ureteral obstruction results in a shift from aerobic to anaerobic renal metabolism. Fatty acid and alpha-ketoglutarate utilization deterio-

Table 2.10: Postobstructive Diuresis

- Loss salt, water after release
  - Bilateral ureteral obstruction or unilateral obstruction with contralateral nephrectomy/poor function
- Associated with azotemia
- Causes
  - Elevated plasma urea
  - Atrial natriuretic factor
  - Damage to intrinsic reabsorptive distal tubular mechanisms
- Treatment
  - Cautious replacement fluids, electrolytes
  - Monitor serum electrolytes

rate significantly, and renal gluconeogenesis is eventually lost. By 6 weeks postobstruction these changes are marked and may be irreversible.

Acute ureteral obstruction may lead to hypertension as a direct result of increased renin secretion. Hypertension in chronic hydronephrosis is independent of renin secretion and is secondary to expansion of the extracellular fluid by sodium and water retention.

Functional Assessment of Obstructive Uropathy

Microscopic or macroscopic hematuria may be noted on urinalysis in patients with renal or ureteric calculi. Bacteriuria signifies urinary infection secondary to stasis.

Urinary obstruction may cause polycythemia, probably as a result of erythropoietin release. Hemoglobin levels may be normal or decreased, depending on the degree of uremia. A polymorphonuclear leucocytosis supports the diagnosis of infection. In postrenal obstruction, the blood urea rises disproportionately to creatinine levels due to increased reabsorption of urea in the obstructed tubules. The ratio of blood urea to creatinine is often above 15. In long-standing obstruction, plasma calcium and phosphate levels fall.

Plain films of the abdomen may reveal opaque calculi and provide an estimate of renal size. Although 95% of renal calculi are radiopaque, they are often difficult to visualize and the usefulness of plain radiographs is therefore limited. Contrast media such as Hypaque, Miokon, and Renografin are excreted from the circulation by glomerular filtration alone. In acute hydronephrosis, there is delay in opacification of the parenchyma by contrast in the tubules (nephrogram phase) and a decrease in size of the kidney. With supervening infection and the development of pyonephrosis, the intravenous urogram (IVU) may show nonfunction or poor visualization.

Retrograde catheterization demonstrates obstructing ureteric calculi. Placement of an indwelling stent in this situation will accomplish renal pelvic drainage and halt deterioration of renal function. Renal ultrasound will confirm the presence of an obstructed urinary tract. Hydronephrosis and thinning of the renal cortex are easily visualized.

Computerized tomography and magnetic resonance imaging provide useful information on the presence of tumors or retroperitoneal causes of obstruction. In some patients, additional information regarding obstruction can be obtained by performing antegrade perfusion pressure measurements (Whitaker test) via an indwelling nephrostomy tube. The increased rate of salt and water reabsorption from the obstructed tubules can be directly monitored by the prolonged passage time of nonreabsorbable radiolabeled agents. The individual contribution of the nephrons in each kidney to overall renal function can be measured with this technique.

CONCLUSION

The four basic renal functions of glomerular filtration, selective tubular reabsorption, tubular secretion, and tubular metabolism maintain the body's physiological balance. Superimposed on this intrinsic regulatory function are multiple extrarenal controls that fine-tune urine production. These include the adrenal cortex and medulla, parathyroid glands, cardiovascular regulatory systems, and the pituitary gland. The end result of many disease states is renal failure accompanied by anuria, acidosis, hyperkalemia, and rising serum urea and creatinine concentrations. The clinician must be able to recognize and treat such disorders at the stage of reversibility (prerenal failure) and prevent progression to established tubular necrosis. This task is compounded by the widespread use of potentially nephrotoxic drugs.

Renal obstruction is increasingly seen by the urologist, and this reflects the aging population. The effects of unilateral versus bilateral or partial versus complete obstruction are now predictable and reproducible. Superinfection in an obstructed renal tract can lead to rapid deterioration of renal function. Postobstructive diuresis can be predicted and appropriate therapeutic intervention initiated.

Each year more knowledge is accrued on renal function. Management of renal disease requires an understanding of renal function. The practicing urologist needs to be aware of current advances in renal function in health and disease.

SUGGESTED READINGS

Gottshalk CW, Lassiter, WE. Micropuncture methodology. In: Orloff J, Berliner RW, eds. Handbook of renal physiology. Washington, DC: American Physiological Society, 1973:129.

Review of techniques employed to glean information on the function of the nephron and its segments.

Porter GA, Bennett WM. Nephrotoxic acute renal failure due to common drugs. Am J Physiol 1981; 241:F1.

Nephrotoxicity of various pharmacologic agents are discussed with particular emphasis on the mechanisms of renal damage and failure.

Kincaid-Smith P. Analgesic abuse and the kidney. Kidney Int 1980; 17:250.

Classic review of effects of commonly used analgesic drugs on renal function.

Leahy AL, Ryan PC, McEntee GM, Nelson AC, Fitzpatrick JM. Renal injury and recovery in partial ureteric obstruction. J Urol 1989; 147(7):199.

Description of an experimental model for partial ureteric obstruction. Role of renal hemodynamic changes is integrated into the pathophysiology of obstructive uropathy.

Brenner BM, Humes HD. Mechanics of glomerular ultrafiltration. N Engl J Med 1977; 297:148.

Multiple mechanisms involved in glomerular filtration succinctly outlined. Excellent review of glomerular physiology.

Laragh JH. Atrial natriuretic hormone, the renin-aldosterone axis and blood pressure-electrolyte hemostasis. N Engl J Med 1985; 313:1330.

Describes hormonal control of blood pressure and electrolytes and discusses the roles of renal and extrarenal hormones.

McDougal WS. Pathophysiology of glomerular dysfunction following ureteral obstruction. Dialogues in Pediatr Urol 1990; 13(6):7.

Concise review of changes in glomerular function that result from obstruction. Roles of prostaglandins and other hormones are described.

Vaughan ED Jr, Gillenwater JY. Diagnosis, characteristics and management of postobstructive diuresis. J Urol 1973; 109:286.

Overview of urologic aspects of postobstructive diuresis. Discussion based on sound pathophysiologic concepts.

Kokko JP, Rector FC Jr. Countercurrent multiplication system without active transport in inner medulla. Kidney Int 1972; 2:214.

Clear description of renal countercurrent exchange multiplier. Simplifies the understanding of kidney secretory and concentrating mechanisms.

Levey AS. Measurement of renal function in chronic renal disease. Kidney Int 1990; 38:167.

Discussion of the various tests of renal function—their limitations, relevance, and applicability to the clinical assessment of renal function.

Kassirer JP. Clinical evaluation of kidney function: glomerular function. N Engl J Med 1971; 285:385.

Focused discussion of glomerular function—its pathophysiology, assessment, and clinical correlations.

Berry CA. Heterogeneity of tubular transport processes in the nephron. Ann Rev Physiol 1982; 44:181.

Excellent review of functional characteristics of nephron segments. Clear discussion of various tubular transport mechanisms.

CHAPTER 3

Ureteral Pathophysiology

Marc Cendron
Grannum R. Sant
George T. Klauber

A clear understanding of ureteral dynamics is essential to an understanding of ureterovesical junction (UVJ) function, obstructive uropathy, and obstructive nephropathy. The urologist is frequently presented with problems in both adults and children that cause upper-tract dysfunction. Upper urinary tract obstruction results in obstructive uropathy and obstructive nephropathy. The uropathy results in structural and functional alterations in the genitourinary tract proximal to the point of obstruction. The diagnostic and therapeutic efforts of the urologist are usually directed to the changes associated with obstructive uropathy, for example, dilated ureter or hydronephrosis. Unrelieved obstruction causes functional and biochemical alterations in the renal parenchyma (nephropathy), which may lead to renal impairment and failure.

Ureters are conduits for the flow of urine from the kidneys to the bladder. Urine flows out of the renal collecting ducts into the minor calyces and then into the renal pelvis. Renal pelvic pressure increases with filling, forcing the urine past the ureteropelvic junction and down the ureter. Intrapelvic pressure, however, remains quite low (1 to 2 mm Hg) under normal conditions. Peristaltic activity enhances the movement of the urine toward the bladder. The ureter and renal pelvis also serve as a modulator to protect the kidney from distal obstruction and backflow.

THE URETER

Anatomy

The ureters are thick, muscular tubes that extend from the kidneys to the bladder. They average 25 to 30 cm in length. The abdominal segment of the ureter descends medially on the psoas muscle and is attached to the posterior aspect of the peritoneum. The gonadal vessels cross the ureters anteriorly. The appendix may overlie the right ureter, and the left ureter is in close relationship to the sigmoid mesocolon. The ureters pass into the pelvic brim by crossing the common iliac arteries. The pelvic segment of the ureter initially courses laterally toward the ischial spine, then converges medially toward the bladder trigone. In the female, the pelvic ureter is in close proximity to the broad ligament of the uterus, the lateral aspect of the cervix, and the uterine artery. The pelvic ureter is at risk for surgical damage during gynecologic surgery, for example, radical hysterectomy.

The blood supply of the ureter is multiple and segmental. The upper ureter is supplied by renal, aortic, gonadal, and aortic vessels, whereas the lower ureter gets its blood supply from the iliac, vesical, obturator, and uterine vessels. The ureteral blood vessels are oriented into ascending and descending branches that run in the adventitial layer. Thus, during donor nephrectomy, a wide swath of adventitial tissues is mobilized so as to ensure an adequate blood supply to the distal end of the transected ureter.

Histologically, the ureter is composed of an inner epithelial layer, a muscular layer, and an outer adventitial layer. The muscular layer is made up of small, smooth muscle cells arranged in two spiral layers, an inner tight spiral and an outer open spiral. Previously, these muscle layers were thought to be circular and longitudinal in orientation. The muscle spirals provide contractility to the ureter. The muscle cells have large surface areas, which allow extracellular calcium to cross the cell membrane easily during excitation. Contractile proteins, actin and myosin, are stored within the cytoplasm. Increased calcium causes contraction of these proteins. The smooth muscle cells of the ureter are syncytial without identifiable neuromuscular junctions. Electrical activity is conducted between cells via low-resistance intermediate junctions or nexuses.

Physiology

Ureteral peristalsis is primarily myogenic, although there are neurogenic and possible endocrine influences (Table 3.1). The nonexcited ureteral smooth muscle cells have a high resting membrane potential (–30 to –70 mV) due to their relative permeability to potassium ions. With excitation, the membrane becomes more permeable to sodium and calcium ions, which enter the cell, depolarize the membrane, and result in an action potential (Table 3.1). The contractile response is promoted by increased cytoplasmic concentrations of calcium acting on actin and myosin. Calcium promotes contractile activity by a complex series of interactions involving calmodulin (a calcium binding protein), myosin

Table 3.1: Mechanisms of Ureteral Peristalsis

Myogenic
- Membrane depolarization: rise in intracellular calcium
- Muscle contraction: calcium, calmodulin, myosin kinase, actin, myosin, ATPase
- Pacemaker cells: minor calyces
- Latent pacemakers in distal ureteral segments

Neurogenic
- Stimulatory: cholinergic, alpha adrenergic
- Inhibitory: beta adrenergic

Hormonal
- Estrogen
- Progesterone
- Glucagon

light chain kinase, adenosine triphosphatase (ATPase), actin, and myosin. The calcium is predominantly derived from the extracellular compartment during membrane depolarization, although there is some contribution from calcium stores in the endoplasmic reticulum.

The ureter undergoes smooth muscle contraction and excitation as well as acting as a tubular propulsive conduit for urine. As the peristaltic wave progresses down the ureter, the intraluminal pressure within the ureter rises from a resting pressure of 0 to 5 cm of water to a pressure of 20 to 60 cm of water (Table 3.2). Peristaltic waves occur 2 to 6 times per minute, with increased frequency during periods of diuresis. The contraction waves progress distally at a speed of 2 to 5 cm/sec. Ureteral propulsion is more a function of wall coaptation than of ureteral shorten-

Table 3.2: Ureteral Dynamics, Propulsion

Laplace's law:

$$\text{Pressure} = \frac{\text{Tension} \times \text{Wall thickness}}{\text{Radius}}$$

Resting pressure 0–5 cm H_2O

Peristaltic pressure 20–80 cm H_2O

Peristalsis 2–6 waves/min

Propagation 2–5 cm/sec

Coaptation
- Segmental
- Bolus propagation

Viscoelastic properties

ing because the ureter shortens only 1 mm for each 10 cm during contraction. Coaptation is a result of ureteral wall tension, which provides a circumferential, centripetal pull with segmental coaptation. Urine trapped between two areas of coaptation becomes a bolus, which is then propagated distally (Figure 3.1). Transection of the ureter and reanastomosis temporarily inhibits the conduction of the peristaltic wave. However, after healing, distal propagation of peristalsis returns.

Although peristalsis is predominantly myogenic, there are neural influences on ureteral contraction and relaxation. Microscopic studies reveal abundant unmyelinated nerve fibers in the ureteral wall. The ureter has excitatory alpha as well as inhibitory beta sympathetic autonomic receptors. The sympathetic supply is T11-12, L1, whereas the parasympathetic supply arises from the vagus and S2-4 sacral segments. Ureteral peristalsis occurs in the absence of innervation, for example, in renal transplantation. Ureteral activity can be modulated by the parasympathetic (cholinergic) and sympathetic (adrenergic) branches of the nervous system. Acetylcholine and other cholinergic agents, such as metha-

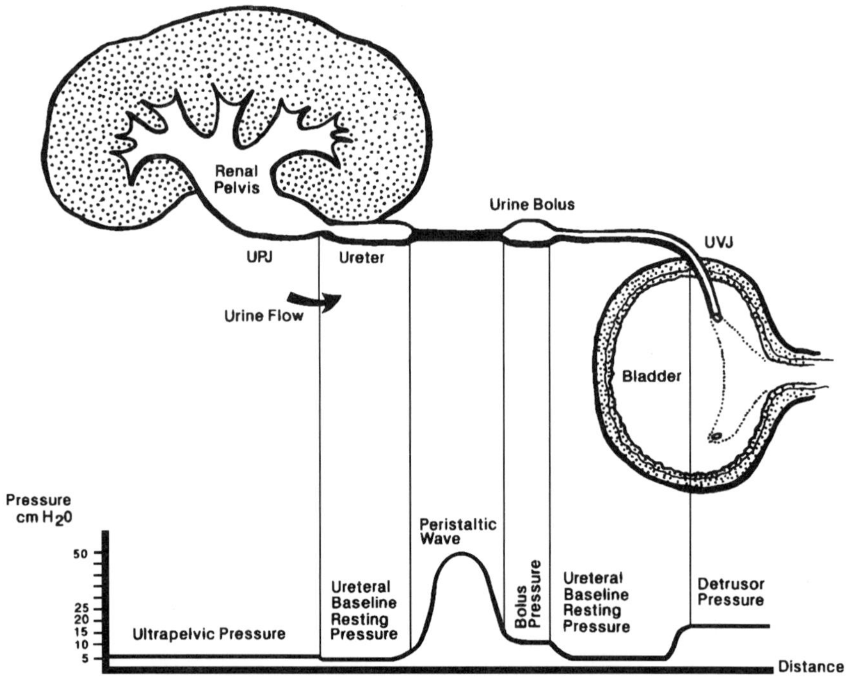

Figure 3.1: Pressure flow relationships in the upper urinary tract.

choline, carbamylcholine, and bethanecol, stimulate ureteral contraction. Alpha-adrenergic agonists (norepinephrine or phenylephrine) also increase the force and frequency of ureteral peristalsis. Beta-adrenergic agonists, for example, isoproterenol, decrease ureteral activity, as do the alpha-adrenergic antagonists phentolamine and phenoxybenzamine.

Clinical use of various pharmacologic agents to treat ureteral disease is limited. Morphine and meperidine (Demerol), for instance, may have an excitatory or spasmogenic effect on the ureter, but their use in treating ureteral colic has been mostly directed toward pain control. A number of pharmacologic agents have theoretical applications, but their side effects or lack of specificity render them virtually useless clinically.

Certain ureteral smooth muscle cells have unstable resting membrane potentials. This results in spontaneous, intermittent membrane depolarization. These "pacemaker" cells, morphologically distinct from the other smooth muscle cells, are thought to reside in the proximal collecting system, especially in the minor calyces (Figure 3.2). The normal pacemaker discharge is about 5 to 6 contractions per minute, but these are damped at the level of the ureteropelvic junction, especially at low urine-flow rates (Table 3.1). Latent pacemakers in the distal ureter (e.g., the ureterovesical junction) may escape the control of the more proximal primary pacemaker in certain pathologic conditions (e.g., obstructive megaureters).

Ureteral dynamics may also be influenced by hormones. Glucagon inhibits ureteral peristalsis, and it has been used to treat ureteral colic. Although the "hydronephrosis" of the second trimester of pregnancy is felt to have a predominant mechanical genesis, hormonal influences may be contributory. Female hormones increase the sensitivity of adrenergic receptors (estrogen → alpha, progesterone → beta). Experimentally, progesterone inhibits peristalsis and causes ureteral dilatation. The bulk of the evidence, however, suggests that the hydronephrosis of pregnancy is due primarily to mechanical factors (Table 3.3).

Ureteral Dynamics

Urine flow, ureteral radius, pressure, and resistance are interrelated. Flow

Table 3.3: Hydronephrosis of Pregnancy: Evidence for Mechanical Etiology

More severe on right side
Does not occur beneath pelvic brim
Does not occur in pelvic kidneys, ileal conduits
Normal ureteral pressures in women
Elevation of uterus reduces hydronephrosis

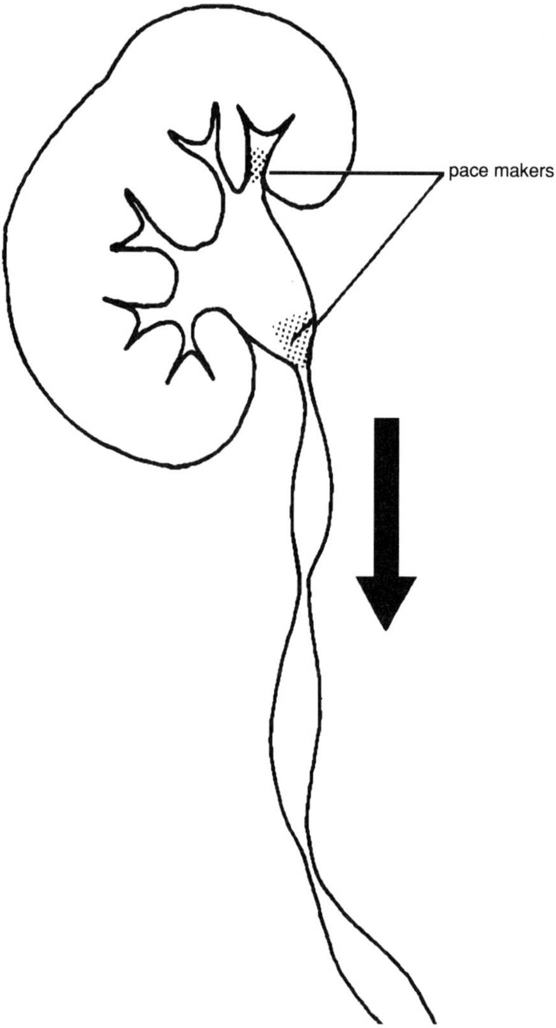

Figure 3.2: Coordinated peristalsis and sites of putative pacemakers. *Reproduced with permission from Blandy J. Lecture Notes on Urology, 4th ed. Oxford: Blackwell Scientific Publications, 1991:42.*

relies on adequate intraluminal pressure and a low resistance. Thus, a minor degree of ureteropelvic junction (UPJ) obstruction may become significant only during diuresis, for example, in patients with UPJ obstruction who develop such symptoms as flank pain after rigorous oral hydration or alcohol intake. Coaptive ureteral dynamics can be predicted from Laplace's equation, which relates intraluminal pressure to wall tension and tubular diameter (Table 3.2). Increases in ureteral diameter (e.g., megaureter, pregnancy) result in reduced intraluminal pressures, reduced coaptation, and impaired urine transport. Tapering of a dilated ureter, as with megaureter repairs, increases coaptation, intraluminal pressure, and urine propulsion. With obstruction or high flow rates (>10 ml/min), tubular diameter increases and flow is reduced. However, these effects are minimized by the intrinsic viscoelastic properties of the ureter.

The UPJ protects the kidney by staying narrow or closed and thus dissipating any back-pressure generated in the ureter. Urine flows down the ureter to reach the ureterovesical junction (UVJ), which acts as a one-way valve system that prevents urine from reentering the ureteral lumen from the bladder. For the bolus of urine to enter the bladder, the intraureteral pressure must exceed the intravesical pressure, which in the normally compliant bladder is low during filling. However, when high intravesical pressures are generated either by a small, noncompliant, hyperactive bladder (a neuropathic bladder) or by high volumes (overdistention from inability to empty due to outflow resistance caused by, for example, benign prostatic hyperplasia), ureteral peristalsis may be significantly impaired. The UVJ may become incompetent, with widening of the submucosal ureteral segment which prevents normal ureteral contraction and inhibits normal transport of urine across the UVJ. Vesicoureteral reflux may also ensue.

Effects of Obstruction on the Upper Urinary Tract

A number of pathologic conditions impair the normal flow of urine from the kidney to the bladder. Obstruction is one of the most common pathologic entities in urology. An obstruction may occur at any point in the urinary tract, from the UPJ all the way down to the urethra, and may be due to extrinsic compression or due to an intraluminal process such as urolithiasis. The main consequence of obstruction is an increase in urine stasis and an elevation of intraluminal ureteral pressure. Obstruction may be acute or chronic. Acute obstruction causes a rapid buildup in pressure of the upper urinary tract with minimal dilatation. Columnation of urine within the ureter and renal collecting system can be demonstrated by intravenous urography.

Obstruction at the UPJ level results in dilatation of the renal collecting system as a consequence of the increase in volume and elevated intrapelvic pressure (>100 cm of water). Causes of UPJ obstruction include congenital malformation, urolithiasis, crossing vessels, compression between vessels, stricture, or tumor. Disorganization of the normal pacemaker activity within the pelvicalyceal area has been reported in association with dilatation of the renal collecting system. Dyscoordinated contractions of the renal pelvis against a fixed obstruction may lead to hypertrophy of the smooth muscles of the renal pelvis. Continued disruption of urine flow past the UPJ may also impair normal peristaltic activity down the ureter. The renal pelvis and calyceal system subjected to outflow obstruction may dilate and become significantly distorted owing to compliance of the renal collecting system.

Trapping of calculi in the upper urinary tract primarily occurs at three distinct anatomic locations: (1) at the ureteropelvic junction (UPJ), (2) where the ureter crosses the iliac vessels, and (3) at the ureterovesical junction (UVJ). Experimental data suggests that the peristaltic wave of contraction may not be propagated across an area of obstruction. A number of factors influence the likelihood of spontaneous passage of ureteral calculi: ureteral spasm and swelling adjacent to the stone, urine hydrostatic pressure proximal to the stone, and size/shape of the stone. Increased hydrostatic pressure proximally facilitates stone passage and is the rationale for recommending hydration in the management of ureteral stones. Prolonged elevation of intrarenal hydrostatic pressure is potentially harmful to the kidney, but it is compensated by the mechanisms of pyelovenous and pyelolymphatic backflow. In acute obstruction, as seen with sudden distal obstruction by small calculi, there may be urinary extravasation via rupture of the calyceal fornices. Relaxation of the spasm adjacent to the stone theoretically facilitates stone passage. Potentially spasmylotic pharmacologic agents include alpha adrenergic antagonists, beta adrenergic agonists, and theophylline. However, their clinical effectiveness has not been demonstrated. Ureteral peristalsis is also reduced by bacterial endotoxins in patients with renal infections, for example, pyelonephritis. This is of clinical importance in patients with ureteral stone obstruction and sepsis in whom spontaneous stone passage may be impaired.

Long-term obstruction to the flow of urine within the ureter leads to proximal dilatation and tortuosity of the affected ureter. The pathophysiologic changes seen within the ureter and collecting system of the kidney vary depending on the degree and duration of the obstruction (Table 3.4). Coincident urinary tract infection also influences these changes. With acute obstruction and continued urine production by the kidney, accumulation of urine will cause a rise in the ureteral intraluminal pressure. Peristaltic activity will transiently increase and then become inefficient as it is unable to overcome the increased pressure. After a few hours of obstruction, the ureteral pressure declines slowly because of changes in intrarenal hemodynamics: decreases in glomerular filtration and in intratubular hydrostatic pressure, with fluid reabsorption by the lymphatic and venous systems.

Table 3.4: Effects of Obstruction

Effects of Obstruction
Determinants
Site
Patient age
Acute versus chronic
Intrinsic versus extrinsic
Completeness
Presence of infection
Unilateral versus bilateral
Preexisting renal function
Renal hemodynamics
Triphasic sequence in renal blood flow (RBF)
Rise in RBF 0–2 hr
Normal RBF 2–5 hr
Fall in RBF >5 hr
Redistribution RBF, GFR
Surface nephrons fall to 70% normal
Juxtamedullary nephrons fall to 50% normal
Effects on nephron
Reduced urine concentration
Reduced urine acidification
Cellular infiltrate
Macrophages
T-lymphocytes

Dilation of the ureter occurs early in the obstructive process. This process also arises in high-urinary-flow states. With dilatation of the ureter, ureteral wall coaptation is inhibited and the dilated ureter becomes inefficient in providing functional contractility. In addition, bacterial infection and release of endotoxin will further inhibit smooth muscle activity at the level of the ureter, further contributing to urinary stasis. Relief of the obstructive process allows decompression of the upper urinary tract. Depending on the duration and degree of obstruction, the renal pelvis and ureter will regain normal tone and function. Dilution of contrast may be noted secondary on intravenous urography because of postobstructive diuresis. The radiographic appearance of the upper urinary tract should return to normal within 3 to 6 months unless the obstruction either occurred early in fetal development or was long-standing, causing permanent distortion of the ureter and renal collecting system.

Increased intraureteral and intrarenal pressures are the first changes in obstruction and result in alterations of renal blood flow (RBF), glomerular filtration rate (GFR), renal tubular function, and kidney morphology;

alteration of kidney morphology is especially marked in developing kidneys (Table 3.4). The changes in renal hemodynamics with obstruction are triphasic. Within the first 0 to 2 hours, there is increased ureteral pressure and RBF, and a slight drop in GFR. Between 2 and 5 hours, tubular pressure plateaus in conjunction with a fall in RBF and GFR. Beyond 5 hours, there is a progressive reduction in RBF and GFR over time to 40 to 50% levels within 5 days. Juxtamedullary RBF decreases to about 30% of normal within 6 hours. The changes in renal blood flow and GFR are mediated by hormones produced by the arachidonic acid, renin-angiotensin, and kallikrein-kinin systems. Vasodilator prostaglandins (PGE_2, PGI_2) and kinins mediate the early increase in renal blood flow. Conversely, the vasoconstrictor activity of thromboxane A_2 (T_xA_2) and the angiotensins predominate in the later stages of obstruction.

GFR is affected by the changes in net ultrafiltration pressure secondary to reduced blood flow and increased intratubular pressure. GFR reduction is greater in surface than juxtamedullary nephrons. GFR changes are usually reversible with short-term obstruction (<30 hours). GFR and RBF changes are variable and depend on the degree/completeness of the obstruction as well as whether the obstruction is unilateral or bilateral.

The major site of insult in obstructive uropathy is the distal nephron (Table 3.4). Urine-concentrating ability is impaired due to inhibition of vasopressin-dependent cyclic AMP. Thus patients with chronic obstruction (e.g., long-standing prostatism) may develop polyuria. Furthermore, the nephron is unable to acidify the urine, with resulting bicarbonate wasting, metabolic acidosis, and hyperkalemia. This is due to a defect in hydrogen ion secretion in the distal nephrons and collecting ducts. These concentrating and acidifying defects can persist after relief of obstruction and result in reduced maximal urinary concentrating ability and nephrogenic diabetes insipidus. In obstructive nephropathy, there is a cellular infiltrate of macrophages and T-lymphocytes, especially in the renal cortex. These cells may release factors that contribute to tubular atrophy and interstitial fibrosis.

The renal effects of obstruction vary with age. Changes are more marked in young children, with alterations in the growth and size of the kidney. Changes in size are greater at earlier ages, and this is important as in-utero nephrogenesis is usually complete by 34 weeks.

Following relief of long-standing, bilateral obstruction, patients may experience a postobstructive diuresis with dramatic loss of salt and water. This is usually seen in azotemic patients, and its multifactorial etiology includes volume status prior to the relief of the obstruction, circulating natriuretic factors including urea, impaired collecting duct sodium and water reabsorption, and the rapid recovery of GFR that follows release of obstruction.

The Effects of Obstruction on the Developing Urinary Tract

Obstructive uropathy varies from mild dilatation of the urinary tract with good renal function to complete distortion of the urinary tract and severely compromised renal function. Obstructive uropathy may be supravesical or infravesical. Supravesical obstruction occurs at various levels: at the infundibulum, at the ureteropelvic junction, at the ureter, or at the ureterovesical junction. Renal infundibular obstruction results in caliectasis and is caused by compression of the infundibulum between vessels (Fraley's syndrome), congenital stenosis, or a hypoplastic infundibulum that prevents adequate calyceal drainage.

The UPJ is the most common site of obstruction in the upper urinary tract. The obstructive process is either intrinsic or extrinsic. Intrinsic obstruction can be due to many factors: (a) kinking of the UPJ as a result of a high insertion of the ureter into the pelvis or by fibrous bands, (b) lack of the normal smooth muscle continuity between the renal pelvis and ureter, or (c) intramural fibrosis. Obstruction may also result from a combination of the above factors and is seldom due to an intrinsic narrowing of the proximal ureteral lumen. Extrinsic compression of the UPJ by aberrant renal vessels is noted in approximately one-third of patients evaluated and treated for UPJ obstruction. However, histologically there is invariably a deficiency of underlying UPJ muscle and fibrous tissue replacement under aberrant crossing renal vessels. Hence, this portion of the ureter must be excised during reconstructive pyeloplasty. UPJ obstruction causes a rise in intrapelvic pressure and a decrease in urinary flow across the UPJ. Dilatation of the renal pelvis accommodates the rise in pressure and results in hydronephrosis. Compliance of the renal pelvis protects the renal parenchyma from the deleterious effects of increased pressures. The natural history of hydronephrosis due to UPJ obstruction diagnosed in the neonatal period is variable, and there is growing evidence that immediate intervention to relieve the obstruction may not be necessary. However, renal function is preserved and may improve if the obstruction is relieved or corrected prior to 6 months of age.

Ureteral dilatation of greater than 7 mm, referred to as megaureter, may be due to obstruction or vesicoureteral reflux. Nonrefluxing, nonobstructed megaureters also occur. Primary obstructed megaureters are associated with aperistaltic distal ureteral segments. A variety of histologic abnormalities have been observed in those distal segments, including an overabundance of muscle fibers in a circular and obstructive configuration and excess collagen deposition. The electron- and light-microscopic findings in the aperistaltic distal ureteral segment are similar to those described in UPJ obstruction. As with UPJ obstruction, the obstruction causes a rise in the intraluminal ureteral pressure and proximal dilatation.

The ureter exhibits significant plasticity and is able to accommodate large volumes of urine at relatively low pressures, thus buffering the kidney from the deleterious effects of back-pressure. Peristaltic waves are not propagated across areas of intrinsic obstruction and may reverse direction and result in retrograde peristalsis. However, persistent stasis of urine and elevated pressure may ultimately jeopardize renal function.

The most common cause of infravesical obstruction in infant males is posterior urethral valves; other causes are obstructing ectopic ureteroceles, anterior urethral valves, urethral agenesis or hypoplasia, and urethral stenosis. In adults, benign prostatic hyperplasia is the most common etiology of bladder-outlet obstruction. The effects of obstruction on the development of the urinary tract are variable and depend on timing, duration, and severity of the obstruction. The pathophysiologic consequences of obstruction occur throughout the urinary tract. The urethra proximal to the obstruction becomes dilated and the bladder wall hypertrophies in response to the increased work needed to overcome the obstruction. This is followed by detrusor hypertrophy, bladder trabeculation, and sacculation. Later, vesicoureteral reflux may develop. Incomplete bladder emptying and urinary stasis in the bladder as well as hydroureteronephrosis may arise with or without reflux. Renal parenchymal damage is often seen in the form of renal dysplasia or interstitial nephritis. In general, upper tract (e.g., ureteral) obstruction is potentially more deleterious to the kidney than infravesical (e.g., prostatic) obstruction. Furthermore, in-utero obstruction is associated with the risk of renal hypoplasia/dysplasia. Three protective mechanisms may help preserve renal function in boys with posterior urethral valves: (1) dilatation of the ureters and renal pelvis, (2) bladder diverticula, and (3) urinary ascites due to leakage of urine at the level of the renal sinus or the bladder. In boys with posterior urethral valves, those with urinary ascites generally have a better prognosis, as do those with a large bladder diverticulum and unilateral rather than bilateral reflux.

A dilated upper urinary tract may occur as the result of obstruction, vesicoureteral reflux, or high urinary flow (overhydration and diuresis). Unfortunately, no single diagnostic tool enables a clear-cut differentiation between obstructive and nonobstructive processes that result in dilatation of the urinary tract. Nonobstructive urinary tract dilatation has many causes (Table 3.5). Dilatation of the collecting system cannot always be equated with obstruction. Conversely, obstruction can be present in the absence of ureteral dilatation, for example, with retroperitoneal fibrosis. Patients with minimal or intermittent obstruction (e.g., mild UPJ obstruction) may have dilated tracts only at times of increased diuresis. Ureters can also become dilated as a result of bladder distension. Persistent dilatation of the upper urinary tract seen in the postnatal

Table 3.5: Causes of Nonobstructive Urinary Tract Dilatation

Congenital
Extrarenal pelvis
Congenital megacalyces
Primary megaureter
Prune-belly syndrome
Pregnancy
Inflammation
Diabetes insipidus
Vigorous diuresis
Bladder distension
Vesicoureteral reflux
Postsurgical
UPJ repairs
Ureteroileal anastomosis
Aortoiliac surgery
Progestational drugs
Retroperitoneal inflammation
Crohn's disease

period has been thought to be due to an early, brief obstruction occurring in the developing urinary tract with subsequent spontaneous resolution, for example, congenital megacalyces. Diagnostic evaluation of the upper urinary tract must identify the cause and severity of the dilatation and determine whether the changes adversely affect renal function. It is often difficult to predict the potential for recovery after correction of the underlying anomaly if the kidney has been damaged.

Evaluation of Upper Urinary Tract Dilatation in Infancy

Prenatal detection of obstruction has allowed prompt postnatal management and improved our understanding of the natural history of a variety of obstructive processes in urology. Most children currently undergoing pyeloplasty for UPJ obstruction have been identified prenatally. However, many neonates with UPJ obstruction seem to undergo stabilization or even improvement in their hydronephrosis.

The common causes of prenatal hydronephrosis are UPJ obstruction (primary or associated with vesicoureteral reflux), obstructive megaureter, vesicoureteral reflux, ectopic ureteroceles, and posterior urethral valves. Multicystic dysplastic kidneys are also frequently diagnosed by in-utero ultrasound. The bladder is enlarged in patients with posterior urethral valves, megacystis-megaureter syndrome, and prune-belly syndrome; it is not visualized in renal agenesis and infantile polycystic kidney disease. Dilated ureters occur with reflux, ureteral ectopia, megaureter, and posterior urethral valves. Dilatation of the urinary tract may be noted as early as at 16 to 18 weeks gestation and warrants careful monitoring. Early, severe dilatation may very occasionally require intervention. Estimation of amniotic fluid quantity (amniotic fluid index, AFI) provides a useful gauge of urine production. Oligohydramnios suggests renal agenesis and infantile polycystic kidney disease, prune-belly syndrome, or posterior urethral valves. Prognosis is poor with the first two and better with early correction of the others. Standards of care for the fetus diagnosed with hydronephrosis are incompletely delineated and are still being established.

Real-time ultrasound is a good screening test to evaluate the degree of dilatation of the renal collecting systems (Table 3.6). It also helps in determining the growth and anatomic appearance of the kidneys and collecting system. Ultrasonographic evaluation should also include an estimation of the bladder volume and wall thickness. Examination of the posterior aspect of the bladder may detect distal ureteral dilation. Color Doppler ultrasonographic assessment of renal vascular resistance (the vascular resistive index) has recently been reported to be potentially useful in the diagnosis of obstruction. Periodic ultrasonography is useful for monitoring patients with

Table 3.6: Fetal Urologic Ultrasonography

Normal Fetal Urinary Tract	*Abnormal Fetal Urinary Tract*
Bladder visible at 14 weeks	Incidence 0.2 to 0.5% all screening ultrasounds
Kidneys visible at 14–18 weeks	20 to 25% all structural abnormalities diagnosed by prenatal ultrasound involve the genitourinary tract
Adrenal visible >30 weeks	Ultrasound best >24 weeks gestation
Ureters not usually visible	UPJ obstruction (40%) (1/2000)
Bladder capacity	Primary
10 ml at 30 weeks	Associated with VU reflux
50 ml at term	Primary obstructive megaureter (20%) (1/10,000)
Fetal sex determination (24 weeks)	Upper pole hydronephrosis with ureteral duplication (10%)
Early visualization external genitalia	Posterior urethral valves (10%) (1/8000)
	Multicystic dysplastic kidneys (1/3000)
	Bilateral renal agenesis (1/4000)
	Ectopic ureterocele or ureter (1/10,000)
	Vesicoureteral reflux (1/100)

hydronephrosis diagnosed in-utero. Follow-up postnatal ultrasounds are misleading if performed within 48 to 72 hours after delivery because the oliguria of the newborn may lessen the degree of hydronephrosis. By contrast, the term fetus has a relatively high urine output, approaching 50 ml/hr 48 to 72 hours after birth. Once in-utero hydronephrosis is discovered, the urologist should become involved in decision-making in conjunction with the parents and the maternal-fetal medicine consultant. Repeat ultrasound scans will identify persistent or worsening hydronephrosis. A careful search should be made for other fetal abnormalities in the nervous system, spine, heart, lungs, and so on. Any fetus with severe bilateral hydronephrosis should be delivered at a tertiary care institution capable of providing prompt, expert evaluation and treatment.

A recommended evaluation algorithm for the fetus diagnosed antenatally with dilatation of the upper urinary tract is outlined in Figure 3.3. Once hydronephrosis or hydroureteronephrosis is established postnatally, further evaluation with a voiding cystourethrogram (VCUG) and a renal functional study is warranted to determine the cause, degree, and extent of the urinary-tract dilatation. The VCUG will identify vesicoureteral reflux and display vesical and urethral anatomy. Hydronephrosis may be secondary to reflux, and up to 15% of infants with a UPJ obstruction

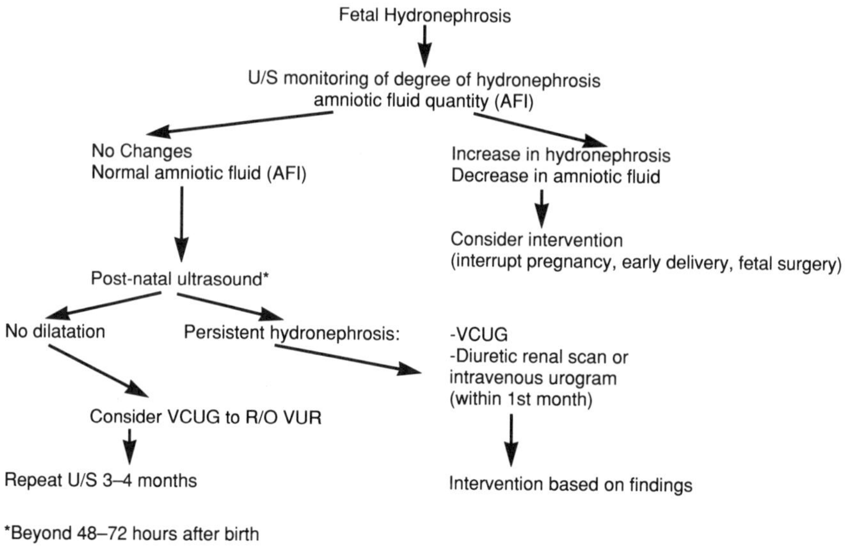

Figure 3.3: Algorithm for the management of prenatal hydronephrosis (U/S, ultrasound; AFI, amniotic fluid index; VCUG, voiding cystourethrogram; VUR, vesicoureteral reflux)

have reflux. Renal functional studies delineate upper urinary tract anatomy and gauge the functional status of the kidneys. Several tests are available, but none provides reliable differentiation of obstructive and nonobstructive processes and none predicts the kidney's ability to respond to therapy. The ideal evaluation of obstruction should assess the efficacy of urine transport within the upper urinary tract. Since the system is compliant and accommodates increasing volumes at relatively low pressures, perfusion tests such as the Whitaker test are not universally reliable in providing clinically relevant data. The diagnosis of hydronephrosis or hydroureteronephrosis is easy using ultrasonography (US), intravenous urography (IVU), or renal nuclear scintigraphy. However, the functional significance of upper-tract dilatation is difficult to assess with these imaging modalities. US does not measure renal function, whereas IVU and scintigraphy provide only relative estimates of renal function.

Diuretic renography is a noninvasive method of assessing renal function and clearance. Following injection of a diuretic (e.g., furosemide), the clearance of radiolabeled contrast is an indirect measure of the degree of functional renal obstruction. Radioisotope clearance half-time ($T^1/2$) correlates with obstruction: $T^1/2 < 10$ minutes is normal; $T^1/2 >$ 20 minutes indicates significant obstruction, and clearance of 10 to 20 minutes is equivocal. Diuresis renography has a variable correlation with the Whitaker test of between 40 and 85%.

Experience has revealed some of the pitfalls of diuresis renography. Poor renal function causes a prolonged $T^1/2$ because of the kidney's inability to respond to the diuretic. The patient's state of hydration, compliance of the collecting system, and the size of the hydronephrotic renal pelvis all influence $T^1/2$ determinations. The larger the renal pelvic volume, the greater the diuretic response needed to clear the system. $T^1/2$ quantitation differs depending on the method of measurement used. It can be measured from the time of injection or response, and it can be actual (reduction to 50% initial activity) or extrapolated. These variances have led to the development of the "well tempered renogram" for use in infants. Patients should be at least 1 month old to reduce the likelihood of immature renal function affecting the results. The bladder is usually catheterized and hydration (dilute saline IV at a rate of 10 ml/Kg for 15 minutes prior to injection of radiopharmaceutical) determined by urine outputs of at least 4 to 5 ml/min.

A number of radiopharmaceuticals are used for renal nuclear scanning (Table 3.7). Technetium-labeled diethylenetriamepentacetic acid (^{99m}Tc-DTPA) is rapidly cleared by glomerular filtration and is used for renal blood flow and functional studies. Technetium-^{99m} dimercaptosuccinic acid (^{99m}Tc-DMSA) is an excellent renal imaging agent. Forty-

Table 3.7: Renal Nuclear Radiopharmaceuticals

Renal Cortical Imaging Agents	*Renal Functional Assessment Agents*	*Predominant Route of Renal Excretion*
Excellent: DMSA	Excellent: MAG_3, OIH	Cortical-bound
Intermediate: GH	Intermediate: DTPA	DMSA 40%
Reasonable: DTPA,	Reasonable: GH	GH 20%
MAG_3, OIH	Poor: DMSA	Glomerular filtration
		DTPA
		Tubular secretion
		OIH, MAG_3

percent is bound to cortical tubular cells, thereby providing good assessment of renal mass, scarring, and parenchymal pathology. Technetium-^{99m} glucoheptonate (^{99m}Tc-GH) combines features of both DTPA and DMSA. Glucoheptonate is excreted mostly by glomerular filtration and, like DTPA, gives information on blood flow, glomerular function, and urinary drainage. About 10 to 20% of injected GH accumulates within tubular cells, allowing some degree of cortical imaging. GH has a lower radiation risk than DMSA. However, it is partially excreted in the bowel, and this reduces the accuracy of renal imaging in delayed scans, especially if renal insufficiency exists.

Iodine-131 0-iodohippuric acid (^{131}I-OIH) is an efficient tubular imaging and function agent. Eighty percent is cleared by tubular excretion and 20% by glomerular filtration. It is an excellent agent for measurement of effective renal plasma flow (ERPF) and tubular cell function. Because ^{131}I emits gamma and beta rays and has a half-life of 8 days, its radiation risk has been reduced by use of iodine-^{123} labeling. ^{123}I-OIH lacks beta emission, has a long half-life (13 hours), and is costly. It is no longer commercially available in the United States.

A new ligand, technetium-^{99m} mercaptoacetylglyclglyclglycl (MAG_3), has been recently introduced. Technetium has a 6-hour half-life, lacks particulate emission, and gives better spatial resolution than OIH. MAG_3 is excreted by both glomerular filtration and tubular secretion, and it has replaced OIH and DTPA scans in many institutions as the radiopharmaceutical of choice in the pediatric age group. The high degree of protein binding of MAG_3 and its smaller volume of distribution contribute to its better imaging quality and minimal background activity. Following the injection of the tracer, images are generated showing arterial perfusion, intrarenal cortical transit, and excretion of the radionuclide into the upper urinary tract. Computer analysis generates time/activity curves of renal uptake and excretion, providing objective quantification of renal function. In addition, wash-out of the radioactive tracer in the urinary tract can be monitored and plotted. The diuretic renogram is helpful in assessing the functional status of the kidney and the degree of obstruction. The evaluation of the dilated urinary tract should be aimed to providing information that will permit rapid treatment of any lesions susceptible of jeopardizing renal function in a permanent manner. This is most important in the pediatric age group.

The Whitaker test is based on the principle that resistance is equal to pressure divided by flow; that is, resistance can be calculated if the flow rate and the pressure required for flow are known. The test measures intrapelvic and intravesical pressures during infusion of fluid into the renal pelvis through a percutaneous catheter (Figure 3.4). The initial enthusiasm for this test was tempered by the realization that a gray zone of indeterminate pressures exists between obstruction and nonobstruction. The test is limited by difficulties in interpretation: low pressure (less than 15 cm H_2O with an inflow rate of 5 ml/min) is indicative of free flow of urine; pressure above 22 cm H_2O is associated with obstruction. The significance of pressures between 15 cm H_2O and 22 cm H_2O is undetermined. Other limitations also exist. The test is invasive, technique-dependent (e.g., needle size, hydronephrotic volume, flow rates) and nonphysiologic. The test is unreliable in patients with large-volume hydronephrosis. Because of its inability to assess renal function and its invasive nature, the Whitaker test is not widely used.

The intravenous urogram (IVU) combines the features of anatomic delineation of the kidneys, calyces, pelves, and ureters with an estimate of the overall function of each kidney. The other tests may surpass the IVU in demonstrating the components of renal form or function, but the IVU provides information about all of them. The utility of the IVU is limited in patients with renal insufficiency because limited contrast concentration provides suboptimal visualization of the collecting system. Urographic contrast agents are rapidly excreted by glomerular filtration and not reabsorbed. Sodium and water reabsorption in the nephron concentrate the contrast and allow its radiographic visualization. Normally, a nephrogram (contrast in the blood vessels, proximal tubules) is seen within 30 seconds of injection and a pyelogram (contrast in the calyces) appears within 2 minutes. Calyceal clubbing and dilatation of the ureters and pelvis are seen in obstruction. The level of obstruction is best ascertained by delayed films. The intravenous urogram provides good anatomic visualization of the upper urinary tract. However, it does not allow objective quantification of renal function. In addition, it is limited by impaired renal function and may be difficult to interpret in the neonatal period.

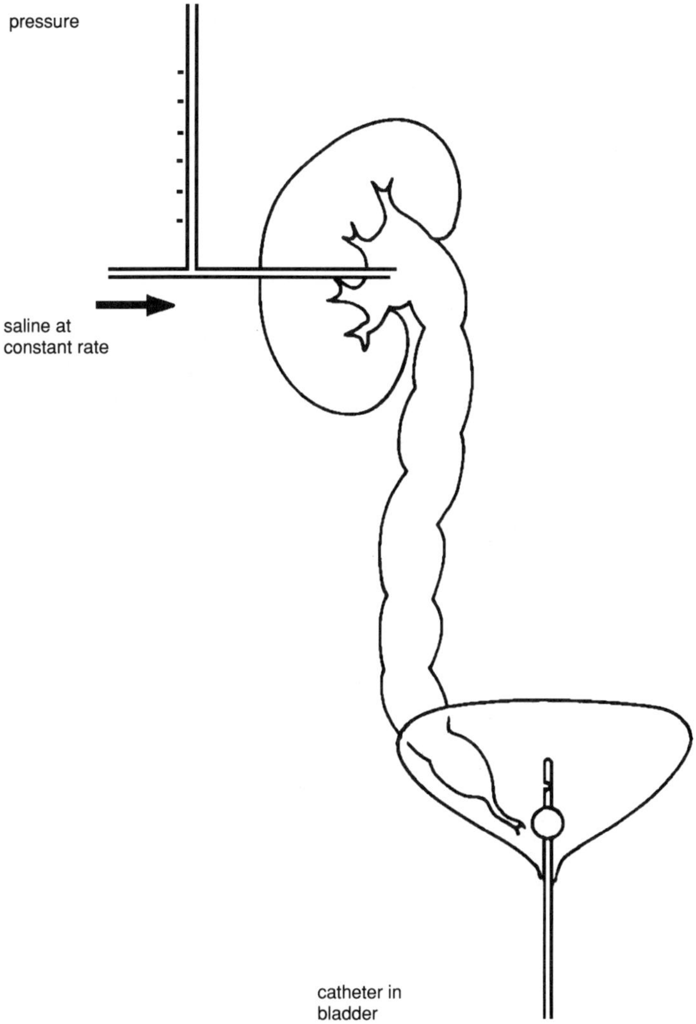

Figure 3.4: Whitaker's test: fluid is run into the ureter at a constant rate and the pressure is measured. *Reproduced with permission from Blandy J. Lecture Notes on Urology, 4th ed. Oxford: Blackwell Scientific Publications, 1991:136.*

VESICOURETERAL REFLUX

The ureterovesical junction (UVJ) normally acts as a one-way valve to prevent retrograde flow of urine from the bladder into the ureters during bladder filling and voiding, when intravesical pressure increases. Vesicoureteral reflux (VUR) is an abnormal condition in which urine regurgitates from the bladder up the ureter in a retrograde fashion. Primary VUR is due to a congenital abnormality of the UVJ that results in incompetence of the valve mechanism. Secondary VUR is associated with anatomical or functional obstruction of the urinary tract, as seen with posterior urethral valves or neurogenic bladder dysfunction.

Historically, the recognition of VUR as a clinical entity occurred in the late 1950s and represents the take-off point for pediatric urology as a specialty. However, as a clinical and pathological entity, reflux is still being actively investigated and remains an area of controversy in terms both of pathophysiology and management. This section presents the salient features of the structure and function of the ureterovesical junction and the pathophysiologic elements of VUR. Current principles of management are then briefly reviewed.

Ureterovesical Junction Anatomy

The anatomy of the UVJ is best understood from a thorough knowledge of the embryologic development of bladder and ureter (see Chapter 1). Events that lead to the elaboration of a normal UVJ include the outpouching (ureteral bud) at the level of the caudal portion of the mesonephric (wolffian) duct during the fourth week of gestation. Growth of the ureteral bud posteriorly and cephalad allows it to join the mesenchymal metanephric blastema, which differentiates into the kidney. The bud remains connected to the caudal portion of the mesonephric duct, from which trigone and bladder neck develop. The mesonephric duct in turn opens into the cloaca. By 8 weeks of gestation, the terminal mesonephric duct and ureteral bud become incorporated into the cloaca. The insertion of the ureteral bud migrates laterally and cephalad as the cloaca develops. The urorectal septum divides the cloaca into an anterior compartment, which forms the body of the bladder, and a posterior compartment, the rectum. Ureteral orifices, trigone, and bladder neck are identifiable in the newly formed bladder by 12 weeks of gestation. Further growth of the bladder determines the final position of the ureter within its wall.

In the mature bladder, the terminal ureter enters the bladder through a posterolateral hiatus to the trigone (Figure 3.5). The ureter courses through the bladder wall toward the trigone at an oblique angle. The distalmost portion of the ureter is attached to the trigone. Histologically, the two spiral muscle layers of the ureter take on a more longitudinal orientation as they enter the bladder wall and fan out to become the trigonal muscle. Waldeyer's sheath, an adventitial layer surrounding the ureteral muscle, provides a useful plane for surgical dissection. Posteriorly, the ureter is backed by detrusor muscle. The lumen of the normal ureter is obliterated at rest by the circumferential pressure of the

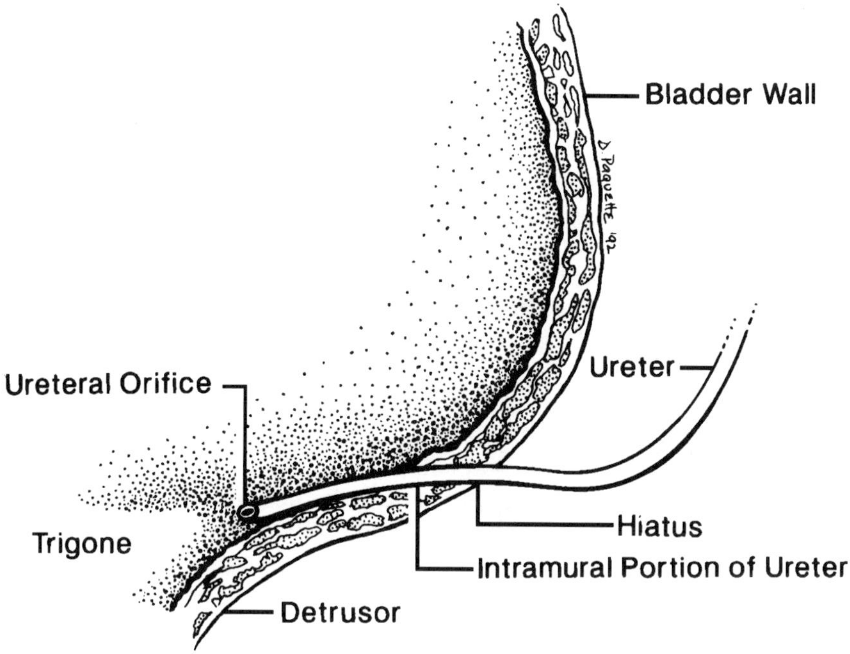

Figure 3.5: Anatomic organization of the ureterovesical junction.

spirally oriented ureteral muscle. The lumen temporarily opens during peristalsis as each bolus of urine passes distally. The UVJ acts as a flap valve as the bladder fills, the submucosal portion of the ureter being compressed against the detrusor muscle by the increasing intravesical pressure. Compression of the ureter can be overcome by peristaltic waves that propel urine down the ureter. The valve mechanism therefore acts passively, although the ureterotrigonal muscle layers contribute to closure of the ureteral orifice.

Vesicoureteral reflux (VUR) is rare in healthy humans. VUR is therefore an abnormal phenomenon, and its exact etiology remains unknown. Traditionally, VUR is thought to be due to a congenital shortening of the suburothelial portion of the ureter. Embryologically, this is caused by an abnormal location of the ureteral bud and lateral ectopia of the UVJ. The normal ratio of suburothelial ureteral length to ureteral orifice diameter was postulated by Paquin to be 4:1 to 5:1 in order to provide an adequate valve mechanism. In the first year of life the normal intravesical ureteral length is approximately 7 mm. This increases to 12 mm by adolescence. Concomitantly, the ureteral diameter grows from 1.4 to 1.9 mm. Lateral ectopia of the ureteral orifice is associated with a shortening of the submucosal ureteral segment, which in turn results in a decreased ratio of suburothelial ureter to diameter of ureter and an incompetent UVJ valve.

An abnormal anatomical organization of the ureterovesical junction is typically seen in bladder exstrophy. The ureters enter the bladder perpendicularly and have virtually no intramural tunnel. This configuration results in VUR in virtually all patients with bladder exstrophy. Hutch contributed to the understanding of VUR by suggesting that a lack of detrusor muscle support or backing is an important factor in the genesis of the reflux. VUR can be induced experimentally by incising the intramural ureter, dividing the trigonal muscle, or by creating a defect in the muscle backing. Several factors, therefore, are responsible for the pathogenesis of reflux. These include (1) configuration and location of the ureteral orifice, (2) increase in intravesical pressure, (3) presence of bladder inflammation causing ureteral edema, (4) paraureteral diverticula resulting from a deficiency in the muscle backing for the ureter, and (5) urinary-tract infections. Any combination of these factors can contribute to reflux. Some authors have proposed that reflux in younger children can be due to an unstable bladder. In this scenario, uninhibited bladder contractions generate high intravesical pressures that exceed the capabilities of an immature UVJ to prevent VUR.

Primary VUR results from an abnormal organization of the UV junction, whereas bladder outflow obstruction and increased intravesical pressure cause secondary reflux. Of men with bladder outlet obstruction due to benign prostatic hyperplasia, 5 to 15% have VUR. VUR is also common in boys with posterior urethral valves. Dysfunctional voiding and neurogenic bladder dysfunction together with uninhibited bladder contractions or detrusor sphincter dyssynergia can result in secondary VUR. Finally, end-stage bladder scarring from chronic inflammation due to bladder calculus, long-term indwelling catheters, tuberculosis, schistosomiasis, radiation cystitis, or chemical cystitis may impair bladder compliance and contractility and result in VUR.

Evaluation of Reflux

The current diagnostic modalities to demonstrate and quantitate vesicoureteral reflux are radiographic or radionuclide voiding cystourethrograms (VCUG or NCUG). In both techniques a urethral catheter is inserted into the bladder and contrast material or radiopharmaceutical material is introduced. The bladder is filled to capacity, and the patient then voids to expel the contrast or radionuclide. The VCUG under fluoroscopy with spot films provides precise anatomical visualization of the urinary tract but allows only "snap-shot" appraisal; the nuclear cystogram may be more diagnostically sensitive. Both procedures have their drawbacks and are technique- and technician-dependent. VUR during bladder filling is known as low-pressure reflux, whereas reflux during voiding is referred to as high-pressure reflux.

The more severe degrees of VUR are associated with upper urinary tract changes. An anatomical system has been proposed by the International Reflux Study in Children (IRSIC) for grading the severity of VUR from grades I to V. Grading is based on the anatomic appearance, at peak voiding pressure, of the ureter, pelvis, renal fornices, and calyces during a standard radiographic VCUG. The grades and the distribution of primary VUR in large population studies are outlined in Table 3.8.

A number of variables must be considered in grading VUR at the time of VCUG. These include the patient's state of hydration, the presence of urinary-tract infections, the bladder pressure generated during filling, the level of patient cooperation, and the pliability of the ureters (especially in neonates) (Table 3.8).

Natural History of VUR

The natural history of VUR varies depending on whether the reflux is primary or secondary. It is likely that the pathological condition is long-standing, especially in patients with primary VUR. Grade of VUR, presence of urinary-tract infection (UTI), age of patient, and intravesical

Table 3.8: Grading of Vesicoureteral Reflux

Primary versus secondary	
Grading system and prevalence	
Gd I, 10%:	ureter only
Gd II, 40%:	ureter, pelvis, calyces; no dilatation
Gd III, 25%:	mild dilatation ureter; minor calyceal blunting
Gd IV, 20%:	moderate dilatation ureter, calyces; papillary impression preserved in majority
Gd V, 5%:	marked calyceal blunting; loss papillary impression; gross ureteral dilatation
Variables in grading reflux	
Technique- and technician-dependent	
State of hydration	
Infection leading to endotoxin-mediated ureteral dilatation	
Degree bladder/micturition pressure	
Reflux may be intermittent	
Patient age	

pressure generated during bladder contraction are all important factors to be considered.

The incidence of VUR decreases with age. Spontaneous resolution of primary VUR is thought to occur as a result of maturation of the UVJ with concomitant lengthening of the intravesical ureter. Several nonrandomized studies have described the resolution of reflux with aging. Lenahan reported spontaneous resolution of VUR in 42% of patients treated conservatively, irrespective of grade; Bellinger and Duckett found resolution of VUR in 63% of patients with grade II VUR, 53% with grade III, and 33% with grade IV. However, in the latter study resolution was documented by only one follow-up study VCUG. Recent studies demonstrate that reflux resolution is not an all-or-none phenomenon. Smellie noted resolution of VUR in 79% of affected ureters (85% of undilated but only 41% of dilated ureters) in a long-term study of children treated with antibiotic prophylaxis for 12 years. Other studies have shown that the rate of VUR resolution is not influenced by occurrence or frequency of UTIs. In a recent study carried out by the Southwest Pediatric Nephrology Study Group, spontaneous resolution of VUR was noted at 2 years in 42% of ureters with grade I reflux, 35% with grade II, and only 12% with grade III. This study documented an increase in the grade of VUR in up to 17% of ureters, irrespective of interim UTIs or bladder dysfunction. This finding demonstrates the evolving picture of VUR and the variability in cystographic findings over time. Lower grades of VUR (III or less) in infants and younger children resolve spontaneously in the majority of patients. Prenatal ultrasound screening is now frequently carried out as part of routine obstetric care, and a number of cases are noted to have fetal urinary-tract dilatation due to VUR. Our approach and understanding of the natural history of VUR may well be altered by such early antenatal diagnosis.

Spontaneous resolution is much less likely in secondary reflux. The treatment of the underlying cause of increased intravesical pressures should provide therapy for VUR. However, persistence of reflux should be expected if the UVJ anatomy is significantly altered.

VUR and Reflux Nephropathy

The effects of sterile reflux on the upper urinary tract, and in particular the human kidney, have not been well characterized. However, the experimental studies of Hodson, Ransley, Ridson, and others have shed some light on the pathophysiology of renal damage secondary to VUR. Bacterial contamination of the renal pelvis in UTIs may lead to intrarenal infection or pyelonephritis, which in turn can cause scarring of the renal parenchyma. This process is referred to as reflux nephropathy (RN).

An important element in the development of renal scarring in patients with VUR is intrarenal reflux (IRR) (Table 3.9). IRR is caused by the structural configuration of the collecting ducts in the renal papillae located at upper and lower poles of the kidney; this configuration allows urine to reflux into the renal collecting ducts (Figure 3.6). A local parenchymal inflammatory reaction can develop with infection, and IRR ultimately leads to interstitial nephritis. This process can destroy the renal parenchyma and cause scarification. The progressive nature of parenchymal injury is thought to be due to the following factors among others: inflammatory reaction caused by autologous tubular antigens or Tamm-Horsfall protein, hyperfiltration, superoxide production, alterations in prostaglandin synthesis. Scarification can be demonstrated by various modalities: ultrasound, nephrotomography, technetium dimercaptosuccinic acid (Tc-DMSA) radionuclide scan or computerized tomographic (CT) scan. Kidney damage similar to reflux nephropathy may also be caused by sterile in-utero reflux associated with the high intrarenal pressures, for example, in patients with posterior urethral valves.

Clinical studies have established that renal scarring is often present when a child first presents for evaluation of either UTI or VUR. Scarring rarely progresses during follow-up and de-novo scarring is unusual, unless the patient has episodes of pyelonephritis. The virulence of the infecting organism and a number of host factors (e.g., blood group antigens and the PI group) influence the rate of renal scarring in experimental animals. However, scarring is a silent process and may occur over a period of time and thus avoid scrutiny. Reflux nephropathy appears to be initiated early, possibly prenatally, and is usually associated with high grades of reflux (Table 3.10). Furthermore, the effects of IRR and infection are greater in immature developing kidneys than in more mature kidneys.

Reflux nephropathy causes significant long-term consequences. Renal functional impairment runs the gamut from impaired urinary concentrating ability, through mild proteinuria, to end-stage renal disease (ESRD). Between 10 and 30% of patients with ESRD have a documented history of VUR, and at least 4% of all long-term patients with VUR

Table 3.9: Intrarenal Reflux (IRR)

Consequence of vesicoureteral reflux
Retrograde flow of urine into ducts of Bellini
Common in compound calyces of upper, lower poles
Leads to reflux nephropathy
Compound or nonconvex papillae
Upper pole > lower pole > mid-zones

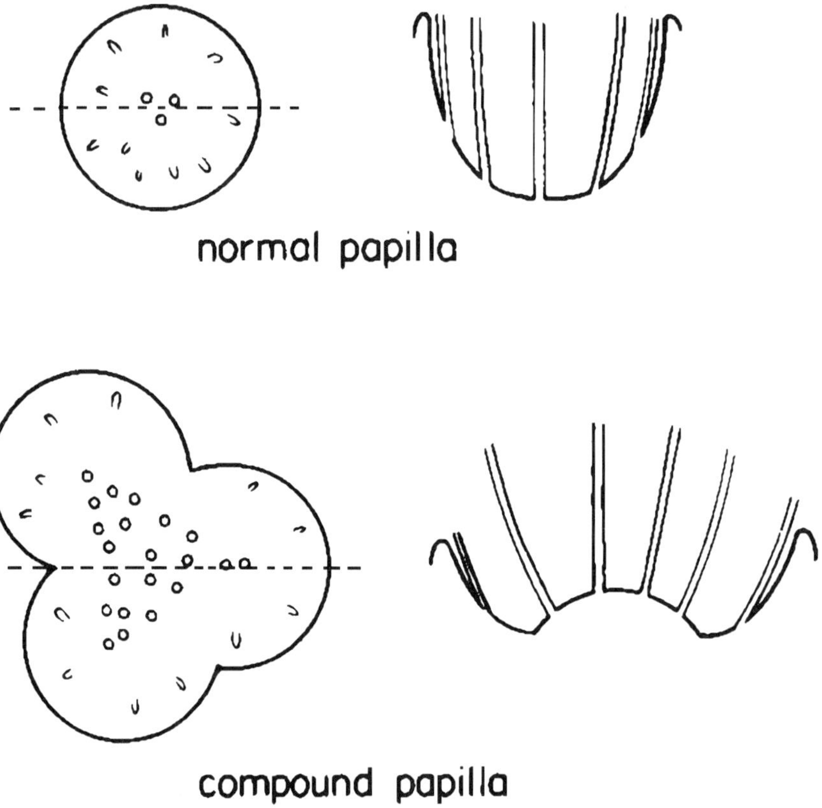

Figure 3.6: In a normal papilla (above) most of the ducts of Bellini will be closed when the pressure inside the calix is increased, but in a compound papilla (below) those that open into the hollow of the crater, formed where the papillae fuse together, have no protective valves. *Reproduced with permission from Blandy J. Lecture Notes on Urology, 4th ed. Oxford: Blackwell Scientific Publications, 1991:35.*

progress to ESRD. Reflux is responsible for ESRD in 25% of children entering dialysis and transplantation programs in Europe.

Hypertension, proteinuria, and azotemia have been reported in patients with reflux nephropathy. A positive correlation between the degree of renal scarring and the development of hypertension exists. Ten percent of children over 6 years of age and adolescents with persistent, severe hypertension have renal scarring; conversely, 50% of adults with renal scarring have varying degrees of hypertension. The pathophysiology of hypertension in patients with renal scarring is probably related to the activation of the renin angiotensin system as seen in the Ask-Upmark kidney.

Table 3.10: Reflux Nephropathy

Clinical and pathologic changes consequent to intrarenal reflux
Renal scarring, e.g., Ask-Upmark kidney
Renal injury due to
  Age of patient
  High pressures
  Infection
Leads to
  End-stage renal disease
    Focal glomerular sclerosis
    Proteinuria
  Hypertension
Common cause of end-stage renal disease in children, adolescents

Occasional reports of urolithiasis in association with primary VUR have appeared in the urologic literature. It is unclear from these reports whether VUR is an etiologic factor in the pathenogenesis of stones; however, VUR allows urea-splitting organisms such as proteus to reach the kidney from the bladder.

Demographics of VUR

The prevalence of primary VUR in the general population is unknown. However, VUR is found in approximately 40% of children and 5% of adults with UTIs who undergo cystographic evaluation. VUR is slightly more frequent in boys than in girls during the first 6 months of life. The paucity of cross-racial studies prevents a clear estimate of VUR by race. However, there is some indication that VUR is infrequent in Afro-American children compared to Caucasian or Asian children. There is a strong familial disposition for reflux. Several studies have shown that VUR is present in between 32 and 45% of asymptomatic siblings of probands with reflux and up to 70% of daughters born to mothers who required antireflux surgery. Screening is therefore recommended for siblings of patients with VUR. The exact mode of inheritance is not well understood, and it is probably multifactorial or polygenic.

Management of VUR

The main principles in the management of VUR are (a) prevention or control of urinary infections and kidney damage and (b) elimination of the reflux, if possible. Most lower grades of reflux resolve spontaneously with time (Table 3.11). Therapy in these patients consists of protecting the kidneys from the effects of bacterial contamination. Continuous

Table 3.11: Medical versus Surgical Treatment of Vesicoureteral Reflux

Few prospective randomized studies
"Considerations" rather than strict indications for surgical treatment
Higher grades reflux less likely to resolve with age
Reflux in women may lead to pyelonephritis during pregnancy
Maternal and fetal complications
Prospective studies
50 to 60% kidneys are scarred at time of diagnosis
Progressive scarring in about 20 to 25%
New renal scars in 10 to 15%
Medical, surgical treatments equivalent
Prevention further renal injury
Later development hypertension, renal failure
Successful treatment with prevention VU reflux no guarantee of sterile urine or prevention of hypertension, further scarring
Surgical treatment strongly considered in Gd IV to V reflux

administration of low-dose prophylactic antibiotics until the radiographic cessation of VUR ensures a sterile urine. This is the conventional form of therapy. Regular monitoring for bacteriuria should be performed in the physician's office or using home-culture kits. Radiologic evaluation should be performed at appropriate intervals, more frequently in younger children and in patients with higher grades of VUR. VCUGs are obtained at 1-to-2-year intervals. Ultrasonographic imaging of the upper tract is required less frequently. Long-term administration of trimethoprim/sulfamethoxazole or nitrofurantoin, at one-third to one-half the therapeutic doses for UTIs, is safe and effective and prevents bacterial colonization of urine in most patients. Antimicrobials should be taken at bedtime in order to provide coverage during times when patients are most likely to retain urine in their bladders. Side effects of chronic trimethoprim/sulfamethoxazole or nitrofurantoin therapy are relatively few. Skin sensitivity and bone marrow depression occur with the former and interstitial pneumonitis/fibrosis in the latter. These conditions are all readily reversible when the antimicrobial is discontinued. Prophylactic antibiotics therapy is discontinued as soon as a negative VCUG (preferably nuclear because of its increased sensitivity) is obtained.

Voiding dysfunction, which is present in a significant number of young female patients with a history of UTI, should always be considered in patients with VUR. Infrequent voiding, leading to bladder distension and urinary stasis, may contribute to or cause a worsening of VUR. Bladder ultrasound evaluation is the best modality for demonstrating increases in bladder thickness, which can be indicative of voiding dysfunction. Bladder retraining and anticholinergic medications are helpful in hastening the resolution of reflux.

VUR in Women

Females in the child-bearing age group represent a distinct population of patients with VUR. Pregnant women are at increased risk for developing bacteriuria and pyelonephritis, with an associated high incidence of premature delivery, low birth weight, and growth retardation. There is no clear explanation for the increase in frequency of pyelonephritis in pregnant women, but several factors are involved, for example, smooth muscle atony with decreased ureteral peristalsis caused by increases in circulating progesterone and mechanical obstruction from the enlarging uterus. Urinary stasis is enhanced, and this encourages bacterial colonization and ascending bacteriuria. There is no evidence that pregnancy causes de-novo VUR. However, VUR in pubertal girls should be considered an indication for corrective surgery, since VUR may predispose to pyelonephritis. Nevertheless, reflux alone does not appear to be the sole factor in the etiology of pyelonephritis. Although successful surgical correction of reflux prevents ascending infections, the overall incidence of the bacteriuria before and after corrective ureterovesical surgery is unchanged. Females with a predisposition to UTIs are also more likely to develop pyelonephritis during pregnancy.

No clinical studies have unequivocally demonstrated that surgical correction of VUR prevents pyelonephritis, although the incidence is clearly reduced. Ostenfield found an increased risk of UTI and fetal loss in patients having undergone surgical repair of reflux during childhood; thus, preexisting urinary tract disease increases the risk of pregnancy and warrants close monitoring. Interestingly, there is no evidence that new renal scars develop in women with either VUR or pyelonephritis or both during pregnancy.

Surgical Correction of Vesicoureteral Reflux

Severe grades of vesicoureteral reflux (grade IV or V), persistent reflux for many years, breakthrough infections, noncompliance with antimicrobial therapy, associated hypertension, and approaching puberty in females are all indications for surgical correction of VUR (Table 3.11). The goal of surgical treatment of VUR is the eradication of reflux. Several surgical techniques achieve this goal, and the best are more than 95% successful when carried out by experienced surgeons. The principles for successful surgical correction of VUR are (1) increasing the length of the suburothelial tunnel to allow for a 4–5:1 ratio between the length of tunnel and the diameter of the ureteral orifice; (2) anchoring the ureteral orifice to the bladder floor; (3) creating a strong detrusor muscle backing for the ureter and preventing a paraureteral outpouching (diverticulum); (4) avoidance of any kinking of the intramural ureter; (5) a tension-free anastomosis between the ureter and the bladder; and (6) preventing new or progressive renal scarring.

The currently popular surgical techniques are the cross-trigonal advancement of Cohen and the modified advancement procedure described by Glenn and Anderson. Both these operations can be performed entirely within the bladder and have largely replaced the intravesical ureteroneocystostomy of Politano and Leadbetter. Some surgeons prefer an extravesical ureteroneocystostomy as described by Lich and Gregoire.

There is considerable debate regarding the indications for surgical correction of VUR. However, patients with higher grades of reflux, documented to be present for at least 3 months, are unlikely to experience spontaneous resolution. Grades IV and V reflux are unlikely to resolve with time and therefore should be treated surgically. Surgery for lower grades of reflux is indicated only when one or more of the previously listed conditions exist.

The complication rates following ureterovesicoplasties are extremely low. Ultrasound examinations are recommended to rule out postoperative UVJ obstruction. The upper tracts usually appear normal within 2 to 3 weeks of surgery, but the ureters, renal pelves, and calyces may remain dilated for up to 6 to 12 weeks after surgery. Dilatation should, however, not exceed the preoperative level. A VCUG done 3 to 6 months after surgery confirms the success of the antireflux operation.

Endoscopic treatment of VUR has received increasing attention recently. The procedure is carried out cystoscopically, with the patient ambulatory and under anesthesia. A small amount of collagen or Teflon is injected at the level of the ureteral orifice in order to create a ball-valve type of antireflux mechanism. The procedure is successful in eradicating VUR in 65 to 80% of patients and is certainly less invasive and more cost-effective. Long-term results are not yet known, but a number of urologists are concerned about use of Teflon paste since it has been shown to migrate and cause a significant local giant-cell inflammatory reaction. Collagen is considered safer for endoscopic treatment of VUR. Long-term studies are still needed to evaluate the ultimate effectiveness of this form of treatment. At present, collagen is not approved by the Food and Drug Administration.

SUGGESTED READINGS

Steinhardt GF. Reflux nephropathy: review article. J Urol 1985; 134:855.

Good summary of the literature regarding reflux nephropathy. Useful references and a nice review of the pathophysiology.

Arant BS. Vesicoureteral reflux and renal injury. Am J Kidney Dis 1991; 18 (5): 491.

In-depth review of VUR from a pediatric nephrologist's viewpoint. Offers the most up-to-date review of the literature concerning VUR and provides some intriguing insights into the management of reflux.

Klahr S. New insights into the consequences and mechanisms of renal impairment in obstructive uropathy (editorial). Amer J Kidney Dis 1991; 18:689.

Concise review of the intrarenal changes in obstructive uropathy. Emphasis on pathophysiology mechanisms.

Weiss RM. Clinical implications of ureteral physiology. J Urol 1979; 121:401.

Excellent overview of ureteral physiology and dynamics, with their clinical applicability.

Lebowitz RL. The detection of vesicoureteral reflux in the child. Invest Radiol 1986; 21:519.

Clear exposition of uroradiologic techniques used to identify and grade vesicoureteral reflux.

Koff SA. Relationship between dysfunctional voiding and reflux. J Urol 1992; 148:1703.

Succinct review of pathogenetic correlation between bladder dysfunction and vesicoureteral reflux.

Whitaker RH. The Whitaker test. Urol Clin North Am 1979; 6:529.

Description of techniques, uses, and limitations of pressure-flow studies in evaluation of the dilated upper urinary tract.

Marchant DJ. Effects of pregnancy and progestational agents on the urinary tract. Am J Obstet Gynecol 1972; 112:487.

Useful review of "hydronephrosis" of pregnancy and effects of female hormones on the upper urinary tract.

Hodson CJ, Maling TMJ, McManamon PJ, Lewis MG. The pathogenesis of reflux nephropathy (chronic atrophic pyelonephritis). Br J Radiol (suppl) 1975; 13:1.

Early paper describing pathogenesis of reflux nephropathy.

Birmingham Reflux Study Group. A prospective trial of operative versus non-operative treatment of severe vesicoureteric reflux: 5 years observation. Br Med J 1987; 295:237.

Paper from Dr. Smellie's group demonstrating no differences in outcomes regarding renal size, renal growth, scar progression, or development of new scars.

Latifpour J, Kondo S, O'Hollaren B, Morita T, Weiss RM. Autonomic receptors in the urinary tract: sex and age differences. J Pharmacol Exp Ther 1990; 253:661.

Careful presentation of current information on autonomic innervation of the ureters and the rest of the urinary tract.

Kaye AD, Pollack HM. Diagnostic imaging approach to the patient with obstructive uropathy. Semin Urol 1982; 11:55.

Presents various uroradiologic approaches to the diagnosis of obstruction. Compares and contrasts limitations and clinical applicabilities.

Conway JJ. "Well-tempered" diuresis renography: its historical development, physiological and technical pitfalls and standardized technique protocol. Semin Nucl Med 1992; 12:74.

Up-to-date review of diuresis renography with special emphasis on standardization and technique.

Eshima D, Taylor A Jr. Technetium-99m (^{99m}Tc) mercaptoacetyltriglycine: update on the new ^{99m}Tc renal tubular function agent. Semin Nucl Med 1992; 12:61.

Review of biology, clearance, and renal handling of MAG_3. Its clinical use is discussed as well as its advantages over other renal nuclear imaging radiopharmaceuticals.

Thomas DFM. Fetal uropathy. Br J Urol 1990; 66:225.

Review of in-utero nephrogenesis and ultrasound recognition of urinary abnormalities. Clear discussion of concepts underlying management of fetal uropathy.

CHAPTER 4

Bladder Function

Simon C. W. Harrison
Paul Abrams

A revolution has taken place over the last 20 years which has resulted in urologists increasingly investigating and treating disorders of the lower urinary tract from a functional, rather than structural, standpoint. The stimulus for this change has been the introduction into clinical practice of urodynamic investigative techniques, a change that has led to a better appreciation of the pathophysiological processes affecting the lower urinary tract. For example, prostatic hypertrophy is now considered in terms of its effect on functional bladder capacity, detrusor instability, voiding bladder pressures, and urinary flow rates rather than in terms of the endoscopic appearances of the prostate, alterations in bladder wall thickness, or the presence of trabeculation.

In parallel with this change in clinical practice, our scientific knowledge of the physiological and pathophysiological mechanisms operating in the bladder and its sphincters has grown dramatically. However, all too often such studies have led to further questions as increasing levels of complexity are demonstrated. It is therefore apparent that the pragmatic approach to the practice of urology that urodynamics offers is set against a scientific jigsaw from which many pieces are still missing.

URODYNAMIC PRINCIPLES AND METHODOLOGY

Urine Storage

The storage phase of the micturition cycle is characterized by the bladder accommodating increasing volumes of urine at low pressures; as long as the pressure within the urethra exceeds that in the bladder, continence is maintained. Failure of the storage mechanisms can lead to renal damage on the one hand and incontinence on the other.

A simple assessment of the storage capacity of the bladder can be made by recording the frequency of micturition and the volume voided on each occasion: the frequency/volume chart or urinary diary. This provides an indication of the volume of urine stored and the diurnal pattern of urine output; nocturnal polyuria is being increasingly recognized as a cause of nocturnal urinary frequency and must not be confused with nocturia commonly present in patients with bladder outflow obstruction.

The behavior of the bladder during filling is objectively examined using the cystometrogram (CMG) (Figure 4.1). Cystometry is generally carried out using twin urethral catheters, one of which is used for bladder filling while the second is attached to a pressure transducer so that intravesical pressure can be continuously monitored. A rectal catheter measures abdominal pressure: subtraction of rectal pressure from bladder pressure gives a pressure record (the detrusor pressure) that reflects the active and passive properties of the bladder wall. Two important abnormalities may be recognized on the filling phase of the cystometrogram: altered bladder compliance and unstable detrusor contractions. A reduction in bladder compliance is reflected in an abnormal increase in intravesical pressure as the bladder volume rises, whereas detrusor instability is characterized by phasic increases in the detrusor pressure, which occur despite the patient's attempt to inhibit micturition.

The function of the urethral sphincter mechanisms can be examined in a number of ways. If a filling cystometrogram is undertaken using radiological contrast media, x-ray screening can be used to determine whether

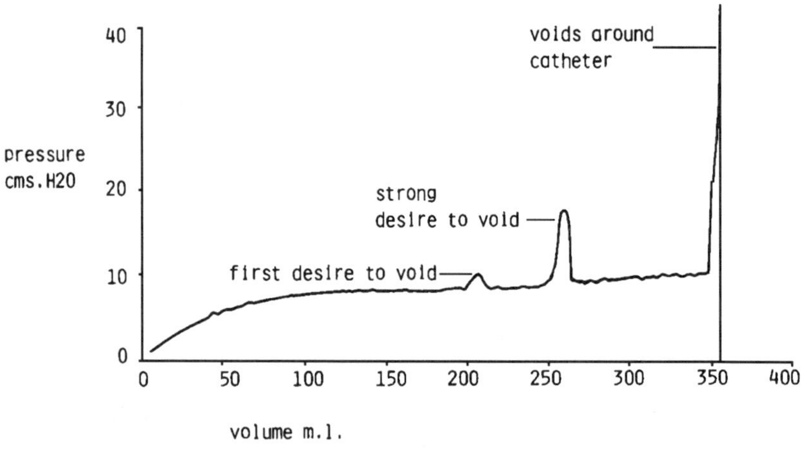

Figure 4.1: Normal cystometrogram. *Reproduced with permission from Blandy J. Lecture Notes on Urology, 4th ed. Oxford: Blackwell Scientific Publications, 1991:157.*

the bladder neck remains closed during filling and during stress events such as coughing and straining; episodes of urinary incontinence will also be observed. A videotape record of the study allows subsequent review. Videourodynamic studies are of particular value in the assessment of the patient with a neuropathic bladder disorder about whom information will be obtained, not only concerning bladder and sphincter function, but also about the possible presence of vesicoureteric reflux, bladder diverticula, and proximal urethral dilatation. The position of the bladder neck and urethra in relation to the pubic symphysis (and therefore the pelvic floor) can also be demonstrated by ultrasound imaging using transvaginal or transrectal probes.

Urethral pressure can be measured using fluid-filled catheters or solid-state pressure transducers. Simultaneous recordings of urethral and intravesical pressure can be made at rest and during repeated stress events; the pressure derived by subtraction of bladder from urethral pressure, the urethral closure pressure, gives a measure of urethral sphincter activity. The urethral pressure is generally recorded along the length of the urethra by slowly withdrawing the pressure-recording catheter from bladder to external meatus, thus producing a urethral pressure profile (UPP). Another technique that can be incorporated into the urodynamic assessment of urethral activity is the electromyographic (EMG) recording of the electrical activity in the external urethral sphincter; the relationship between sphincter activity and other urodynamic parameters can then be examined.

Micturition

The voiding phase of the micturition cycle occurs when a sustained increase in intravesical pressure occurs while urethral pressure falls (Figure 4.2). The urethral closure pressure becomes negative as the bladder empties. The bladder is completely emptied within an appropriate time period, a process reflected by measurement of the urinary flow rate (UFR). Abnormalities of the voiding phase of the micturition cycle may lead to inadequate bladder emptying as a result of a failure of detrusor contractile mechanisms or as a result of an obstruction to the bladder outflow tract.

The urodynamic evaluation of micturition is most commonly undertaken by measurement of the urinary flow rate. Urine is voided into a flow meter, which generates a printout of the urinary flow rate with time; sequential flow rates are necessary in order to ensure representative measurements. Uroflowmetry is usefully combined with an ultrasound assessment of the residual volume of urine (PVR) that remains in the bladder after micturition. Both the pattern of the flow recording and the absolute values of the flow rate may indicate an abnormality. A reduction in

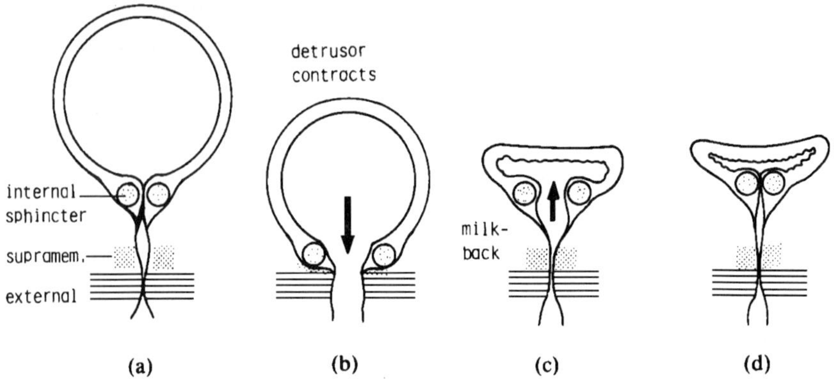

Figure 4.2: Sequence of events in micturition. The full bladder (a) is closed off by the internal, supramembranous, and external sphincters. As the detrusor contracts, the trigone descends (b) and the sphincters relax. After the bladder is emptied (c), urine above the external sphincter is milked-back into the bladder by the action of the supramembranous sphincter, before the internal sphincter contracts (d). *Reproduced with permission from Blandy J. Lecture Notes on Urology, 4th ed. Oxford: Blackwell Scientific Publications, 1991:156.*

the maximum flow rate (often combined with impaired bladder emptying) may be sufficient grounds on which to base a decision to operate on a patient with presumed prostatic hyperplasia, but it must be stressed that obstruction cannot be diagnosed with certainty using this test alone.

Bladder outflow obstruction is diagnosed urodynamically by the demonstration of a high intravesical pressure during voiding and a low urinary flow rate. Failure of detrusor contraction will produce a low-pressure, low-flow picture. Pressure/flow recordings are usually obtained following a filling cystometrogram; the filling catheter is removed, leaving the intravesical and rectal catheters in-situ, and the patient voids into a flow meter. The use of radiological screening and videotape recordings provides additional information, particularly regarding the site of any outflow tract obstruction. A summary of the clinical indications for urodynamic investigations is given in Table 4.1.

The Limitations of Urodynamic Investigations

Correct interpretation of urodynamic investigations is possible only if the limitations of such studies are appreciated. Failure to note the deficiencies of current urodynamic investigative techniques may lead to inappropriate treatment decisions and inevitably poor results.

One of the fundamental criticisms of urodynamic investigations is

Table 4.1: Clinical Indications for Urodynamic Investigations

Method	*Indication*
Frequency/volume chart	All patients with lower urinary tract symptoms
Serial flow rates plus residual urine estimates	Suspected bladder outflow obstruction or detrusor failure Urinary-tract infection Urinary frequency and/or urgency Neuropathic bladder
Filling cystometrogram	Urinary frequency and/or urgency Mixed stress/urge incontinence Enuresis persisting after puberty
Pressure/flow studies	Equivocal bladder outflow obstruction Suspected detrusor failure
Video-urodymanics	Neuropathic bladder Obstruction of undefined site Unproven or complicated stress incontinence Postprostatectomy incontinence
Urethral pressure profilometry	Selected patients with stress incontinence Postprostatectomy incontinence

the fact that they are unphysiological and, as such, may not accurately reflect lower urinary tract function. Much energy is being directed to the quest for newer techniques that bear a closer resemblance to the natural situation. Ambulatory bladder pressure monitoring (the "bladder Holter") is such an example; natural bladder filling and normal patterns of physical activity are incorporated into the design of the investigation. Noninvasive monitoring methods remain the unachieved ideal.

Psychological stress can undoubtedly affect lower urinary-tract function. This should be minimized by performing studies in a suitable environment, with adequate time available and with a positive staff attitude. However, artifactual results, such as the intermittent stream of the anxious voider, may nevertheless be seen, accompanied by the potential for misdiagnosis and inappropriate management.

Any diagnostic investigation must be reproducible if it is to be of clinical value. Most urodynamic investigations examine a single voiding cycle, which carries the risk of sampling error. Some measurements vary widely from cycle to cycle so that, for example, the volume of residual urine should be considered a qualitative rather than a quantitative measurement. Multiple urinary flow studies should be performed to ensure consistent results. In contrast, cystometrography is usually carried out on a single fill/void cycle. Experience with repeat examinations and with ambulatory monitoring suggests that a single cycle is usually representative, although this may not be the case in patients with neurogenic bladder disorders, in whom repeated cycles should be examined.

Other factors that must be considered when interpreting urodynamic studies include the type of monitoring equipment and catheters used, the medium (e.g., fluid or gas) used for bladder filling, the temperature of the medium, the rate of filling, the position of the patient during the study, and whether the patient is taking medications that can affect bladder function. Although these factors are universally important, the urodynamic response of the neuropathic bladder is particularly dependent on investigation methodology such that the filling cystometrogram obtained with a fast filling rate may be indistinguishable from that obtained with the bladder being filled slowly. Although urodynamic investigations produce objective results, there is no doubt that the quality of the data produced is dependent on the details of technique used to carry out the study.

CONTINENCE MECHANISMS AND SPHINCTER FUNCTION

Urinary continence is dependent on both urethral and bladder function. Disorders of the sphincter mechanisms are considered in this section; abnormalities of bladder function that lead to incontinence are examined later. Although the male and female sphincter mechanisms are broadly similar, they are subject to different insults, so that the pathophysiological processes that lead to incontinence differ between the sexes.

The bladder neck in men consists of a definite circular ring of smooth muscle fibers, whereas in women the bladder neck muscle lies in oblique and longitudinal orientations. Sphincteric function of the female bladder neck may depend more on the elasticity of the tissues than on muscle contraction. The distal sphincter in both sexes is made up of a thin inner layer of smooth muscle, which may serve to shorten the urethra during micturition. A circular layer of slow-twitch striated muscle cells (the rhabdosphincter) forms the most important component of the distal or external striated sphincter mechanism. The striated muscle of the pelvic floor includes periurethral muscle slings, which provide visceral support and contribute a short-term occlusive force on the urethra.

Sphincter competence depends on both passive and active processes (Table 4.2). The urethral mucosa and submucosa provide pliable tissues that, when compressed, form a urine-tight mucosal seal; atrophy of these tissues due to estrogen deficiency may be a factor in postmenopausal female incontinence. Other passive mechanisms include the transmission of intra-abdominal pressure to the proximal urethra and the occlusive

Table 4.2: Continence Mechanisms in Women

Urethral mucosal seal
Transmission intra-abdominal pressure to proximal urethra
Elasticity urethral wall
Muscle contraction: bladder neck, external sphincter

forces that are produced by the elasticity of the urethral wall and sphincters. Active muscle occlusion of the urethra occurs at the level of the bladder neck and external urethral sphincter. In men, muscular occlusion of the prostatic and bulbar urethra may occur, but it is not of significance in preserving continence except in the prevention of postmicturition dribbling.

Sphincter-Weakness Incontinence in the Female

Incontinence due to sphincter weakness in the presence of normal bladder function in the female may arise as a result of different pathophysiological processes. These include failure of transmission of intra-abdominal pressure to the proximal urethra, deficiency of bladder neck or distal sphincter mechanisms, periurethral fibrosis, and episodic urethral relaxation (the unstable urethra).

Stress urinary incontinence is commonly accompanied by demonstrable descent of the bladder base in relation to the pelvic floor. The abnormality may be obvious on clinical examination or may be demonstrated using radiological or ultrasound examinations. Bladder base descent results in the proximal urethra lying at the level of, or below, the pelvic floor muscles; raised intra-abdominal pressure therefore leads to an increase in intravesical pressure without any compensating increase in intraurethral pressure and the consequent risk of leakage during stress events. This can be demonstrated using the stress urethral pressure profile, in which sudden increases in intravesical pressure (produced by the patient coughing repeatedly) result in the urethral closure pressure dipping at these moments. Bladder base descent may have other effects that compromise sphincter function. Urethral shortening may decrease the length of the high-pressure zone in the urethra and reduce the efficiency of sphincter contraction. The relationship between bladder neck descent and incontinence is, however, complex, because it is recognized that some women with prolapse are continent. Deficient sphincteric activity must therefore accompany the visceral prolapse in these women if stress incontinence is to develop.

The thesis that descent of the bladder base relative to the pelvic floor is a key factor in the development of stress incontinence is supported by the fact that the most reliable surgical techniques for its correction are designed to correct this anatomical abnormality. The Burch colposuspension and the Marshall-Marchetti-Krantz and Stamey procedures all result in effective bladder neck elevation. Improved intra-abdominal pressure transmission may not be the only factor leading to restoration of continence. Urethral lengthening and increased urethral resistance may be additional effects of these operative procedures.

The role of the bladder neck in preventing stress incontinence is controversial. Radiological studies show that 50% of women have an incompetent bladder neck on coughing, while anatomical studies in women reveal a lack of a clearly defined circularly oriented smooth muscle sphincter as is seen in men. In those women in whom urine is held up at this level, it has been argued, urethral closure is the result of the passive effect of the elastic fibers seen on anatomical studies of the region.

Failure of the distal urethral sphincter in patients with stress incontinence may develop as a result of several different processes. Childbirth results not only in prolapse of the bladder and urethra but also in denervation of the pelvic floor musculature. The deficiency in sphincter function that coexists with descent of the bladder neck in parous women with stress incontinence may therefore be a result of anatomical distortion of the urethra and damage to the innervation of the distal sphincter mechanism. However, stress incontinence also occurs in women without bladder neck prolapse or previous pregnancies; some of these women are described as having a congenital short urethra, but the etiology of their incontinence remains obscure.

In other women, sphincter failure is the result of periurethral fibrosis, which effectively converts a supple, muscular tube into a rigid conduit. Such patients may have had repeated surgical procedures, radiotherapy, or pelvic trauma. A further group of patients have been identified as having abnormal, phasic episodes of urethral sphincter relaxation in the absence of detrusor contractions. This pattern of activity has been termed urethral instability, but the cause, though presumed to be neurological, remains obscure.

The relationship between activity of the periurethral pelvic floor musculature and urethral function is not entirely clear, although the principal role of the pelvic floor is to provide visceral support. Contraction of the pelvic floor produces a short-term occlusive force on the urethra, which is liable to fatigue. This effect may be of importance during stress events, and improving function in these muscles by means of pelvic floor exercises may be the only treatment required in some women with stress incontinence.

In clinical practice, urodynamic investigations cannot reliably predict the success of bladder neck repositioning procedures. For example, urethral pressure profile studies exhibit considerable overlap between the normal and stress-incontinent populations in terms of maximal urethral closure pressures and functional profile length measurements; statistically, the populations can be shown to differ with regard to these parameters, but values for any individual are not diagnostic. This lack of understanding of the pathophysiology of sphincter incontinence underlies some of the deficiencies in diagnosis and explains the poor results in up to 20% of women surgically treated for incontinence.

The principles of treatment of genuine stress incontinence involve attention to several factors. Physiotherapy to the pelvic floor musculature should be considered before surgical intervention is contemplated. The aim of surgery is to restore the position of the bladder neck so that the proximal urethra lies in an intra-abdominal position and urethral length is restored. In patients who fail to respond to bladder neck repositioning or in whom primary sphincter weakness is believed to be the predominant factor causing their incontinence, attention should be given to providing a compressive force on the urethra; this can be provided by a sling procedure, periurethral buttressing (for example, using Teflon or collagen), or, in severe cases, using an artificial urinary sphincter. Finally, periurethral fibrosis may require a combination of urethrolysis and the interposition of adhesion-preventing, vascularized tissue such as omentum or labial fat between the urethra and the vagina and/or pubic symphysis.

Sphincter-Weakness Incontinence in the Male

The mechanisms causing sphincter failure in men are different from those in women. The bladder neck is a clearly defined smooth muscle sphincter whose principal role may be the prevention of retrograde ejaculation of semen but which nevertheless is the level at which continence seems to reside on radiological screening of normal men. The distal sphincter mechanism is separated from the bladder neck by the prostatic urethra, which is represented by an age-related prostatic plateau on urethral pressure profilometry. The distal sphincter provides the zone of highest pressure and lies at the apex of the prostate. The fixation of the bladder neck is more secure in men since the prostate is anchored by strong ligamentous attachments (puboprostatic ligaments), and the integrity of the pelvic floor is not compromised by childbirth. Direct damage to the sphincter, or its innervation, is therefore the main cause of male stress incontinence.

Clinical experience clearly demonstrates that an intact bladder neck or an intact distal sphincter mechanism is adequate to maintain complete urinary control. This is demonstrated on the one hand by patients undergoing prostatectomy or incision of the bladder neck, in whom reliance is placed solely on the distal sphincter, and on the other hand by patients whose distal sphincter is destroyed at the time of a pelvic fracture and whose subsequent urethral reconstruction depends on the bladder neck for continence.

Stress incontinence in neurologically intact men occurs only when both bladder neck and distal sphincter mechanisms have been injured. Clinically, this is most commonly seen in patients with postprostatectomy incontinence but may also occur in patients with prostatic cancer whose tumor has directly invaded the external sphincter or its nerve supply. The operative techniques of prostatectomy, either by open or transurethral approaches, are designed to minimize the risk of distal sphincter damage. However, the sphincter is at risk because of its close anatomical relationship to the apex of the prostate. The mechanism of injury may be by traction on the sphincter in delivering the apices of the lateral lobes during an open procedure or by direct resection of sphincter muscle (or electrical injury to the muscle or its nerve supply by injudicious use of diathermy) during a transurethral prostatectomy. Occasionally, residual tissue following prostatectomy mechanically prevents mass sphincter closure. Such patients can be rendered continent by resection of the residual tissue.

Some men with postprostatectomy stress incontinence achieve some improvement with pelvic floor exercises. However, significant leakage requires surgical correction. In contrast to the situation in women, the primary principle of treatment is passive urethral compression. This is most satisfactorily achieved using an artificial urinary sphincter.

BLADDER FUNCTION

During the very early stages of bladder filling, urine is accommodated by the unfolding of the bladder wall (Table 4.3). Relaxation of the detrusor smooth muscle then allows the bladder wall to stretch in a viscoelastic

Table 4.3: Bladder Functions

Urine Storage		*Bladder Emptying*
Bladder accommodation		Bladder muscle contraction
Urethral pressure greater than bladder pressure		Urethral pressure less than bladder pressure
Bladder neck closed at rest and during stress		Opening and funneling of bladder neck
Laplace's law		
Bladder	$P = \frac{2T}{R}$	Absence of obstruction

P, detrusor pressure; *T*, tension per unit width of bladder wall; *R*, radius of bladder.

manner. The detrusor is composed of interlacing smooth muscle bundles, which contract as a unit to increase intravesical pressure and so empty the bladder. The attachment of the detrusor to the base of the bladder may cause the muscle to have a secondary action, that of pulling open the bladder neck.

Failure of the bladder's functions of storage and emptying are common clinical problems. A minority of patients have demonstrable neurological disease (see section on the neurogenic bladder), but most will be neurologically intact. This section examines the pathophysiological background of several important clinical conditions in which bladder function is disordered.

Detrusor Instability

Detrusor instability is a urodynamic diagnosis made on cystometrography and is characterized by phasic increases in detrusor pressure during filling despite attempts to inhibit micturition (Table 4.4). Patients may be asymptomatic or experience urgency of micturition with associated frequency and, in severe cases, incontinence. Although formal diagnosis requires urodynamic studies, a clinical diagnosis is often made by inference in patients with typical symptoms who respond to appropriate pharmacologic treatment.

Table 4.4: Detrusor Instability

Classification

Idiopathic, most common
Neuropathic (detrusor hyperreflexia)
Obstruction-related, e.g., benign prostatic hyperplasia (BPH)

Possible Causes

Failure of maturation of CNS control mechanisms
Low detrusor levels of inhibitory vasoactive intestinal peptide (VIP)
Abnormal enkephalin-mediated inhibitory neurotransmission
Denervation supersensitivity

Treatment

Psychotherapy/biofeedback
Anticholinergics
Surgery (cystoplasty)

Instability in BPH

Occurs in 40 to 50%
Disappears following prostatectomy in 70 to 80%

Detrusor instability in patients with neurological disease is termed detrusor hyperreflexia (see below). It also occurs in association with bladder outlet obstruction, for example, benign prostatic hyperplasia, and is discussed further under that heading. In the absence of neuropathy or outflow obstruction, detrusor instability is usually termed idiopathic. This label obscures the fact that research has produced a number of interesting findings, though not a clear pathophysiological explanation, for the phenomenon.

The normal micturition reflex in characterized by a fall in urethral pressure followed by contraction of the detrusor muscle and bladder emptying. An identical sequence of events occurs during unstable bladder contractions. This observation suggests that unstable bladder contractions represent coordinated reflex patterns of activity that have escaped from the normal inhibitory influences of the central nervous system. This failure to control the micturition reflex may represent occult neurological disease; opiate antagonists have been shown to worsen instability, suggesting an abnormality of enkephalin-mediated inhibitory pathways. Alternatively, instability can be regarded in behavioral terms. Infant bladders fill and empty on an automatic cycle; conscious control is established during childhood toilet training. Failure of this learning process leaves the micturition reflex under incomplete control and can lead to unstable bladder contractions.

Concentrations of the inhibitory neuropeptide, vasoactive intestinal polypeptide (VIP), are lower in the bladder wall of patients with bladder instability than in that of controls. This might indicate a peripheral etiology for detrusor instability but represents no more than an interesting observation, as the precise role of VIP in the neural control of the detrusor is unknown.

Clinical experience with urodynamic investigations suggests that the prevalence of idiopathic detrusor instability increases with age, but epidemiological confirmation of this observation is not available. The mechanism for the association between aging and instability is not clearly defined, but histologic studies have demonstrated that the cholinergic innervation of the detrusor muscle becomes less dense with age. Alterations in detrusor innervation occur as a consequence of bladder outflow obstruction (see below); this suggests a common etiology of detrusor instability in outlet obstruction and aging. Despite these observations and theories, the term idiopathic detrusor instability remains appropriate.

Most women with incontinence have either genuine stress incontinence or urge incontinence associated with detrusor instability. However, a significant minority have both types of incontinence (mixed incontinence). This complicates management because procedures to reposition the bladder neck have an unpredictable effect on bladder behavior. Some patients develop more severe instability postoperatively and remain incontinent. It is not clear whether the apparent deterioration is due to instability being uncovered as a result of the bladder being able to fill to increased volumes or whether deterioration is a direct effect of the surgery, perhaps related to the introduction of a degree of bladder outflow obstruction.

Nocturnal enuresis in childhood can be regarded in most cases as a failure of bladder sensation to break into the sleep pattern; improvement occurs as the central nervous system matures, perhaps with the help of reinforcement in the form of an enuresis alarm or a reward system such as a star chart. In addition, enuretic patients tend to have an impaired ability to concentrate urine at night. However, the presence of daytime symptoms of frequency and urgency or bed-wetting occurring after puberty defines a group of patients in whom detrusor instability is the likely underlying cause.

The treatment of detrusor instability is based on several different strategies (Table 4.4). The concept that instability is caused by a failure of central control of the micturition reflex has led to interest in the use of psychotherapy in this context. The intensity of therapy varies from a simple explanation of the condition coupled with the patient monitoring progress with frequency/volume charts to hypnotherapy, biofeedback regimes, and intensive in-patient bladder training programs. Excellent short-term response rates have been reported, although few studies give data on symptom control over longer periods.

Another approach involves disruption of the peripheral bladder innervation with the aim of breaking the overactive reflex. This is most commonly undertaken using anticholinergic agents; the primary motor innervation of the detrusor muscle is cholinergic, so that such drugs serve to partially uncouple the muscle from its nerve supply. Anticholinergic drugs with additional sites of action (such as oxybutynin) appear to be the most effective agents, perhaps because their activity is less readily overcome by homeostatic mechanisms. Surgical approaches to the disruption of the micturition reflex include selective sacral neurectomy, phenolization of the pelvic plexus, and bladder transection. These techniques have failed to gain wide acceptance because good early responses are followed by symptom relapse over several months in many patients.

A few patients have severe, intractable symptoms from detrusor instability and may be considered for more major surgical intervention. The clam enterocystoplasty has proved successful in the treatment of such cases. The interposition of a length of ileum into the bladder wall has the effect of disrupting the mechanical integrity of the bladder, thus rendering contractions of the bladder wall inefficient; the procedure may have an additional denervating effect.

BLADDER OUTFLOW OBSTRUCTION

A precise urodynamic definition of bladder outflow obstruction is not available, but the key findings are increased intravesical pressure during micturition combined with a reduction in the urinary flow rate. These two parameters can be related, to derive urethral resistance, but the clinical use of urethral resistance factors has proved unreliable in practice. Despite this problem, urodynamic investigations have proved invaluable in diagnosing obstruction and defining its effects.

Obstruction to the bladder outflow tract develops as a consequence of many conditions, of which benign prostatic hyperplasia, bladder neck dyssynergia, carcinoma of the prostate, and urethral stricture are the most common. The effects of obstruction are both structural and functional.

Studies in humans and animal models have demonstrated that obstruction leads to detrusor muscle hypertrophy and hyperplasia; these changes are accompanied by an increase in the connective-tissue content of the detrusor as a result of collagen deposition between and within muscle bundles. On a macroscopic level, trabeculation may be seen as muscle bundles hypertrophy and the bladder mucosa herniates between the bundles to form saccules and diverticula. The mechanism by which these changes occur is not clear but might be expected to relate to increases in intravesical pressure (and therefore bladder wall tension); trabeculation is most commonly seen in patients whose bladders are both obstructed and unstable and therefore exposed to high intravesical pressures both during filling and during voiding.

Obstruction usually leads to a reduction in the maximal urinary flow rate, although this measurement must be related to normal values for the patient's age, sex, and volume voided. Sufficient detrusor compensation for the degree of obstruction is sometimes seen, with the result that the maximal flow rate remains in the normal range (as a result of an increased voiding pressure); pressure/flow studies are required in patients whose clinical picture suggests outflow tract obstruction but who have normal flow rates. Detrusor muscle hypertrophy and hyperplasia relate to the increased intravesical pressures observed in outlet obstruction, but additional changes in the contractile properties of the detrusor also develop. The obstructed detrusor has been shown to exhibit a reduction in its ability to maintain a rapid contraction; a reduced speed of shortening of detrusor fibers may explain why some patients fail to recover a normal flow rate after surgery to correct their outflow obstruction. Detrusor fatigue toward the end of micturition is thought to be a cause of incomplete bladder emptying, which leads to the development of persistent residual urine.

The obstructed bladder frequently exhibits abnormalities in the filling phase of the micturition cycle. An increase in the end-fill pressure may be seen with an associated fall in bladder compliance; this change may relate to the infiltration of the bladder wall with increased quantities of connective tissue or to impairment of the hypertrophied detrusor muscle fibers' ability to relax during filling. Furthermore, a large number of studies have shown that patients with bladder outflow obstruction frequently exhibit detrusor instability during filling and that this unstable bladder behavior is a common cause of symptoms. It has been argued that obstruction and instability may be associated simply because both are common conditions in the elderly and therefore coexist in many cases; this explanation can be refuted only if urodynamic studies of the population at large fail to demonstrate a similar rate of instability in nonobstructed and obstructed individuals or if a mechanism can be shown to link the two conditions. A number of clinical and experimental observations suggest that the relationship between instability and obstruction is not simply due to chance.

It has been repeatedly demonstrated that relief of outflow tract obstruction will render an unstable bladder stable in approximately 70% of cases. Although the effect of surgery may be to interrupt the overactive reflex pathway, it seems probable that the effect is due to relief of obstruction, since denervating procedures have been generally ineffective in the long-term treatment of idiopathic instability. Furthermore, the denervating effect of a bladder neck incision or prostatotomy is unlikely to be significant.

It has been suggested that the overactive reflex giving rise to unstable bladder contractions may be the result of a high level of sensory input into the spinal cord due to changes in the bladder wall, such as increased wall tension during filling. The increased sensory input may combine with age-related failure of the central inhibitory pathways to suppress unstable contractions.

An additional factor in the genesis of detrusor instability in the obstructed bladder is detrusor denervation. A reduction in the density of the cholinergic nerve supply to the obstructed detrusor has been demonstrated in both humans and animal models. Furthermore, animal models of outflow tract obstruction have demonstrated urodynamic changes that mirror those of detrusor instability in humans; since detrusor instability relates to a loss of conscious control over bladder contractions, this term should not be applied to the changes seen in animal studies. Pharmacological studies have shown that detrusor denervation causes the muscle to become supersensititve to cholinergic and other agonists; this change is greater in men with instability than in those with stable bladders. It has been suggested that this supersensitivity causes instability, but this simplistic explanation fails to explain what stimulus triggers activity in the damaged nerve supply. It has been shown that blocking the spinal reflex pathway abolishes instability in the obstructed patient. In addition, the bladder's innervation is complex, and it may be the pattern of nerve loss among different types of nerves (sensory and motor, inhibitory and excitatory) that determines the overall urodynamic behavior of the bladder. Cholinergic nerve loss also arises as a result of aging, thereby suggesting that instability might develop in the elderly by the same process as in bladder outflow obstruction. If denervation and instability are related, could reinnervation explain the fact that many bladders revert to stable behavior after relief of outflow obstruction? This is a possibility, since axonal, rather than cell body, loss has been observed, thereby leaving open the possibility for axon regeneration.

Chronic urinary retention results when bladder emptying becomes inefficient and the volume of residual urine becomes large. High intravesical pressures and ureteric obstruction at the level of the intramural ureter can lead to upper tract dilatation and renal impairment. Why painless bladder decompensation occurs is not clear, but sensory- and motor-nerve failure are possible mechanisms.

THE INNERVATION OF THE URINARY BLADDER

Neuroanatomy

The parasympathetic, sympathetic, and somatic nervous systems all contribute to the innervation of the lower urinary tract. Parasympathetic fibers (S2, 3, 4) run in the pelvic nerve to the pelvic and vesical plexuses before entering the bladder; parasympathetic ganglia are found in these plexuses and in the bladder wall (Table 4.5). Sympathetic nerves derive from thoracolumbar spinal levels (T11, 12; L1, 2) and pass through the sympathetic trunk to reach the inferior mesenteric ganglion. From here fibers pass in the hypogastric nerves to the pelvic plexus and bladder (Table 4.5). Sympathetic relays are found in the inferior mesenteric ganglion and in the pelvic plexus. The somatic nervous system supplies the periurethral pelvic floor musculature via the pudendal nerve.

Sensory information from the bladder is largely derived from free nerve endings that act as tension receptors and relay to the spinal cord via the pelvic and hypogastric nerves. Within the cord, information from bladder afferents is integrated with that from other viscera and somatic

Table 4.5 Autonomic Innervation of the Lower Urinary Tract

Parasympathetic	*Sympathetic*
S2, 3, 4 roots	T11, 12; L1, 2 roots
↓	↓
Pelvic nerve	Inferior mesenteric ganglion
↓	↓ Postganglionic
Ganglia in pelvic plexus and bladder wall	Hypogastric nerves
↓ Postganglionic	↓
Smooth muscle	Smooth muscle

sources and projected to the brain stem centers that coordinate the micturition cycle. Cells in the medulla, pons, and midbrain have been found to relate to bladder and sphincter function, and these areas receive additional, complex inputs from the cerebral cortex, cerebellum, hypothalamus, and basal ganglia.

Descending pathways converge on the sacral micturition center, which lies in the intermediolateral grey matter and ventral horn in the sacral cord. Preganglionic parasympathetic neurones have their cell bodies in this center. The motor neurones that supply the external urethral sphincter lie in Onuf's nucleus in the ventral horn of the sacral cord.

Neurophysiology of Urine Storage

Studies in animals suggest that micturition is suppressed until bladder filling reaches a set point determined by centers above the level of the pons. Higher centers, therefore, determine when micturition is appropriate, and they provide an inhibitory influence on the brain stem mechanism reflex during urine storage. Further inhibitory mechanisms in animals include a brain stem storage reflex, a spinal reflex (which is served by pelvic nerve afferent fibers and has efferent fibers running in the sympathetic supply to the bladder), and inhibitory circuitry in the sacral spinal cord centers.

In addition to these central storage processes, there are peripheral adaptations to urine storage (Table 4.6). There is evidence that the parasympathetic ganglia act as filters and discharge only in the face of high levels of activity in the preganglionic neurones; this effectively blocks low-level preganglionic activity from causing premature detrusor excitation. The ganglia are also exposed to inhibitory influences from sympathetic fibers. Finally, inhibitory mechanisms are at work in the wall of the bladder; a direct sympathetic inhibitory innervation to the detrusor has been identified in the cat. The situation in humans is less clear, since lumbar sympathectomy appears to have little influence on bladder function in human subjects.

Table 4.6 Neurophysiology of Micturition

Urine Storage	*Urine Expulsion*
Central storage reflexes	Central reflexes in brain stem, spinal cord
Peripheral processes	Peripheral processes
Sympathetic inhibition of parasympathetic ganglia	Parasympathetic mediated detrusor contraction
Sympathetic alpha-adrenergic stimulation of bladder neck	Somatic relaxation of external sphincter
Sympathetic beta-adrenergic inhibition of bladder contractility	Sympathetic relaxation of bladder neck smooth muscle
Increased somatic tone in external sphincter	

The male bladder neck is under sympathetic control and remains closed during bladder filling. In women, the bladder neck has a relatively sparse adrenergic innervation and appears to be a less significant sphincter. The external sphincter is tonically active under the influence of its somatic nerve supply. An increase in intravesical pressure is matched by an increase in sphincter tone as a result of activity in sacral-cord–based reflex; sphincter activity is also under the influence of the pontine nucleus.

Neurophysiology of Micturition

The timing of micturition is determined by centers above the brain stem; these centers also coordinate the activities that precede and accompany bladder emptying (Figure 4.3). When micturition is appropriate, the brain stem micturition reflex can be activated. In the cat, stimuli leading to bladder contraction include bladder and urethral distension; afferent fibers in the pelvic, hypogastric, and pudendal nerves transmit information to relays in the spinal cord and hindbrain. As a result of activity in these afferent pathways (particularly those carried in the pelvic nerves), stimulation of the brain stem centers leads to activation of the descending pathways in the lateral columns of the spinal cord and subsequent stimulation of the sacral parasympathetic nucleus. High levels of activity in the preganglionic parasympathetic fibers cause the parasympathetic ganglia to switch from an "off" to "on" pattern of activity, with firing of postganglionic fibers resulting in detrusor contraction (Table 4.6). The postganglionic nerves terminate as a plexus that surrounds the smooth-muscle cells of the detrusor and stimulates muscle contraction.

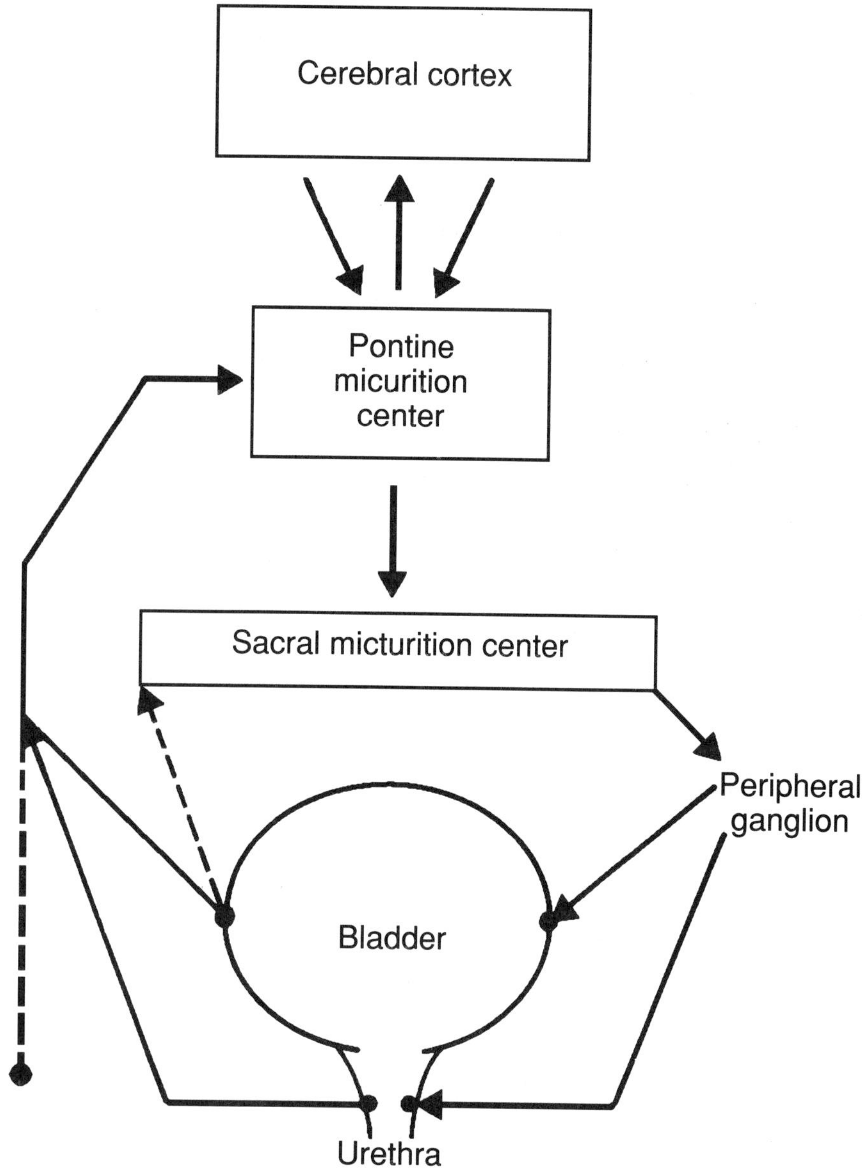

Figure 4.3: The micturition reflex, schematic representation. *Reproduced from Webster G, Kirby K, King L, et al eds. Reconstructive Urology Vol 1. Boston: Blackwell Scientific Publications, 1993:28.*

The bladder neck opens as a result of relaxation of its smooth muscle and the effect of detrusor contraction pulling open the sphincter. The external sphincter relaxes immediately prior to and during micturition, perhaps in response to activity in a spinal reflex as described in the cat.

Neurophysiology of Neurotransmission

Knowledge of the neurotransmitters involved in the control of the micturition cycle is incomplete, although more is known about transmitters in peripheral pathways than those in the central nervous system (Table 4.7). Experimental studies have demonstrated the involvement of endogenous opiates in the central inhibition of micturition.

Excitatory neurotransmission in the parasympathetic ganglia involves the release of acetylcholine from preganglionic fibers, which stimulates nicotinic receptors on the postganglionic neurones. Inhibitory influences from the sympathetic system are mediated by norepinephrine acting on alpha-receptors. Enkephalin-containing nerves also exert an inhibitory effect at this site.

The major excitatory neurotransmitter stimulating contraction of

Table 4.7: Autonomic Innervation and Neurotransmitters

Cholinergic receptors

- Muscarinic (bladder muscle)
- Nicotinic (skeletal muscle and autonomic ganglia)

Adrenergic receptors

- Alpha 1,2 (smooth muscle contraction)
- Beta 1,2 (smooth muscle relaxation)
- Bladder body: beta > alpha
- Bladder base: alpha > beta

Neurotransmitters

- Acetylcholine (Ach)
- Norepinephrine (NE)
- Nonadrenergic, noncholinergic (NANC)
  - Inhibitory
    - Endogenous opioids
    - Vasoactive intestinal polypeptide
    - Gamma-aminobutyric acid
  - Excitatory
    - Adenosine triphosphate (ATP)

detrusor smooth muscle in humans is acetylcholine, which acts on muscarinic receptors. In other animal species, noncholinergic, nonadrenergic transmission is also important. Whether acetylcholine is the only transmitter involved in the human is the subject of debate; secondary transmitters may be of importance in modulating cholinergic transmission. Neurotransmitters that have been shown in various species to have a role in inhibiting detrusor contractions include norepinephrine (acting on beta-receptors), vasoactive intestinal polypeptide (VIP), and gamma-aminobutyric acid (GABA).

The circular, smooth muscle sphincter of the male bladder neck is supplied by both cholinergic and adrenergic nerves; contraction of this muscle is mediated by norepinephrine acting on alpha-receptors (Figure 4.4). The major transmitter involved in contraction of the striated-muscle component of the external sphincter (the rhabdosphincter) is acetylcholine, which acts via nicotinic receptors.

NEUROGENIC BLADDER DYSFUNCTION

Disordered urinary function can be caused by a wide variety of neurological diseases. Deranged bladder function may lead to minimal symptoms or cause major morbidity and even mortality. The aim of management is

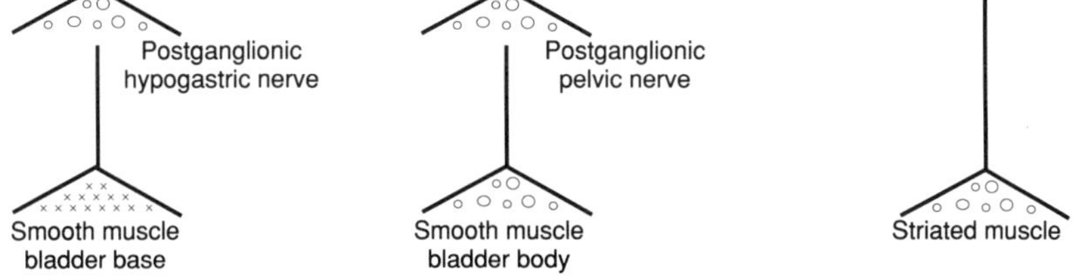

Figure 4.4: Preganglionic and Postganglionic Neurotransmitters.
(Dots: Acetylcholine-neurotransmitter at somatic motor fibers, all preganglionic autonomic fibers, and parasympathetic postganglionic fibers; Xs: norepinephrine-neurotransmitter at postganglionic sympathetic fibers.) This simplified outline does not include details of probable secondary neurotransmitters that may be coreleased with acetylcholine or norepinephrine or be found in separate, nonadrenergic, noncholinergic neurons.

twofold: prevention of upper tract damage with its risks of renal failure, and preservation of continence and the patient's quality of life. Consideration is given to some of the important causes of neurogenic bladder dysfunction.

Spinal Cord Injury

The level and extent of spinal cord injury determine the pattern of abnormal detrusor and sphincter activity. Injuries may be partial or complete, and treatment must be based on the urodynamic behavior of the lower urinary tract rather than a prediction based on anatomical considerations such as the level of injury. Furthermore, as in many neurological conditions, the urodynamic picture changes over time so that periodic reevaluation is essential to proper management.

Injury to the sacral cord or its roots leads to paralysis of the detrusor muscle and associated sphincter weakness, since the excitatory innervation to detrusor and sphincter is damaged. The storage capacity of the bladder is generally satisfactory, although bladder compliance may be reduced. Poor compliance is seen as an abnormal increase in detrusor pressure for a given volume increment; compliance relates to both active contraction and the pressure properties of the bladder wall. Sphincter weakness may lead to stress incontinence, which, if severe, may require the insertion of an artificial urinary sphincter. Bladder emptying is impaired because of absent or weak detrusor contractions. In addition, emptying (for example, by straining) may be hindered by contraction of the distal sphincter, a phenomenon called isolated distal sphincter obstruction. This abnormality can lead to the paradoxical occurrence of sphincter weakness incontinence during filling and obstruction due to sphincteric contraction during voiding. The cause of isolated distal sphincter obstruction is not clear, although an abnormal pattern of sphincter reinnervation with adrenergic fibers is a possible cause. If bladder emptying by straining or abdominal compression is unsuccessful, the bladder can be satisfactorily emptied by regular, clean, intermittent, self-catheterization.

The immediate result of a spinal injury is depression of neuronal activity below the level of the lesion: spinal shock. The result of spinal shock is a flaccid, noncontractile bladder, which leads to painless retention of urine and an overdistension injury to the bladder. In order to prevent retention and its associated risks of incontinence, sepsis and renal failure, the bladder should be decompressed during spinal shock by either permanent or intermittent catheterization. The return of neural activity below the lesion is incremental and may take weeks or months.

Lesions above the level of the sacral cord will produce, after the period of spinal shock, an uncoordinated pattern of bladder and sphincter activity. The bladder and sphincters remain under the control of the spinal reflexes that have remained intact and, in animal models, new reflex pathways emerge. However, not only is voluntary control lost but also the coordination between the fragments of preserved reflex activity. The urodynamic problems posed by such injuries affect both the storage and emptying functions of the bladder. Accurate urodynamic diagnosis is particularly dependent on careful attention to the details of the urodynamic investigation. For example, the bladder should be filled at a slow rate on top of any residual urine since emptying the bladder prior to filling can alter bladder behavior.

In the filling phase, detrusor hyperreflexia (i.e., detrusor instability in a patient with neurological disease) is commonly seen, and this may limit the storage capabilities of the bladder. Treatment strategies to improve storage include the use of anticholinergic agents, which block the effect of acetylcholine on detrusor smooth muscle, and the use of augmentation cystoplasty procedures, which incorporate segments of bowel into the bladder wall. The latter serves both to increase bladder volume and to dissipate the effect of hyperreflexic detrusor contractions.

Voiding is also affected by suprasacral lesions because of abnormal detrusor and sphincter function. Reflex detrusor contractions are seen to occur either spontaneously or in response to such stimuli as suprapubic tapping, but voiding is frequently obstructed at the level of the distal, striated sphincter. This failure of coordinated sphincter relaxation, detrusor-sphincter dyssynergia, usually takes the form of phasic sphincter contractions that occur as the detrusor contracts (Figure 4.5). The reflex contraction of the full bladder appears to lead to a guarding reflex response from the sphincter rather than the relaxation pattern that typifies normal micturition. The occurrence of detrusor–sphincter dyssynergia is related to the level of the cord injury; the abnormality is more common with high lesions, (i.e., cervical or high thoracic injuries) (Table 4.8). Bladder emptying may be further impaired by poorly sustained detrusor contractions. Dyssynergia at the level of the bladder neck is rare in spinal cord injured patients.

The high-pressure bladder in the female generally leads to incontinence since urethral resistance is relatively easily overcome by powerful detrusor contractions. In contrast, high intravesical pressures and poor bladder emptying may be seen in men, since they appear to have less of a urethral safety-valve effect. The upper urinary tract is therefore exposed to increased pressures and the potential of renal damage.

Some patients with suprasacral cord injuries can stimulate reflex detrusor contractions by a variety of maneuvers, for example, tapping the

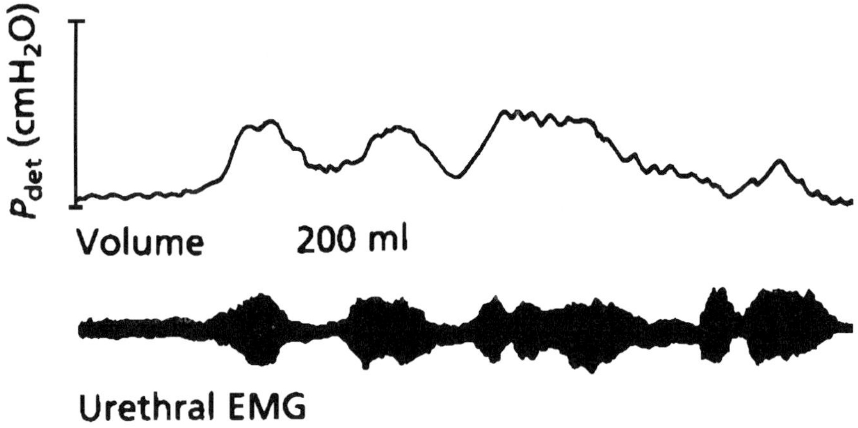

Figure 4.5: Detrusor–sphincter dyssynergia in quadriplegia. *Reproduced with permission from Blandy J. Lecture Notes on Urology, 4th ed. Oxford: Blackwell Scientific Publications, 1991:132.*

abdominal wall; if detrusor–sphincter dyssynergia is not severe, the bladder may be satisfactorily emptied by this technique. If reflex voiding is unsatisfactory, the bladder can be emptied by intermittent self-catheterization. If this is not feasible, it may prove necessary to render the patient incontinent by external sphincterotomy in order to protect the upper renal tract.

Table 4.8 Detrusor–External-Sphincter Dyssynergia

High thoracic, cervical cord lesions
High detrusor voiding pressures
Urinary-tract infection
Vesicoureteral reflux
Obstructive uropathy
Calculi
Renal failure
Treatment
Lower bladder pressures by:
Anticholinergics
Catheterization
External sphincterotomy
Prevent infections, calculi

Autonomic Dysreflexia

Patients with spinal cord lesions above the T6 neurological level may suffer from an abnormal pattern of autonomic activity in response to visceral or somatic stimulation below the level of injury. This syndrome, termed autonomic dysreflexia, is most commonly seen in response to bladder distension (Table 4.9). Sensory input to the isolated segment of spinal cord results in a high level of activity in the sympathetic nervous system supplied by this part of the cord. Below the level of the injury, vasomotor reflex activity causes vasoconstriction, which leads to an increase in blood pressure and produces the typical pounding headache; the hypertensive response can be life-threatening. The increased blood pressure is detected by the carotid sinus and aortic arch baroreceptors, which trigger regulatory reflex activity above the injury level. Thus, vagal responses lead to bradycardia, while vasodilatation and sweating are seen above the level of the cord lesion. These responses are largely ineffective in reducing the blood pressure, and resolution of the crisis depends on removal of the precipitating stimulus, for example, by bladder drainage or fecal disimpaction. Additional treatment with antihypertensive agents may be required if these simple measures are not effective.

The Effects of Pelvic Surgery on the Bladder

Radical surgery to the rectum or uterus puts the pelvic autonomic nerves at risk from surgical damage and therefore holds the possibility of subsequent lower urinary tract dysfunction. The nerve fibers most at risk are the preganglionic parasympathetic nerves (injury to which results in a decentralized bladder) and the sympathetic hypogastric nerves. In addition, anatomical distortion of the pelvic viscera after such surgery may further compromise bladder function. The majority of surgical injuries to

Table 4.9: Autonomic Dysreflexia

Uncontrolled sympathetic response to stimulation below level of cord lesion
High spinal cord lesions, usually above T6
  ↑ Blood pressure, ↑ pulse, sweating, headaches
Cause
  Dyssynergia
  Overdistended bladder (e.g., blocked catheter, retention with dyssynergia)
  Distended rectum/sigmoid
  Painful stimuli below level of lesion (e.g., pressure sores)
Treatment
  Relieve precipitating factors
  Pharmacologic lowering of blood pressure

the pelvic nerves are partial and followed by varying degrees of reinnervation. Therefore, urodynamic abnormalities evolve and vary over time in these patients.

The most common feature seen with pelvic plexus injuries is difficulty in voiding or urinary retention. The parasympathetic drive to the detrusor is diminished so that bladder emptying is inefficient, and this may be exacerbated by distortion of the urethra as a result of the surgery. In some cases bladder compliance is reduced, probably because of an imbalance between the damaged sympathetic and parasympathetic influences on the detrusor. Sphincter denervation may lead to sphincter weakness and associated incontinence, particularly in the presence of a large residual urine volume.

Treatment is directed at improving bladder emptying; this may be achieved by clean, intermittent self-catheterization. An alternative approach is to lower outflow tract resistance by urethrotomy or transurethral prostatectomy; although such procedures can be effective, they carry a risk of further compromising sphincter function and should therefore not be undertaken lightly.

In addition to the clear-cut autonomic nerve injuries discussed above, hysterectomy is frequently blamed for a variety of symptoms complexes. It must be stressed that hysterectomy is so frequently undertaken that a significant proportion of women presenting with lower tract symptoms will have had such a procedure. The operation undoubtedly carries the potential for nerve damage, alteration of pelvic anatomy, and changes in the hormonal environment; but carefully controlled, prospective studies of the effects of hysterectomy are needed before the pathophysiological consequences of the operation can be properly evaluated.

Multiple Sclerosis

Bladder dysfunction and incontinence are common features in multiple sclerosis, and the resultant difficulties are frequently exacerbated by impaired mobility. Because the sites of demyelination in the central nervous system are variable, the effects of the disease on the lower urinary tract are unpredictable, although typical patterns of abnormality can be recognized.

The most common abnormality seen in multiple sclerosis patients is detrusor hyperreflexia. It appears likely that interruption of spinal tracts and the emergence of abnormal reflex pathways (as in spinal cord injury) along with damage to the inhibitory mechanisms of the centers above the brain stem cause the hyperreflexia. Disruption of reflex pathways may also lead to a breakdown of coordination between detrusor and sphincter so that detrusor–sphincter dyssynergia may also occur. Other abnormal findings that may be seen less often include detrusor acontractility and urethral instability; the latter abnormality is seen as episodic urethral relaxations occurring in the absence of detrusor activity and may lead to incontinence.

One particular difficulty seen in the immobile woman with multiple sclerosis is the development of a wide-caliber, patulous urethra. This abnormality, usually seen in patients treated by indwelling catheter, may develop as a result of severe hyperreflexia leading to repeated catheter expulsion (despite an inflated balloon) and sphincter paralysis due to denervation. Treatment includes suprapubic catheterization with urethral closure or, alternatively, urinary diversion.

Urinary Incontinence in the Elderly

No pathophysiological processes leading to loss of urinary control are specific to the geriatric population, but many conditions become more common with advancing years and several etiological factors frequently coexist in older patients. It is particularly relevant to interpret investigations and to tailor treatment in the context of the patient environment as a whole, while avoiding the danger of undertreatment simply on the basis of age.

Dementia, from whatever cause, will lead to a loss of appreciation of the social requirements of micturition and, eventually, the apparent loss of awareness of lower urinary tract function. Regular toileting may be successful in preserving continence, but permanent urinary drainage is frequently indicated. Cerebrovascular accidents frequently lead to urinary retention in the initial phase, presumably by a mechanism analogous to spinal shock. Subsequent continence may be endangered by loss of social appreciation, impaired mobility, and the development of detrusor hyperreflexia.

Parkinson's disease, also common in the elderly, appears to be associated with the development of detrusor hyperreflexia, which is probably related to the loss of inhibitory influences on micturition from the diseased basal ganglia. The picture is frequently complicated by immobility, depression, and effects of medication, and coexisting urinary tract disorders such as bladder outflow obstruction. Diabetic autonomic neuropathy is also seen, particularly in the older diabetic, and leads to loss of bladder sensation and chronic urinary retention; urinary-tract infections, a reduced flow, and overflow incontinence are typical sequelae.

The prevalence of bladder outflow obstruction (due to prostatic hyperplasia or carcinoma) and detrusor instability (whether primary or secondary to obstruction) increases with age and may require treatment. The presence of detrusor instability in the elderly has been shown to be associated with reduced cortical perfusion, suggesting that the abnormality may be a reflection of global neurological deterioration. Other factors that may complicate management are postmenopausal changes in the urethra, the effects of medication (particularly diuretics), urinary-tract infection, and constipation. Finally, it is now recognized that some patients (particularly in the older age groups) may have a reversal of the normal circadian pattern of urine production, with consequent difficulties regarding urinary frequency or incontinence at night; nocturnal polyuria, which can be diagnosed by the use of a frequency/volume chart, may be caused by mobilization of fluid from the extremities in some patients and an abnormal pattern of production of antidiuretic hormone in others.

CONCLUSION

The understanding of the pathophysiology of disorders of the urinary tract has improved dramatically with the introduction into clinical practice of urodynamic techniques. Treatment is now administered in an increasingly rational manner as it is possible to define bladder and sphincter function accurately during bladder filling and emptying. Urodynamics is, however, a developing field, and new techniques (such as long-term ambulatory monitoring) promise to add further diagnostic sophistication.

Although urodynamic investigations allow descriptive diagnoses to be made in most patients with lower urinary-tract symptoms, this should not mask the fact that understanding is as yet lacking as to the precise mechanisms causing conditions such as detrusor instability. It is to be hoped that advances in knowledge in these areas will herald further improvements in treatment.

An important area of recent interest is that of neurotransmission in the autonomic nervous system. The likely contribution of secondary neurotransmitters in bladder and sphincter function holds out promise for more effective pharmacotherapy as drugs with multiple actions, or combinations of drugs, are developed.

SUGGESTED READINGS

Mundy AR, Stephenson TP, Wein AJ. Urodynamic principles, practice and application. Edinburgh: Churchill Livingstone, 1984.

Excellent text reviews urodynamic methodology and its application to functional disorders of lower urinary tract.

Fletcher TF, Bradley WE. Neuroanatomy of the bladder-urethra. J Urol 1978; 119:153.

Concise account of neuroanatomy of lower urinary tract.

Blaivas JG. The neurophysiology of micturition: a clinical study of 550 patients. J Urol 1982;127:958.

Important paper presenting clinical data to support the concept of micturition being coordinated at the level of the brain stem.

DeGroat WC, Kawatani M, Hisamitsu T, et al. Neural control of micturition: the role of neuropeptides. J Auton Nerv Syst Suppl 1986;369.

Review from major group involved in physiological and pharmacological research into micturition. Gives valuable insight into the increasing complexity of neural mechanisms now becoming apparent.

Lucas MG. Urinary incontinence: pathology and principles of treatment. In: Chisholm GD, Fair WR, eds. Scientific foundations of urology. 3rd ed. Chicago: Yearbook Medical Publishers, 1990:324.

Useful discussion of pathophysiology of incontinence and treatment strategies.

Snooks SJ, Badenoch DF, Tiptaft RC, Swash M. Perineal nerve damage in genuine stress urinary incontinence. An electrophysiological study. Br J Urol 1985;57:442.

Evidence that damage to the innervation of urethral and periurethral striated muscle may be seen in women with genuine stress incontinence.

Chalfin SA, Bradley WE. The etiology of detrusor hyperreflexia in patients with infravesical obstruction. J Urol 1982;127:938.

Experimental study suggesting that activity in prostatic sensory nerves may have a role in causing disordered bladder function in patients with bladder outflow obstruction.

Speakman MJ, Brading AF, Gilpin CJ, Dixon JS, Gilpin SA, Gosling JA. Bladder outflow obstruction: a cause of denervation supersensitivity. J Urol 1987;138: 1461.

Experimental evidence that bladder outflow obstruction leads to damage to the parasympathetic nerve supply to the detrusor muscle.

Foote J, Yun S, Leach GE. Postprostatectomy incontinence: pathophysiology, evaluation and management. Urol Clin North Am 1991;18:229.

Good review covering most aspects of the condition.

Thomas DG, Lucas MG. The urinary tract following spinal cord injury. In: Chisholm GD, Fair WR, eds. Scientific foundations of urology. 3rd ed. Chicago: Yearbook Medical Publishers, 1990;286.

Discussion of the neurological basis of lower urinary-tract dysfunction in spinal cord injury coupled with description of clinical problems that arise and their investigation.

Trop CS, Bennett CJ. Autonomic dysreflexia and its urological implications: a review. J Urol 1991;146:1461.

Comprehensive account of pathophysiology and management of autonomic dysreflexia.

CHAPTER 5

Benign Prostatic Hyperplasia

Grannum R. Sant
John P. Long

Benign prostatic hyperplasia (BPH) represents the most common neoplastic condition in men. BPH is the source of most urinary complaints in men over 50 years of age, and it is probably the most common abnormality seen in the typical urologic practice. After the age of 30, the incidence of BPH rises dramatically, and all men eventually develop this condition if they live long enough. The time-honored treatment for BPH is surgical, and up to 20 to 30% of men with symptomatic BPH require prostatectomy to relieve their symptoms. In the United Kingdom, 35,000 to 40,000 transurethral prostatectomies (TURPs) are performed annually. In the United States, BPH is second only to cataracts among conditions requiring surgery, and this translates into nearly 400,000 prostatectomies annually at an estimated cost of nearly 4 billion dollars. The economic and health service implications of BPH are significant, especially with the increasingly aged population in both developed and developing countries.

In recent years, significant effort has been directed toward the introduction of nonsurgical approaches to the treatment of bladder outlet obstruction secondary to BPH. The widespread prevalence of BPH, the socioeconomic impact of its treatment, the low but definite mortality/morbidity of prostatectomy, and a better understanding of the etiology and pathogenesis of BPH have fueled these developments. This chapter summarizes current information pertaining to the pathophysiology, pathogenesis, and new treatment modalities of BPH.

ANATOMY AND EMBRYOLOGY OF THE PROSTATE

During the third month of fetal gestation, endodermal buds proliferate and penetrate into the condensed mesenchymal mass of the urogenital sinus to form the prostate gland, with its characteristic epithelial and stromal components. The prostatic mesenchyme, the primary target of androgenic stimulation by dihydrotestosterone (produced from testosterone), induces proliferation of the endodermal glands and ducts, and the prostate is well differentiated by the 16th week of gestation.

The main blood supply of the prostate is the prostatovesicular artery, a branch of the inferior vesical artery. Terminal urethral branches penetrate the bladder neck at the 5 and 7 o'clock positions, and capsular branches course along the posterolateral margins of the prostate gland. The prostatic veins join the deep dorsal vein of the penis to form Santorini's plexus in the puboprostatic space. The prostate is enveloped by Denonvillier's fascia posteriorly, the endopelvic fascia with its condensed puboprostatic ligaments superiorly, and the pelvic fascia laterally. The nerves to the corpora cavernosa arise from the autonomic pelvic plexus and traverse the lateral pelvic fascia posterolaterally before entering the corpora. The primary lymphatic drainage of the prostate is the obturator nodes in the pelvis.

The prostate is composed of smooth muscle, epithelial glands, and fibrous and connective tissue. It is enveloped by a capsule (true capsule) of condensed tissue and divided into lobules by fibrous sheaths. The lobules drain into tubules and ducts, which drain into the urethra at the level of the verumontanum. The anterior fibromuscular component of the gland blends with the smooth muscle fibers of the bladder, and the distal prostate urethral segment is surrounded by the external striated sphincter. Destruction of the smooth muscle ring (internal sphincter) surrounding the proximal prostatic urethra is the cause of retrograde ejaculation following transurethral prostatic resection (TURP).

The urethra courses through the prostate and divides the gland into ventral (anterior) fibromuscular and dorsal (posterior) glandular segments. Midway between the base and apex of the prostate gland, the urethra angulates ventrally at about 35°.

PHYSIOLOGY OF THE PROSTATE

The primary functions of the prostate are support and promotion of male insemination and fertility and protection against bacterial infections of the lower urinary tract. The basal output of prostatic fluid is 20 to 80 μl per hour. During ejaculation, there is more than a 2000-fold increase in volume and production of 3.0 to 3.5 ml of semen, consisting of spermatozoa, seminal vesicle fluid, prostatic fluid, and secretions from Cowper's gland and glands lining the urethra.

Spermatozoa comprise less than 1% of the ejaculate. The initial segment of the ejaculate is rich in sperm and prostatic secretions, whereas the later fraction contains a high proportion of fructose, which is produced by the seminal vesicles. Prostatic secretion is mediated by cholinergic innervation from the pelvic and hypogastric nerves, whereas contraction is mediated by the alpha-adrenergic nerves. Prostatic fluid, 15 to 30% of the ejaculate, contains products synthesized, stored, and secreted by prostatic acinar cells as well as substances transported from the serum.

Within about 5 minutes of ejaculation, semen coagulates into a semisolid gel, which then liquifies spontaneously after 10 to 20 minutes. Coagulation is a function of seminal vesicle proteins, and liquefaction is due to plasminogen activators and a seminal neutral protease (seminin) present in prostatic fluid. Citrate, a major component of prostatic fluid, with concentration 500 to 1000 times greater than that of plasma, maintains the osmotic equilibrium of seminal fluid and is a good transport medium for spermatozoa. Prostatic secretion is rich in polyamines (mainly spermine), cholesterol, lactate dehydrogenase, and lipids. The primary polyamines are putrescine, spermidine, and spermine-(cationic molecules synthesized from ornithine). Aldehydes released from the enzymatic breakdown of spermine give semen its characteristic odor. The polyamines regulate seminal clot formation, and they may have antibacterial properties. The functions of the various secretory products of the prostate are summarized in Table 5.1.

Zinc is a major cationic component of prostatic fluid, and prostatic zinc concentrations are the highest in the human body. Zinc, actively transported into the prostatic ducts from the serum, has definite antibac-

Table 5.1: Physiology of the Normal Prostate

- Normal ejaculate volume 3.0 to 3.5 ml
  - Seminal vesicles 50%
  - Prostate 15 to 30%
  - Cowper's, urethral glands 5%
- Main functions of prostatic fluid
  - Sperm support
  - Reproduction
  - Antibacterial
- Major prostatic secretory products
  - Zinc (antibacterial factor)
  - Citrate (sperm transport)
  - Spermine (odor; cell proliferation)
  - Lipids (sperm production)
  - Seminin (semen liquefaction)
  - Prostate specific antigen

terial properties (prostatic antibacterial factor PAF) in men. Seminal fluid has bactericidal activity against common gram-positive and gram-negative uropathogens. Prostatic fluid in elderly men and men with chronic bacterial prostatitis (CBP) has reduced antibacterial activity and reduced zinc levels.

The predominant proteins secreted by the prostate gland are prostatic acid phosphatase (PAP, prostatic specific antigen (PSA), and prostatic specific protein (beta-inhibin). PSA is a serine protease with both chymotrypsin and trypsin-like activities and it plays a role in lysis of the ejaculate clot.

HISTOLOGY AND ANATOMY OF BENIGN PROSTATIC HYPERPLASIA

The definitive research of McNeal on the anatomic and histologic origins of BPH has contributed to our current understanding of prostatic histogenesis and the development of BPH. The internal architecture of the adult prostate is characterized by four morphologically distinct lobes (Table 5.2). The largest, or peripheral zone (PZ), consists of 70% of the mass of the glandular prostate. Ducts draining the PZ arise and extend

Table 5.2: Histologic Characteristics of BPH

BPH growth phases
Microscopic
Macroscopic
"Clinical" (prostatism)
Microscopic BPH
Stromal nodules in periurethral tissue
Epithelial hyperplastic nodules in transition zone
BPH cell growth doubling times
4 to 5 years: 30 to 50 years
10 years: 50 to 70 years
100 years: > 70 years
Stromal versus epithelial elements
Stroma:epithelium ratio in normal prostate = 2:1
Stroma:epithelium ratio in BPH = 5:1
40% prostatic stroma = smooth muscle
Prostatic compartments
Central zone
Peripheral zone
Anterior fibromuscular stroma
Transition zone
Periurethral zone

from posterolateral recesses on either side of the urethral wall from the verumontanum distally to the external sphincter. The central zone (CZ) is the next largest and is cone-shaped, with the base forming most of the base of the prostate and the apex located at the verumontanum. Its ducts arise in a small area immediately surrounding the ejaculatory duct openings. The third largest zone, the anterior fibromuscular stroma, lacks glandular tissue and consists of a cap of connective tissue.

The transition zone (TZ) is the smallest lobe, consisting of only 2% of the total prostatic volume. The TZ ducts arise from discrete areas in the proximal prostatic urethra just distal to the caudal margin of the internal sphincter. Intimately associated with the TZ is the periurethral region, a tiny area of the prostate made up of minute ducts and acini scattered within the preprostatic sphincter and draining into the posterior aspect of the proximal urethra. The site of origin of BPH appears to be limited to the tissues—the transition and periurethral zones—located along the axis of the proximal urethra between the bladder neck smooth-muscle sphincter and the verumontanum.

The prostatic autonomic nervous system has been investigated by characterization of neuroreceptor binding sites, tissue assays of neurotransmitters and neuropeptides, and evaluation of the response of prostate smooth muscle to pharmacologic agents. The prostate gland—normal and BPH—has been evaluated by quantitative morphology, point-counting stereology, immunohistochemistry, and color-assisted computerized analysis. Recent studies indicate that BPH is primarily a stromal process associated with significant smooth muscle hyperplasia (Table 5.2). The overall ration of stroma to epithelium in BPH is approximately 4:1 to 5:1, with the smooth muscle proportion of the hyperplastic stroma being approximately 40%. By comparison, the ratio of stroma to epithelium in normal prostates is only about 2:1.

The dynamic (see below) component of bladder outlet obstruction due to BPH is related to the tone and tension of prostatic smooth muscle in the stroma and the "surgical" capsule. Muscarinic cholinergic (MCh), alpha$_1$-adrenergic, and alpha$_2$-adrenergic receptors have been identified in the human prostate. MCh receptors, the most abundant, are localized predominantly to the epithelium. Their absence from prostatic smooth muscle suggests that they have an insignificant role in the pathogenesis of BPH. Alpha$_1$-adrenoreceptors are localized to the stromal elements. The roles of alpha$_2$-adrenergic and dihydropyridine (calcium-linked flux mechanisms) receptors are not clearly defined. The alpha$_1$-amino acid peptide, endothelin 1, a potent mediator of smooth muscle contraction, has been immunoenzymatically identified in prostatic epithelium, but its role in the pathogenesis of BPH is currently unclear.

PATHOGENESIS OF BPH

BPH is a hyperplastic process characterized by increased numbers of prostatic cells and increased DNA synthesis. Although the mechanisms underlining the pathogenesis of BPH have yet to be established, extensive histologic analysis provides a clearer picture of BPH development. BPH is best conceptualized as progressing through two phases: pathologic and clinical (Table 5.2). The TZ nodules develop earlier and are larger, with branching of small ducts from existing ducts and the development of a new ductal/glandular system reminiscent of embryonic development. This suggests that the origin of BPH may be due to a reawakening during adulthood of the embryonic inductive potential of the prostatic stroma.

Pathologic BPH is divided into two stages: microscopic and macroscopic (Figure 5.1). The earliest microscopic nodules of BPH, which develop between 30 and 50 years of age in tiny glands located along the periurethral zone, consist of new foci of glandular hyperplasia that arise from preexisting periurethral ducts. The expansion of these microscopic nodules is limited by the surrounding internal sphincter, but some ducts escape outside the distal margins at the verumontanum to extend into the transition zone. Other ductal structures may proliferate toward the bladder

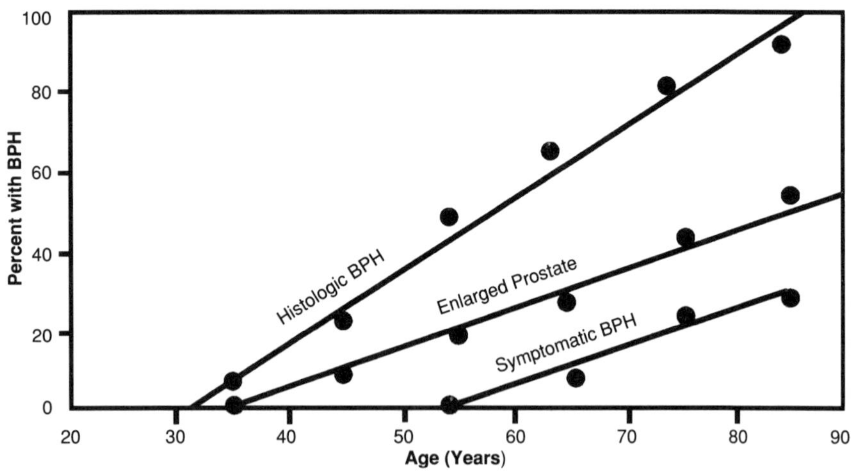

Figure 5.1: Relationship between histologic, clinically detectable, and clinically symptomatic BPH

lumen in the posterior aspect of the proximal urethra, and their enlargement causes the classical median lobe of clinical BPH. Most of the periurethral micronodules are stromal, while the early nodules forming in the transition zone are primarily glandular. It is believed that periurethral foci of BPH maintain their stromal composition during proliferation, whereas TZ foci of BPH acquire a mixed glandular and stromal configuration.

Coincident with and following the establishment of microscopic disease in the TZ, the TZ itself undergoes a diffuse enlargement with maintenance of the internal lobar architecture. Curiously, this enlargement is not felt to be secondary to the proliferation of the microscopic nodules. Although the TZ nearly doubles in size between the ages of 50 and 70, BPH tissue accounts for only approximately 15% of this increased mass. The reasons for this are unknown.

ETIOLOGY OF BPH

The causes of BPH are imprecisely defined, and multiple factors influence the growth characteristics of the prostate gland. However, aging and the presence of androgens, especially dihydrotestosterone, are essential factors for the development of BPH.

Dihydrotestosterone Hypothesis

A widely recognized feature of BPH is its dependence on functioning testes. Castration or hypopituitarism occurring in men prior to age 30 prevents the development of histologic BPH. Moreover, castration (used as a therapy for BPH in the nineteenth century) in adults produces prostatic involution and a reduction in gland volume of 50 to 75%. It is obvious, therefore, that androgens have at least a permissive role in the development of BPH (Table 5.3).

The hypothalamic–pituitary–testes–prostate axis creates the appropriate hormonal milieu for androgen production (Figure 5.2). Pulsatile hypothalamic release of the decapeptide, luteinizing hormone releasing hormone (LH-RH), stimulates pituitary release of luteinizing hormone (LH), which reaches the testes via the peripheral circulation and binds to surface receptors on Leydig cells to stimulate testosterone (T) biosynthesis. Within prostatic epithelial cells, dihydrotestosterone (DHT) is formed from testosterone by the action of a nicotinamide-adenine dinucleotide phosphate (NADP) dependent enzyme, 5-alpha-reductase. DHT then binds to specific prostatic epithelial cell androgen nuclear receptors to produce DNA synthesis and cell growth and proliferation (Table 5.4).

Evidence that BPH may be caused by DHT comes from patients with a genetically linked male pseudohermaphroditism syndrome due to

Table 5.3: Hormonal Influences on BPH

Androgen Dependence
Castration causes prostatic shrinkage
BPH does not develop in men castrated before puberty
BPH does not develop in men with 5-alpha-reductase deficiency
Androgen receptors and prostatic dihydrotestosterone levels are high in BPH
Estrogen Dependence
Increased ratio free estradiol: free testosterone
Estrogens produced by aromatization circulating androgens (androstenedione, testosterone)
Estrogens promote stromal hyperplasia
Estrogens increase androgen receptor levels in prostatic epithelial cell nuclei
Estrogen receptors present in stromal cell nuclei
Increased liver synthesis of sex hormone binding globulin

5-alpha-reductase deficiency (Table 5.5). Affected individuals have 46XY karyotypes. Females are normal, but boys with this autosomal recessive genetic disorder are unable to metabolize T to DHT. At birth, they have ambiguous genitalia, a small penis, hypospadias, small atrophic prostates, and cryptorchidism. At puberty, serum levels of T rise with resultant testicular descent and normal penile and scrotal development. However, the prostates remain small, male pattern baldness does not develop, and beard growth is negligible. These observations suggest that certain androgen-sensitive tissues (e.g., testes) respond to T whereas others (e.g., prostate) require DHT for growth and differentiation.

The major circulating plasma androgen is testosterone, more than 90 to 95% of which is derived from the testicles. The remaining 5% comes from direct synthesis of other C_{19} steroids (e.g., androstenedione, dehydroepiandrosterone) by the adrenals, or peripheral conversion, by aromatization, of these steroids to testosterone. Over 98% of circulating plasma testosterone is protein-bound to albumin and sex hormone binding globulin (SHBG). "Free" testosterone enters prostatic cells by diffusion and leads to cellular growth, proliferation, and differentiation.

Two isoenzymes (type 1, type 2) of 5-alpha-reductase have been identified on the basis of biochemical, pharmacologic, and genetic criteria. The type 2 isoenzyme is active at acidic pH, expressed in high levels in the prostate, sensitive to finasteride (Proscar), and is encoded on chromosome 2. A cytosine mutation in exon 5 of the 5-alpha-reductase gene of chromosome 2 has recently been reported in male pseudohermaphro-

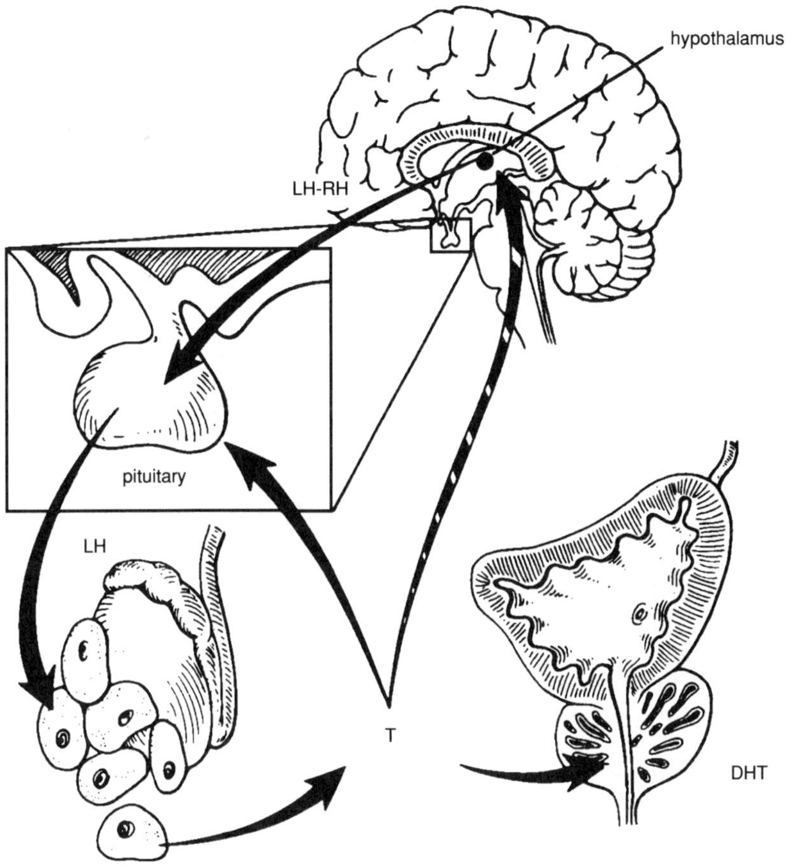

Figure 5.2: The hypothalamus–pituitary–testes–prostate hormonal axis. T, testosterone; LH, luteinizing hormone; LH-RH, luteinizing hormone-releasing hormone; DHT, dihydrotestosterone.

dites. The type 1 isoenzyme is insensitive to finasteride, is found at low levels in the prostate, and is encoded on chromosome 5.

DHT represents over 90% of nuclear-bound steroids in prostatic epithelial cells and has an androgen-receptor affinity that is 4 to 5 times greater than that of testosterone. DHT levels are significantly higher in the prostate than in other organs, and these levels are maintained with advancing age in spite of declining serum testosterone levels (Table 5.4). Initial studies found higher levels of DHT in BPH tissue than in age-matched normal prostates. However, this difference is artifactual, result-

Table 5.4: Theories of the Etiology of BPH

- Appropriate milieu
  - Aging
  - Androgens
- T–DHT hypothesis
  - 5-alpha-reductase enzyme
  - Androgen receptors in prostatic cells
  - Rise in intraprostatic DHT levels
  - Rise in cellular DNA synthesis, proliferation
- Estrogen hypothesis
  - Rise in estrogen levels with age
  - Fall in free testosterone levels
  - Rise in serum sex hormone binding globulin
- Epithelial–stromal interaction (Cunha)
  - Prostatic mesenchyme induces glandular epithelial hyperplasia
  - Reawakening of embryonic prostatic organogenesis in presence of androgens
  - Paracrine prostatic growth factors produced by stromal cells lead to promotion of epithelial hyperplasia
- Cell death
  - Cell replication balance
  - Rise in growth factors
  - Rise in oncogenes
  - Fall in suppressor genes
  - Rise in transforming growth factor beta
  - Inhibited by estrogens which lengthen life span of prostatic cells
- Stem cell therapy
  - Rise in production of differentiated prostatic cells (amplifying, transit cells)

ing from the comparison of DHT levels in fresh BPH tissue with those in normal, but frozen, prostate tissue harvested from cadavers. Normal prostate tissue has levels of DHT identical to those of fresh, age-matched BPH tissue. Moreover, 5-alpha-reductase enzymatic activity in BPH tissue is similar to that in age-matched normal prostatic tissue.

Estrogen Hypothesis

In men, 70 to 90% of circulating plasma estrogens are derived from the peripheral conversion of androstenedione and testosterone to estrone and estradiol via the aromatase reaction (Figure 5.3). The C_{19} androgenic steroids are converted to C_{18} estrogenic compounds by removal of the 19-methyl moiety and formation of an aromatic (or phenolic) steroid A ring. The increasing prevalence with age coincides with the shift in the ratio of androgen to estrogen in favor of estrogens. With aging, although the hypo-

Table 5.5: 5-Alpha-Reductase Deficiency

XY chromosomal karyotype
Autosomal recessive inheritance pattern
Ambiguous genitalia
Severe hypospadias
Blind-ending vaginal pouch
Normal pubertal masculinization
Absence of frontal (male-pattern) baldness
Normal libido, sexual identity, sperm production
Nonpalpable prostate—no development of BPH
Two isoenzymes (I, II)

thalamic–pituitary stimulus is unchanged, Leydig cell responsiveness to luteinizing hormone (LH) is reduced. This leads to reduced plasma testosterone levels, further magnified by increased levels of serum testosterone-estrogen–binding globulin (TeBG) produced by the liver. Free estradiol levels remain relatively unchanged, thereby producing an increase in the overall ratio (up to 40%) of serum free estradiol to free testosterone (Table 5.3).

Experimental evidence indicates that estrogens may have an important role in the genesis of BPH (Tables 5.3 and 5.4). Canine BPH differs from human BPH in many respects: It is predominantly epithelial rather than stromal, is not divided into zones, and is uniform rather than nodular. An estrogen receptor has been identified in the prostate, and estrogens are preferentially accumulated in the stroma of human hyperplastic prostate tissue. Prostatic stromal hyperplasia can be induced in dog and monkey prostates by the administration of aromatizable androgens, and the hyperplasia can be reversed by aromatase inhibitors such as atamestane. In dogs, estrogen induces prostatic stromal growth and collagen production and increases the expression of androgen receptors. This suggests that estrogens may exert their action via the androgen rather than estrogen receptors. However, these findings have not been clearly demonstrated in men, and the evidence for the role of estrogens in BPH development remains circumstantial. The shift in the ratio of serum estrogen to androgen occurs well after the usual age of onset of microscopic BPH disease. More studies into the role of estrogens in the genesis of BPH are needed.

Stromal/Epithelial Interactions (Embryonic Reawakening)

Prostatic stromal elements may play a role in the regulation of prostatic epithelial cell growth. Autopsy studies indicate that the initial lesions in BPH consist of tiny periurethral gland budding. These new glands exhibit a budding pattern that is nearly identical to that seen during the

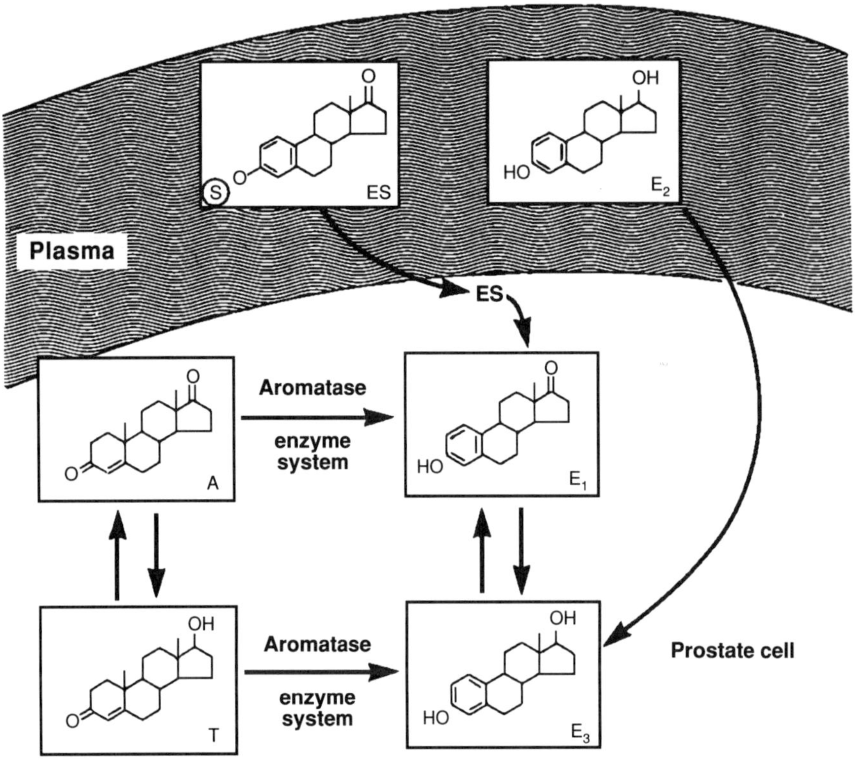

Figure 5.3: Aspects of estrogen synthesis and metabolism by prostate cells. A, androstenedione; E_1, estrone; E_2, estradiol-17β; ES, estrone sulfate; T, testosterone. *Reproduced with permission from Blandy J. Lecture Notes on Urology, 4th ed. Oxford: Blackwell Scientific Publications, 1991:46.*

embryonic development of ducts and acinar systems. Since new duct and acinar systems should not be developing in the adult prostate, these histologic findings have led to the hypothesis that BPH arises as a result of an "embryonic reawakening" of stromal factors responsible for the induction of prostatic epithelial growth (Table 5.4).

Cunha has demonstrated that prostatic epithelial development is dependent on androgen-sensitive, stromal mediators. Murine urogenital sinus mesenchymal cells, when coincubated with intact male murine bladder cells, will induce these cells to proliferate, bud, and acquire a distinctly prostatic appearance. This inductive process is androgen-dependent. Furthermore, media extracts derived from human bone marrow or prostatic fibroblasts can induce in cultured human prostatic carcinoma cells a proliferative response 3 to 10 times more potent than other known mitogens. Thus, it appears that intact stromal elements usually serve to keep normal epithelial cells differentiated, whereas in the embryonic, or perhaps neoplastic, state, these elements are turned off or inactivated and result in epithelial cell dedifferentiation.

Growth factors, peptide molecules that affect cell division and differentiation, have been identified in normal and hyperplastic prostatic tissue. Intensive investigations of these growth factors, such as basic fibroblast growth factor (BFGF), tumor growth factor beta (TGF-β), tumor growth factor alpha (TGF-α) and others, are underway (Table 5.6). Epidermal growth factor (EGF) and basic fibroblast growth factor (B-FGF), both expressed in BPH tissue, have mitogenic effects on the prostatic epithelium. Another growth factor, transforming growth factor beta (T_RGF-β), inhibits cellular mitotic activity, and reduced levels/expression may be a factor in the genesis of prostatic hyperplasia. Growth factors may act on the cells in which they are produced (autocrine) or nearby cells (paracrine). Both stromal and epithelial cells are capable of producing growth factors that bind to specific membrane receptors and release activated kinases with resultant calcium release, protein phosphorylation, and DNA production. Inhibitory growth factors, for example, TGF-β work in reverse and result in cell death.

Stem Cell Theory

An equilibrium or steady state exists between proliferating and dying cells in living organs. Prostatic growth is the result of such a balance between cell replication and cell death. This balance is dependent on hormonal factors (testosterone, dihydrotestosterone, estrogens), growth factors (mitogens, inhibitors), aging, suppressor genes, and oncogenes, for example, c-fos oncogene (Table 5.4). Estrogens, in the presence of

Table 5.6: Major Putative Prostatic Growth Factors

Fibroblast growth factor beta (FGF β)
Rise in BPH, stromal tissue
Epidermal growth factor (EGF) (prostatropin)
Rise in prostate cancer
Transforming growth factor alpha (T_RGF α)
Low levels in BPH
30% homology with EGF
Transforming growth factor beta (T_RGF β)
Rise in BPH
Inhibits epithelial cell mitosis/proliferation

androgens, inhibit prostatic cell death in dogs; this leads to hyperplasia, which is associated with a significant (up to one-third) reduction in DNA synthesis. Thus, BPH may be the result of reduced cell death rather than increased proliferation.

The control over this steady state may reside in the number of prostate stem cells—cells capable of unlimited self-renewal. Stem cells give rise to daughter cells, which acquire increasingly differentiated phenotypes with succeeding generations. A spectrum probably exists in the prostate between stem cells (i.e., more undifferentiated with high proliferative potential) and daughter cells, which are generally more differentiated but have less proliferative potential. Issacs and Coffey have suggested the existence of three prostatic cell types: stem cells, amplifying cells, and transit cells, each with progressively diminished proliferative capacity. BPH may be the result of an imbalance in the normal number of proliferative cells among the total cell population of the prostate.

Experimental studies in dogs suggest that at least 50% of the stem cells of the prostate develop before adulthood. Furthermore, high doses of exogenous androgens administered to normal male pups during the adolescent period are capable of inducing increased numbers of stem cells. These data support the contention that the maximal complement of prostatic stem cells is reached by adulthood and that these stem cells serve as the basis for repopulating the entire gland under the influence of androgens later in life.

Although stem cells may be increased in human BPH tissue compared to normal prostate tissue, the etiology for such cellular imbalance is unknown. Stem cells in normal prostate tissue or BPH have not been isolated or identified. However, there is indirect support for this hypothesis in that the rate of regrowth of BPH tissue in humans following pharmacologic castration and then resumption of normal androgen levels is three times faster than normal.

EPIDEMIOLOGY AND NATURAL HISTORY OF BENIGN PROSTATIC HYPERPLASIA

The prostate undergoes little change in size between birth and puberty. Thereafter, a rapid growth spurt ensues. From age 12 to 30, the prostate mass increases about 1.6 g/yr to reach the average adult weight of 20 ± 6 g. Autopsy studies have provided information on the age-specific prevalence of microscopic BPH (Table 5.7). Microscopic BPH has a 10% prevalence in the fourth decade, and the prevalence increases steadily with age. By the sixth decade, 50% of men have microscopic BPH, and over 90% of men in the 80s have histologic BPH. Studies in Scandin-

Table 5.7: Natural History of BPH

"Rule of 50s"
- 50% of men develop histologic BPH by age 60
- 50% of men with histologic BPH develop macroscopic BPH
- 50% of men with macroscopic BPH develop "symptomatic" BPH

50-year-old man has a 25 to 30% lifetime chance of requiring a prostatectomy for BPH

BPH progression is variable
- Time lag of 5 years between histologic and macroscopic BPH

Watchful waiting in BPH
- Symptom stabilization/improvement, 50 to 60%
- Urinary retention, 1 to 2% per year
- Azotemia, obstructive uropathy, 1 to 2%
- Urinary-tract infection, risk unknown

avian, European, and Far Eastern countries confirm that BPH occurs early in life and that most men develop histologic evidence of BPH if they are blessed by longevity.

The increasing age-prevalence of BPH is generally associated with increased tissue mass. However, not all patients with histologic BPH have palpably enlarged glands. The age-specific prevalence of macroscopic BPH (palpably enlarged gland by digital rectal examination) increases with age, but at a lower rate than microscopic or histologic BPH. In fact, only 50% of glands with microscopic BPH progress to macroscopic BPH, and there is a lag time of approximately 5 years (Table 5.7). The mean weight of prostates without microscopic BPH is 20 ± 6 g and of those with BPH is 33 ± 16 g.

Macroscopic BPH results from a marked increase in size of microscopic BPH nodules. Growth occurs mainly in the inner areas of the gland. The surrounding tissue that becomes compressed and stretched over the growing adenoma is the "prostatic capsule," a pseudocapsule rather than a true, anatomic capsule. Estimates of prostatic size by digital rectal exam (DRE) and transrectal ultrasound (TRUS) indicate that macroscopic disease develops in the sixth decade. Interestingly, this growth spurt appears to be rapid and lasts only 5 to 7 years before slowing down and reaching a plateau. After this, macroscopic disease may continue to grow, but at a much slower rate compared to that seen during the transition from microscopic to macroscopic disease. The cell-population doubling time for BPH has been estimated to be 4.5 years between ages 31 and 50, 10 years at age 50, and over 100 years at age 70.

Using prostatectomy rates as a proxy for the incidence of clinical or symptomatic BPH, it appears that 50% of men with enlarged prostates develop prostatism. Since only 50% of men with microscopic BPH develop macroscopic disease, it follows that only 25% of men with histologic BPH ultimately require surgical intervention, for example, prostatectomy (Table 5.7). This estimate is in agreement with information from such epidemiologic studies as the Longitudinal Normative Aging Study. However, prostatectomy rates are unreliable guides to the incidence of clinical BPH. Prostatectomy rates in the United States vary up to threefold in geographically defined areas. Patients have varying thresholds for seeking medical attention for their voiding symptoms, as do their primary care physicians for urologic referral and consultation. Furthermore, the urologic indications for and the timing of prostatectomy vary significantly.

The natural history of BPH is poorly understood. Available data are sparse and somewhat anecdotal. Several observational studies of untreated BPH exist, but they vary regarding the definition of BPH, duration of follow-up, response criteria, and other parameters. However, they suggest that if men with "prostatism" are followed for 1.5 to 3 years, a significant number (up to 50%) experience stabilization or improvement of symptoms in the absence of medical intervention (Table 5.7). Not all foci of microscopic BPH progress to macroscopic disease; neither does every man with macroscopic disease develop prostatism. The exact mechanisms by which pathologic BPH progresses to symptomatic BPH require further study, and this is being addressed on numerous fronts: molecular biological, epidemiological, clinical, outcomes, and quality-of-life.

Untreated prostatism may lead to significant complications, for example, urinary-tract infection, retention, renal failure secondary to ureteral obstruction, and bladder decompensation. However, the true incidence of these complications in men with untreated BPH is unknown. A Veterans Administration prospective, randomized clinical trial comparing prostatectomy to "watchful waiting" documented a low incidence of these complications. Consistently predicting whether an individual BPH patient will progress to clinical BPH, develop complications, or remain stable is impossible. This dilemma clearly impacts on treatment planning. A primary goal of current clinical and scientific studies of BPH is the recognition and differentiation of patients prone to develop complications versus those who stabilize or improve without treatment. Predictors of failure are the presence of moderate to severe trabeculation and large postvoid residuals (over 100 to 150 ml) (Table 5.7).

CLINICAL MANIFESTATIONS

Prostate size does not predict the type or severity of symptoms of BPH: Some men with large glands have minimal symptoms, whereas others with small "fibrotic" glands can be very symptomatic. Clear distinctions exist between the histologic development of BPH, the physiologic effects of prostatic enlargement and obstruction, and symptomatic BPH. This paradox is due, in part, to the underlying mechanisms of urinary obstruction. Symptoms are due to urethral obstruction as well as to alterations in bladder function.

Urinary obstruction in BPH has both dynamic and static (or mechanical) components (Table 5.8). Dynamic obstruction is due to prostatic smooth muscle tone, whereas static obstruction is caused by the mechanical (bulk) effect of the prostatic adenoma that narrows the urethral lumen. The prostatic surgical capsule, composed of muscular and fibrous elements, is a useful surgical landmark during transurethral prostatectomy and serves as the enucleation plane during open (retropubic or transvesical) prostatectomy. An elastic, expansile capsule allows prostatic expansion with minimal urethral compression, whereas increased capsular tension, possibly adrenergically mediated, retards expansion and leads to compression of the posterior urethra. The smooth muscle cells in the bladder neck, prostatic adenoma, and prostatic surgical capsule are richly innervated by alpha$_1$-adrenoreceptors, which mediate a marked contractile response. "Prostatism" in men with small prostates is likely secondary to dynamic obstruction, since these glands frequently have a histologic predominance of smooth muscle and stromal elements. Static obstruction is more common in patients with palpably enlarged prostates or median lobe hyperplasia, which causes a ball-valve obstruction at the bladder neck.

The symptoms of BPH are classified as obstructive or irritative. Irritative symptoms such as nocturia, frequency, urgency, and dysuria are urodynamically characterized by uninhibited bladder contractions, re-

Table 5.8: Pathophysiologic Correlates of Symptomatic BPH

- Symptoms secondary to
  - Dynamic obstruction 2° increased muscle tone in prostate
  - Mechanical obstruction 2° glandular volume, bulk
- Symptoms variable, depend on
  - Size of prostate
  - Muscle tone in prostate capsule, stroma
  - Detrusor muscle function
  - Prostatic infarcts
  - Miscellaneous factors
    - Prostatitis
    - Concomitant medications
- Obstructive versus irritative voiding symptoms

duced bladder capacities, and loss of bladder compliance. In animals, these urodynamic alterations parallel changes in the viscoelastic properties and increased collagen levels in the bladder detrusor (Table 5.9) Detrusor instability in BPH is caused by two factors, the aging process itself and infravesical obstruction, which is associated with increased collagen deposition and reduced detrusor contractility. Instability, present in more than 50% of symptomatic patients, resolves in about 75% of men within 12 months of prostatectomy. No reliable preoperative test is capable of predicting postoperative resolution of detrusor instability. Detrusor instability may be due to postjunctional supersensitivity consequent upon partial denervation. Renervation of postganglionic parasympathetic axons is slow, and this explains the sometimes long period (up to 1 year) of persistent frequency and urgency following prostatectomy. Prolonged, unrelieved obstruction can cause irreversible damage to the bladder innervation and smooth muscle. Molecular biologic techniques have demonstrated changes in contractile proteins and cytoskeletal proteins in the obstructed bladder. Neurotrophic factors (e.g., nerve growth factors) are increased in obstruction and may cause alterations in detrusor function.

Symptoms of prostatism may be unrelated to outflow obstruction (either tone or bulk) but secondary to alterations in the contractile properties of the bladder smooth muscle. Experimentally, the earliest response to obstruction is smooth muscle hypertrophy with an increase in muscle mass. As trabeculations develop, detrusor collagen and extracellu-

Table 5.9: Detrusor Muscle Response to Outlet Obstruction

Increased collagen deposition
Increased muscle mass
Changes in cytoskeletal contractile proteins
Detrusor activity
- Compensated
- Decompensated
- Instability

Detrusor instability
- 60 to 70% of men with BPH
- Secondary to obstruction and aging
- Causes
  - Parasympathetic denervation hypersensitivity
  - Earlier stretching tension receptors
  - Direct sensory input from adenoma
  - Change of bladder innervation from predominantly beta to alpha$_1$-adrenergics

lar matrix deposition increased the number of acetyl-cholinesterase containing (parasympathetic) nerves decreases.

Obstructive symptoms include hesitancy, difficulty in initiating voiding, intermittency (interruption of urinary flow), terminal dribbling, poor urinary stream, and a feeling of incomplete bladder emptying. Unrelieved obstruction can lead to bladder decompensation, urinary retention, high postvoid residual volumes, and upper tract (ureters and kidney) dilatation. Residual volumes do not correlate with symptom severity or urodynamic findings in BPH, and they are widely variable even in individual patients. Indeed, some men with marked BPH have little or no postvoid residuals.

Acute retention is the indication for prostatectomy in about 20% of patients who undergo surgery for BPH. Some men develop acute urinary retention while taking alpha-adrenergic drugs (such as cough medicines and nasal decongestants), which increase prostatic smooth muscle tone to the point where it combines with baseline BPH to cause retention. Factors such as alcohol, cold temperatures, and immobility may precipitate retention in men with partial degrees of prostatic obstruction.

A number of conditions contribute to the symptoms of BPH (Table 5.8). The enlarging hyperplastic prostate may outgrow its blood supply, and this leads to prostatic infarcts. Serum prostate specific antigen (PSA) levels are frequently elevated in men with acute urinary retention because of prostatic infarction. Up to 85% of BPH patients presenting with acute urinary retention have prostatic infarcts, compared to only 3% of men having prostatectomy for other indications. In addition to infarcts, other conditions commonly found in BPH specimens include prostatic calculi, foci of acute and chronic inflammation, and granulomatous nodules. These conditions may (acutely or gradually) push some patients over the edge from baseline asymptomatic BPH to symptomatic obstruction. Some men with chronic retention (postvoid residuals of greater than 300 ml) develop overflow incontinence. Occasionally, silent dilatation of the upper tracts (hydroureter, hydronephrosis) or increased levels of serum creatinine (azotemia) and renal insufficiency result. Unattended, this process may progress to renal failure. This dreaded complication of BPH is rare, occurring in less than 1% of patients undergoing prostatectomy. The azotemia associated with chronic retention can develop insidiously and is a cause of postobstructive diuresis when treatment is instituted with catheter drainage.

The risks of urinary-tract infection (UTI) and urosepsis in BPH have not been adequately studied in either longitudinal cohort or treatment outcome studies. Urinary stasis associated with increased PVRs may increase the risk of UTIs, but the magnitude of this risk is unknown. However, clinical experience suggests that the risk of serious UTIs is probably very low.

The symptoms of BPH are subjective and highly variable, and they can vary capriciously over time. A perplexing issue in BPH is the complex relationship between prostate size, symptom type, and severity. No correlation has been found between symptom severity and palpable enlargement of the prostate; factors other than size contribute to infravesical prostatic obstruction. In an effort to standardize and quantitate the symptoms of BPH, a number of symptom scoring systems have been developed, for example, the Boyarsky, the Maine Medical Assessment Program, and the Madsen-Iverson. The recent explosion of interest in the nonsurgical treatment of BPH and watchful waiting protocols has highlighted the paucity of data on the natural history of untreated BPH and the clinical outcomes following prostatectomy. The American Urological Association (AUA) has recently adopted a BPH symptom index, which can reliably predict symptom variation that correlates with treatment outcomes. This index improves on previous scoring systems because it is self-administered and includes questions concerning the effects of symptoms on quality of life. The major utility of these scoring systems will be the study of treatment outcomes and the natural history of untreated BPH.

Most men undergo prostatectomy to alleviate their urinary symptoms and improve the quality of their lives. Very few require surgery for objective indications such as intractable UTIs, obstructive uropathy, renal failure, or urinary retention.

TREATMENT OF BPH

Transurethral prostatectomy (TURP) is the most widely performed surgical treatment for clinically significant BPH. Surgical mortality and morbidity are low, and most patients report significant postoperative improvement of symptoms. The effectiveness of prostatectomy has only recently been questioned and objectively assessed. Its morbidity, mortality, efficacy, and dollar costs are now receiving increasing attention. Mortality is low (about 0.2%), but morbidity is not insignificant. Common complications include urinary infection, epididymitis, impotence, incontinence, and the need for transfusions. Furthermore, outcome studies reveal that about 20% of patients fail to achieve improvement in their voiding symptoms following prostatectomy and 15% of patients require reoperation for stricture, bladder neck contracture, recurrent "prostatism" or other problems within 8 years of surgery. These factors have fueled the search for less invasive and nonsurgical treatments (Table 5.10). Since most men (more than 90%) with prostatism have mild, non–life-threatening symptoms, they are becoming increasingly interested in nonsurgical forms of therapy.

Table 5.10: BPH Treatment: Alternatives to TURP

Watchful waiting
Surgical
  Prostatic urethral stents
  Hyperthermia
  Thermotherapy
  Lasers
  Cryosurgery
  Focused external heat (pyrotherapy), shock waves, ultrasound
  Balloon dilatation
Pharmacologic
  Hormonal
    Antiandrogens
    Androgen ablation
    Aromatase inhibitors
  Alpha-adrenergic blockers
  Cholesterol-lowering drugs
    Macrolide antifungal drugs (e.g., Candicidin)
    Metabolic inhibitors (e.g., Clofibrate)
  Phytotherapy
    Plant extracts
  ? Growth inhibitors

The surgical alternatives to TURP focus on less invasive or minimally invasive procedures. With the exception of the transurethral incision of the prostate (TUIP) and prostatic stents, these new techniques involve potentially expensive technologies such as hyperthermia, thermotherapy, lasers, balloon dilatation, and cryosurgery, which are targeted toward prostatic tissue destruction and posterior urethral and bladder neck dilatation—effects similar to those of a TURP or TUIP. New insights into the pathogenesis of BPH have led to the introduction of noninterventional, pharmacologic therapies that cause tissue shrinkage and/or reduction of prostatic and bladder neck smooth muscle tone. The treatment goal is achieved by reduction of prostatic mass or improvement in the outlet diameter of the bladder neck and prostatic urethra.

NEW NONPHARMACOLOGIC TREATMENT

Balloon Dilatation

Balloon dilatation of the prostate is a relatively noninvasive treatment with a low complication rate. Dilatation to 25 to 35 mm (75 to 105 F diameter) for periods of 10 to 15 minutes at pressures of 3 to 4 atmospheres has been studied. The mechanisms of action of balloon dilatation are incompletely defined but include stretching of the prostatic capsule, attenuation of alpha$_1$-adrenergic receptors, compression of the prostate with enlargement of the prostatic urethral lumen, glandular ischemia, and splitting of the anterior prostatic commissure. The bladder neck is usually preserved along with normal antegrade ejaculation. The low morbidity of balloon dilatation plus the fact that it can be done with local anesthesia/sedation makes it attractive. However, long-term results are disappointing, and a recent study suggests that it is no better than cystoscopy alone. Contraindications to balloon dilatation include the presence of a median lobe, a prostate over 30 to 35 g, retention (acute, chronic), detrusor instability, or prostatitis. The current consensus is that balloon dilatation is not recommended for definitive treatment for BPH.

Prostatic Stents

Intraurethral endoprostatic stents (temporary and permanent) have been used as alternatives to TURP, especially in sick elderly men for whom surgery is unsuitable. Two groups of intraprostatic stents have been used clinically: intraurethral, nonepithelialized, hollow metal (stainless steel, gold-plated) spirals, and extraurethral, epithelialized, expandable, permanent stents made of such materials as titanium or stainless steel super alloy. Although the epithelialized stents have less risk of migration, infection, and encrustation, they cannot be removed after 2 months because of their tissue fixation and epithelialization. Intraprostatic stents do relieve obstruction, but their long-term efficacy and safety have not been adequately studied.

Hyperthermia/Thermotherapy

Heat is known to selectively destroy neoplastic cells. The internal architecture of normal cells and their ability to increase their blood supply in response to a hyperthermic stimulus makes them resistant to heat. Temperatures over 45° C damage both normal and neoplastic cells, whereas between 40 and 45° C only neoplastic cells are destroyed. The relative vascular deficiency of prostatic hyperplastic tissue suggests that BPH tissue may be thermosensitive. Two thermal techniques are used to treat BPH, hyperthermia and thermotherapy. With hyperthermia, temperatures of 42 to 45° C are achieved by the use of transrectal or transurethral probes. No significant tissue necrosis or gland shrinkage is seen, and serum PSA levels do not change. This suggests that prostatic epithelial cells are largely unaffected by these temperatures and explains the less-than-exciting efficacy of this form of treatment.

Transurethral heating of the prostate to temperatures between 45 and 50° C—thermotherapy—achieves tissue coagulation and necrosis with a resultant rise in serum PSA. Periurethral infarction leads to tissue sloughing and swelling, which may cause posttreatment urinary retention. The prostate gland shrinks following thermotherapy, and urinary flow rates are generally improved. Although hyperthermia and thermotherapy are safe and relatively cheap, and do not require hospitalization, their long-term effectiveness is still under scrutiny. These techniques may well have a place in the therapeutic armamentarium, especially for younger men with small glands and less than severe symptoms.

Lasers

Lasers have been used to perform transurethral prostatic incision (TUIP) or prostatectomy. Laser prostatectomy compares favorably with conventional electrocautery prostatectomy. The recent development of side-firing, or open-fiber, lasers has led to the introduction of laser-induced prostatectomy. Temperatures of between 70 and 100° C are produced in the prostate, and the laser energy is focused using real-time ultrasound sector scanning. The transurethral ultrasound-guided laser-induced prostatectomy (TULIP procedure) utilizes a neodymium: yttrium aluminum garnet (Nd:YAG) laser delivery system. General or regional anesthesia is required, but no irrigation (e.g., glycine) is needed. The morbidity of the TULIP procedure is low, and the treatment outcomes in initial studies are encouraging. This modality of treatment may eventually impact the treatment of BPH.

Cryotherapy

Cryotherapy has been tried in the treatment of BPH. Early studies in the 1960s used a transurethral probe with cooling to –140 to –190° C. This technique resulted in formation of an "ice-ball" at the tip of the probe, and treatment for 4 to 15 minutes caused tissue necrosis and sloughing. Because of the need for prolonged catheterization, and for the passage of sloughed tissue, and because of complications such as ureteral injury and prostate-rectal fistula due to the imprecise control of the cooling zones, cryotherapy fell into disrepute. Recent improvements in technology and the more precise control of cooling using ultrasound visualization of the probe tips and ice-balls may renew interest in this form of treatment for BPH. Cryosurgical techniques have recently been successfully applied to this treatment of prostatic cancer, with minimal morbidity and excellent control of prostatic mass destruction.

Other Techniques

Other techniques currently being considered and applied for BPH treatment include focused extracorporeal pyrotherapy (heat), focused extracorporeal shock-wave therapy, and focused ultrasound. These techniques are in the early stages of development and studies of their efficacy, safety, and cost are eagerly awaited.

NEW PHARMACOLOGIC TREATMENT

Androgen Deprivation

The androgen-dependence of prostate growth suggests a role for antiandrogen therapy in the treatment of prostatism (Table 5.11). Luteinizing hormone-releasing hormone (LH-RH) agonists have great affinity for anterior pituitary LH-RH receptors. Synthetic LH-RH agonists administered in a continuous, nonpulsatile fashion cause down-regulation of these receptors, with cessation of follicle-stimulating hormone (FSH) and LH secretion within a few weeks and a fall in serum testosterone to castrate levels (<50 μg/dl). The small amount of circulating androgens produced by the adrenals is insufficient to maintain prostatic hyperplasia, and the end result is shrinkage of the prostate.

LH-RH agonists used to treat BPH include buserelin, nafarelin acetate, leuprolide acetate, and Zoladex. In general, these drugs cause a 25 to 30% decrease in prostatic gland volume after 3 to 6 months of treatment, and 30 to 40% of men report subjective and/or objective (i.e., uroflow) symptomatic improvement (Table 5.11). The androgen-

Table 5.11: Androgen Suppression in BPH

- Hormonal agents
  - Antiandrogens
  - GnRH analogues
  - 5-alpha-reductase inhibitors
  - Progestins
  - Cyproterone acetate
- Results of treatment
  - 20 to 30% reduction in prostate volume by 6 months
  - 30% symptom score/uroflow improvement
- Drug side effects
  - GnRH analogues
    - Impotence, reduced libido, hot flashes
  - Antiandrogens (e.g., flutamide)
    - Gynecomastia, breast tenderness, diarrhea
  - Finasteride
    - Low incidence sexual dysfunction
    - Fall in serum PSA

responsive epithelial component of BPH is primarily affected by the decrease in androgenic stimulation accompanied by epithelial involution and gland shrinkage. Morphometric evaluation of the prostate after LH-RH agonist treatment shows 40% epithelial and 20% stromal regression rates. The reduced serum testosterone levels that result from LH-RH analogue therapy adversely affect libido and potency. These effects are reversible once treatment is discontinued. Hot flushes, gynecomastia, and headaches also occur. LH-RH agonists are viable alternatives to prostatectomy in selected patients, for example, men already impotent or sexually inactive. New depot preparations (monthly, 2 to 3 monthly) will lessen the frequency of injections and make LH-RH agonists more attractive as therapeutic agents for BPH.

Flutamide, a nonsteroidal antiandrogen that blocks androgen receptor binding of DHT, has been used to treat BPH. Treatment outcomes with regard to symptom improvement, gland size reduction, and improved flow rates are comparable to those seen with LH-RH agonists. However, libido and potency are preserved in the majority of men, although breast pain, gynecomastia, and gastrointestinal side effects occur. Serum testosterone levels are not reduced. The sparing of libido/potency is due to the lack of progestogenic activity because of flutamide's nonsteroidal structure.

Studies of LH-RH agonists and flutamide have been done in small groups of patients and without controls. All these agents, except flutamide, induce hypogonadism and adversely affect potency and libido. Casodex and Nilutamide, nonsteroidal antiandrogens related to flutamide, are of potential benefit in BPH. Casodex has fewer side effects than flutamide and can be administered in single daily doses.

Five-Alpha-Reductase Inhibitors

The critical roles of dihydrotestosterone (DHT) and 5-alpha-reductase in prostatic growth and epithelial cell replication are well established (Figure 5.4). This realization led to a search for a drug that would competitively inhibit 5-alpha-reductase, reduce prostatic intracellular DHT, and cause prostatic shrinkage without compromising libido or potency.

Finasteride (Proscar), a 4-azasteroid inhibitor that lacks androgen-receptor affinity, is a potent, reversible inhibitor of 5-alpha-reductase that causes a reduction in plasma and prostatic DHT levels within 1 week. Serum testosterone levels are unchanged, and sexual potency and libido are unaffected in the vast majority of patients.

Clinical studies underscore the utility of finasteride for the treatment of BPH (Table 5.11). In a 12-month study, therapy reduced prostatic size by about 20%, lowered serum DHT levels by greater than 60%, and

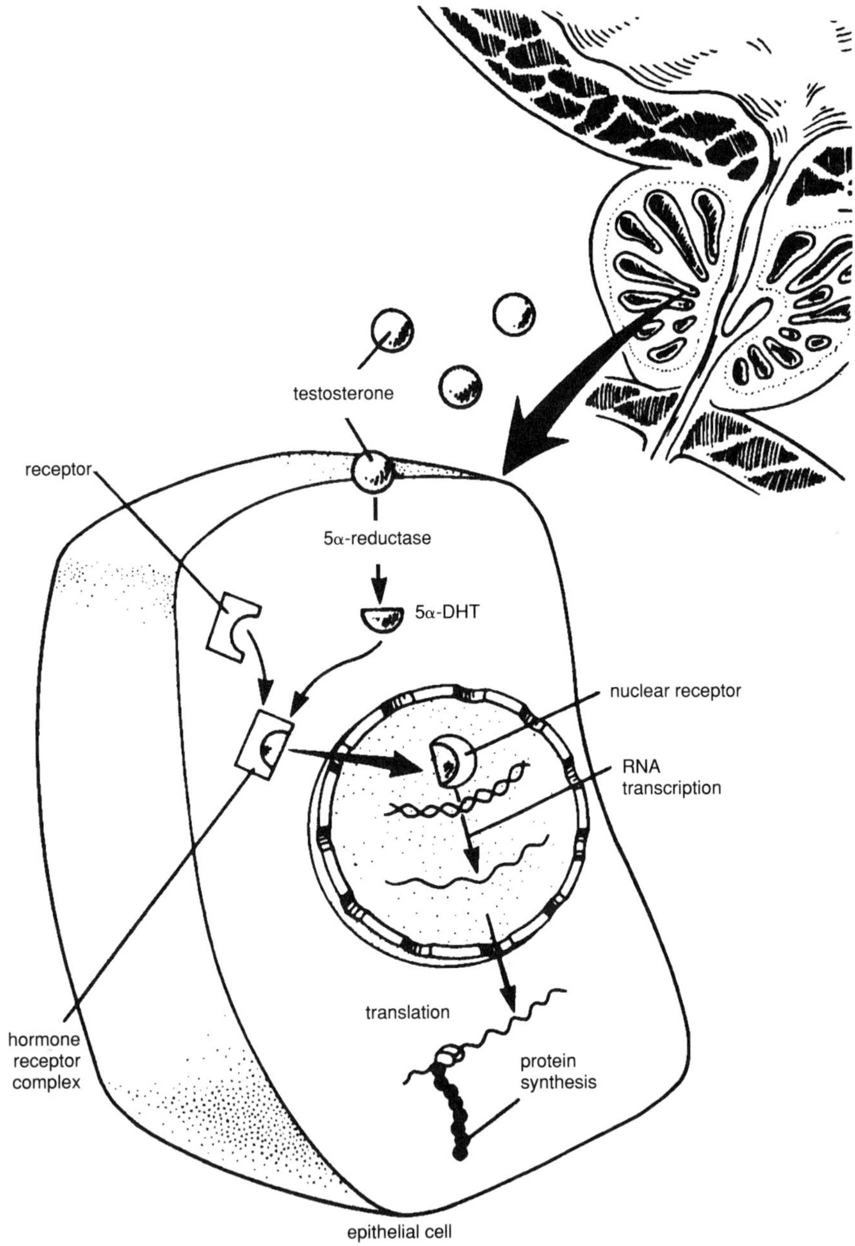

Figure 5.4: Conversion of testosterone to dihydrotestosterone by the enzyme 5-alpha-reductase in the prostatic epithelial cell.

lowered serum prostate specific antigen (PSA) levels by about 50%. Symptoms, assessed by symptom scores, are improved and uroflows statistically improved. About 30% of patients experience favorable improvement in their symptoms and modest improvements in their urinary flow rates. Decreased libido and impotence occur in about 5% of patients, but potency returns after the medication is stopped. There are no antiandrogenic actions such as nipple tenderness, gynecomastia, or altered spermatogenesis. The prostatic shrinkage probably reflects the action of finasteride on the glandular epithelial component of BPH rather than on the fibromuscular stroma. It may well be that patients with minimal stromal hyperplasia will respond better to finasteride.

An extract from the dwarf palm tree (Serenoa repens B) has antiandrogenic and 5-alpha-reductase inhibitor properties and has been used in certain European countries to treat BPH. Other synthetic 5-alpha-reductase inhibitors are currently being developed and undergoing Phase I and II clinical trials.

Because BPH is predominantly a stromal disease, it may be inferred that most BPH glands would shrink in response to stromal rather than epithelial inhibition. This coincides with the reported shrinkage rates of only 20 to 25% in long-term clinical studies with finasteride. Finasteride also reduces prostate-specific antigen levels by about 50%. However, the potential effects of 5-alpha-reductase inhibitors on the development, recognition, and progression of prostatic cancer are unknown.

Alpha Adrenergic Blockers

The $alpha_1$-adrenergic innervation of the abundant prostatic stromal and smooth-muscle elements in the surgical capsule and stroma accounts for the tension in the prostate and contributes to the dynamic component of BPH obstruction. $Alpha_1$ receptors are abundant in the bladder base and prostate but sparse in the bladder body. Experimental and clinical studies have confirmed the contribution of the adrenergic receptors to the pathophysiology of BPH, and alpha-adrenergic antagonists are capable of reducing prostatic urethral resistance and affecting the dynamic component of BPH resistance (Table 5.12).

The initial 1976 clinical report on the use of alpha blockers in BPH used phenoxybenzamine, a nonselective alpha blocker. Although subsequent studies support the role of alpha blockers in the treatment of BPH, many were deficient in their study designs, using nonspecific entry criteria, short-term follow-up, ill-defined outcome measures, and large drop-out rates. More recent studies of selective alpha blockers, performed in prospective, multicenter, placebo-controlled trials, have avoided these pitfalls.

Table 5.12: Alpha-Blocker Therapy for BPH

Rationale for use
Increased alpha-adrenergic activity in stroma, smooth muscle
Alpha-adrenergic innervation
Dynamic component of outlet obstruction
Drugs used
Nonselective blockers
Selective $alpha_1$ blockers
Short-acting drugs (e.g., prazosin)
Longer acting drugs (e.g., Hytrin)
Treatment results
No significant change in prostate volume
30 to 50% improvement in uroflow, symptom scores
Hypotension uncommon in normotensive patients

Terazosin (Hytrin) is a long-acting, selective $alpha_1$-adrenergic antagonist that is used for the treatment of hypertension. Its long half-life is an advantage over other available alpha blockers and leads to better compliance. Phase II and phase III studies confirm the safety and efficacy of terazosin treatment for men with BPH. Symptom scores (both obstructive and irritative), urine flow rates, and global patient assessment parameters are significantly improved. Improvement is maintained after more than 2 years of therapy, and side effects are minimal. Adverse effects, headache, asthenia, and dizziness/postural hypotension, are minor (<5 to 10%) and reversible. Overall, average improvement in flow rates are seen in about 30%, and between 45 and 70% report symptomatic improvement (Table 5.12).

Prazosin (Minipress) is a short-acting, selective $alpha_1$-adrenergic antagonist. In the short term (up to 4 weeks) it is beneficial in alleviating the symptoms of BPH, increasing uroflow and reducing postvoid residual. However, long-term placebo-controlled studies have shown that prazosin is not significantly better than placebo. Another drawback is the "first-dose phenomenon," which can cause troublesome postural hypotension if the dose is not slowly titrated upward over 4 to 7 days.

Multicenter, randomized, placebo-controlled studies have been done with other selective $alpha_1$-blockers, for example, Alfuzosin and YM617 (a Japanese drug). In general, these blockers are well tolerated and adverse side effects are mild, reversible, and similar to those of placebo. The clinical and urodynamic responses to alpha blocker therapy are dose-related, and Terazosin appears to be more efficacious than YM617 or Alfuzosin. Other selective blockers being evaluated include Doxazosin (a selective blocker with a longer half-life than Terazosin), Thymoxamine, Indoramin, and Nicergoline.

Long-term alpha-adrenergic antagonist therapy does not cause shrinkage of prostatic smooth muscle or a reduction of prostate volume. There is no significant association between treatment response and baseline measurements such as prostatic volume, flow rate, or symptoms score. Currently, alpha-blocker treatment is attractive for men with moderate symptoms, those without absolute indications for surgery, and those who are poor surgical risks. These drugs may also be useful to treat acute retention and avoid the risks of surgery in the nonelective setting. The best $alpha_1$ blocker for BPH treatment has not been identified, nor has the optimal candidate for treatment been defined. Unlike the antiandrogens or LH-RH analogues, alpha blockers do not affect libido or potency or cause hot flashes or gynecomastia. Alpha blockers may well have an additive effect to that of the 5-alpha-reductase inhibitors in the treatment of BPH. They relax prostatic smooth muscle and reduce dynamic obstruction, whereas finasteride shrinks prostatic glandular tissue and reduces the mechanical component of obstruction. A current Veterans Administration hospitals study in the United States should provide information on single- versus double-drug therapy for BPH.

Aromatase Inhibitors

The increasing prevalence of BPH with age is paralleled by an increase in the serum ratio of estrogen to androgen, and the role of estrogens in the pathogenesis of BPH has been experimentally confirmed in animals. In men, estrogens are produced by the extratesticular production of estrone and estradiol from androstenedione and testosterone, respectively. Aromatase, a cytochrome P450-dependent enzyme responsible for the above reaction, is widely distributed in the prostate, especially the periurethral zone, and other reproductive tissues. Androstenedione causes stromal hyperplasia in animals, and this can be reversed by administration of an aromatase inhibitor. These experimental data have led to the use of aromatase inhibitors for BPH treatment.

Ketoconazole and aminoglutethimide are nonselective aromatase inhibitors. Both have been used to treat prostatic carcinoma, and their side effects are well known. Ketoconazole (an antifungal agent) has the potential for serious hepatic toxicity, whereas aminoglutethimide causes depression, gynecomastia, and other side effects. Atamestane, a new selective aromatase inhibitor (1-methyl-androsta-1, 4-diene-3, 17-dione, or 1-methyl-ADD), antagonizes the stromal hyperplasia and BPH induced by estrogens in experimental animals. The aromatase inhibitors, atamestane and testolactone, are currently being studied, and clinical results should be available in the near future.

Another approach to antiestrogen therapy of BPH is the use of estrogen-receptor antagonists. The antiestrogen, tamoxifen, unfortunately has intrinsic estrogenic activity, which limits its potential role in BPH treatment. A new agent, 1C1 183720, has more estrogen-blocker activity than tamoxifen and no estrogenic activity. This compound may be useful in treatment. Multicenter, placebo-controlled, double-blind studies are currently being performed and should provide a definitive answer regarding the efficacy of antiestrogens (e.g., receptor blockers, inhibitors of synthesis) in the management of BPH.

Other Medical Treatment

Drugs used to treat hypercholesterolemia have been used to treat BPH. Candicin, however, did not show efficacy in controlled trials. Likewise, bromocriptine—an antagonist of prolactin—has been used without effect on the prostate.

A number of plant extracts, for example, permixon, have been tried on the basis of the theory that the phytosterols in these plants, particularly the sitosterols, affect prostatic growth by a direct cytotoxic effect, reduced liver synthesis of sex hormone binding globulin, or weak alpha-reductase activity. Currently, phytotherapy or treatment with the plant extracts, is believed to be no more beneficial than placebo treatment for the treatment of symptomatic BPH.

CONCLUSIONS

The treatment of benign prostatic hyperplasia (BPH) is currently being revolutionized. New, nonsurgical forms of treatment are being introduced with good, short-term results. A better understanding of the pathophysiology and pathogenesis of BPH will undoubtedly lead to other pharmacologic treatment modalities. Future studies of BPH will need to address a variety of critical issues (Table 5.13).

The natural history of untreated prostatism has not been studied adequately, although available data suggest that symptom improvement and stabilization are not uncommon. Information from watchful waiting protocols will provide more reliable data on the course of untreated prostatism and affect the treatment algorithm for prostatism.

For patients who need prostatectomy for relief of infravesical obstruction in BPH, a variety of minimally invasive approaches to prostatic shrinkage/destruction are being used, and new technologies are on the horizon. By the dawn of the twenty-first century, the treatment of BPH will be clearly different from the current approaches. Fewer men will undergo prostatectomy, and more will be treated pharmacologically or with minimally invasive surgical techniques.

Table 5.13: Future Study of BPH

Unresolved medical treatment issues
Long-term safety, efficacy
$Alpha_1$ blockade versus androgen suppression
Combination treatment
Duration of response
Long-term costs, compliance
Alternative device therapies
Cost issues
Efficacy and safety
Watchful waiting protocols
Better knowledge of natural history of BPH
Allow selective intervention
Drug, device, observation studies require
Use of AUA/WHO symptom scoring
Quality-of-life issues
Randomized studies

SUGGESTED READINGS

McConnell JD. Androgen ablation and blockade in the treatment of benign prostatic hyperplasia. Urol Clin North Am 1990; 17:661.

Excellent review of androgen dependence in BPH. The hormonal rationale for antiandrogen treatment is addressed and treatment results summarized.

McNeal J. Pathology of benign prostatic hyperplasia: insight into etiology. Urol Clin North Am 1990; 17:447.

Insightful account of development of BPH, with particular reference to the zonal anatomy of the prostate. The author has made significant contributions to our understanding of prostatic anatomy and histology in BPH.

Gup DI, Shapiro E, Baumann M. Autonomic receptors in asymptomatic and symptomatic BPH. J Urol 1990; 143:179.

Study of the influence of $alpha_1$-adrenoreceptors in the pathogenesis of BPH. Symptomatic and asymptomatic men were studied.

Shapiro E, Hartanto V, Lepor H. Quantifying the smooth muscle content of the prostate using double-immunoenzymatic staining and color-assisted image analysis. J Urol 1992; 147:1167.

Sophisticated analysis of the area density of smooth muscle and other stromal elements in BPH. Confirms earlier morphometric evaluations and firmly indicates that human BPH is a predominantly stromal disease.

Habenicht U-F, El Etreby MF. Rationale for using aromatase inhibitors to manage benign prostatic hyperplasia: experimental studies. J Androl 1991; 12:385.

Review of the role of estrogens in the pathogenesis of BPH and the rationale for the use of aromatase inhibitors for treatment. The experimental literature dealing with estrogens in BPH is succinctly summarized.

Gormley GJ, Stoner E, Bruskewitz RC, et al. The effect of finasteride in men with benign prostatic hyperplasia. N Engl J Med 1992; 327:1185.

Describes a controlled 12-month study of the 5-alpha-reductase inhibitor, finasteride, in men with BPH. The drug reduces prostate size and improves urinary flow rates and symptom scores.

Barry MJ. Epidemiology and natural history of benign prostatic hyperplasia. Urol Clin North Am 1990; 17:495.

Succinct review of the various aspects of the epidemiology and natural history of BPH. Interesting observations pertaining to watchful waiting observation protocols.

Berry SJ, Coffey DS, Walsh PC, Ewing LL. The development of human prostatic hyperplasia with age. J Urol 1984; 132:474.

Early study emphasizing the rising incidence of microscopic BPH with age. BPH develops in the majority of men by age 60. However, histologic BPH is not paralleled by gland enlargement or the development of symptoms.

Davies P, Eaton CL. Regulation of prostatic growth. J Endocrinol 1991; 131:5.

Roles of steroids, steroid receptors, and polypeptide growth factors in the pathogenesis of BPH are discussed. Prostatic growth and the development of BPH and prostatic cancer is a complex process with multiple, interrelated inputs (stimulating and inhibitory).

Lepor H, Meretyk S, Knapp-Maloney G. The safety, efficacy and compliance of Terazosin therapy for benign prostatic hyperplasia. J Urol 1992; 147:1554.

A 24-month study of the utility of terazosin for the treatment of symptomatic BPH. Safety and compliance issues are discussed together with the drug's overall therapeutic effect. Terazosin is a useful drug for BPH, especially in younger men with mild to moderate symptoms.

Chung LWK, Cunha GR. Stromal-epithelial interactions. II: regulation of prostatic growth by embryonic urogenital sinus mesenchyme. Prostate 1983; 4:503.

Experimental demonstration of stimulation of epithelial prostatic cells by cells of stromal origin. Such epithelial reawakening, mediated by stromal autocrine factors, may contribute to the development of human BPH.

Jacobs SC, Story, MT, Sasse J, Lawson RK. Characterization of growth factors derived from the rat ventral prostate. J Urol 1988; 139:1106.

Biological activity of prostatic growth factors are discussed and their potential role in the development of BPH addressed.

Roos NP, Wennberg JE, Malenka DJ, et al. Mortality and reoperation after open and transurethral resection of the prostate for benign prostatic hyperplasia. N Engl J Med 1989; 320:1120.

Important study addressing the treatment outcomes following prostatectomy for BPH. It was instrumental in redirecting the attention of urologists to the results of prostatectomy, the natural history of BPH, and the outcomes after treatment.

CHAPTER 6

Male Infertility

John P. Pryor

Male fertility depends on the satisfactory integration of a series of physiological events starting with semen production and ending with fertilization of the oocyte. This process may be interrupted voluntarily, by pathological changes, or by adverse factors in the female partner. The essence of fertility management is to establish a prognosis, or the chance of the partner conceiving in a given period of time–be it 1 year with normal intercourse or 1 cycle of assisted conception. In order to make such a prognosis, it is necessary to have a sound understanding of the pathophysiology of infertility. The choice of treatment is made on the basis of the chances of it improving the prognosis, and in many instances the couple is faced with several options that are less than ideal. The infertile couple needs to be acquainted with the chances of success, the risks associated with the various forms of treatment, and the costs of such treatment.

Most couples expect to be fertile, and failure of the wife to conceive causes stress. Some societies attach a social stigma to being childless, and the problem is usually perceived as being due to the female partner. In all societies, however, men are devastated if they are found to be the cause of the infertility. Generally, about 10% of the population are involuntarily infertile. Male factors predominate as the cause of the infertility in about 25% of couples, combined male and female factors are present in a further 25%, and the problem is purely female in another 25% of patients. The cause for the infertility is unexplained in the remaining 25% of couples. The precise cause varies in different series and is dependent on the diagnostic techniques used and geographical location. The main etiological factor that influences the outcome is the proportion of the population studied who have genital tract infections.

The processes involved in normal fertility may be summarized as sperm manufacture, maturation, and storage; accessory gland secretion and ejaculation; sperm transport in the female tract; and fertilization and embryo development. Interference with any of these may cause infertility, and some factors may act at more than one stage.

SPERM MANUFACTURE

Normal Spermatogenesis

The testis must be developed normally in order for there to be normal spermatogenesis. The man must have a normal chromosome pattern (XY), and the testes should be descended into the scrotum (see Chapter 1). During childhood the testes are small and the seminiferous tubules are solid cordlike structures containing primitive spermatocytes and Sertoli cells. The seminiferous tubules gradually acquire a lumen as the spermatocytes differentiate after the age of 6 years.

Testicular size increases significantly during puberty (Table 6.1); this increase is driven by hormonal changes: an elevation of the levels of both luteinizing hormone (LH) and follicle stimulating hormone (FSH) (Figure 6.1). These hormones consist of about 115 amino acids, have a molecular weight of about 30,000 d, and are produced by gonadotroph cells of the adenohypophysis. Gonadotrophic releasing hormone (GnRH), produced by the hypothalamus, is under both hormonal and neural control. The releasing hormone stimulates the anterior pituitary to produce LH and FSH. There is still some debate as to whether there are one or two releasing hormones, and it is likely that much of the molecule is common to both hormones. Luteinizing hormone is made available to the Leydig cells of the testis by means of LH receptors on the surface of the cells. Many other chemicals have now been shown to have an effect on Leydig cell function and the production of testosterone from cholesterol. The steps in the process are shown in Figure 6.2; each stage requires the appropriate enzyme.

The final conversion of testosterone to dihydrotestosterone requires 5-alpha-reductase, and a deficiency of this enzyme is associated with abnormalities of the genitalia. Circulating testosterone may be protein-bound, but little evidence suggests that it is necessary in clinical practice to measure the free testosterone levels. Circulating testosterone acts on the hypothalamus to provide a negative feedback mechanism (Figure 6.3) and maintain the circulating testosterone level within the normal range

Table 6.1: Increase in Testicular Size at Puberty

Age (Years)	10	11	12	13	14	15	16	17	18	19	20
Testicular Volume (ml)	1	1.5	3	6.5	11	13	14	15	17	18	20

After Prader

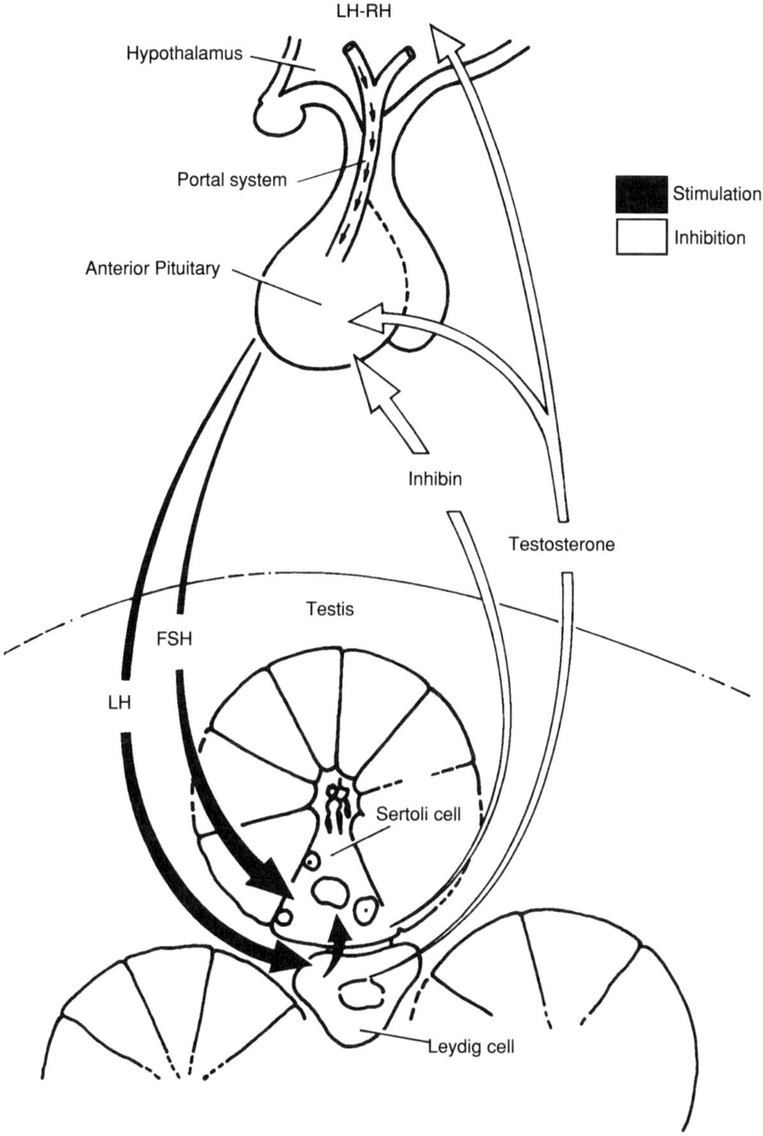

Figure 6.1: Hypothalamic–pituitary-gonadal axis. *Adapted from Marrs R. Assisted Reproductive Technologies. Boston: Blackwell Scientific Publications, 1993:30.*

(10 to 35 nmol/L). In contrast, FSH acts through the Sertoli cells to stimulate the germ cells to manufacture sperm. Another hormone called

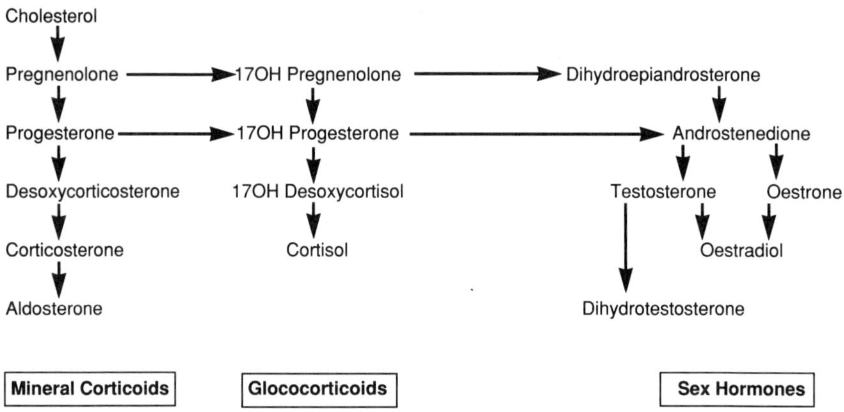

Figure 6.2: Metabolic pathway for androgen production

inhibin is produced by the Sertoli cells once spermatogenesis proceeds to the spermatocyte stage and is the feedback mechanism to regulate FSH production. Inhibin is a protein, not a steroid. An elevated FSH level is a bad prognostic sign in any man with infertility as it suggests some degree of testicular failure to produce sperm.

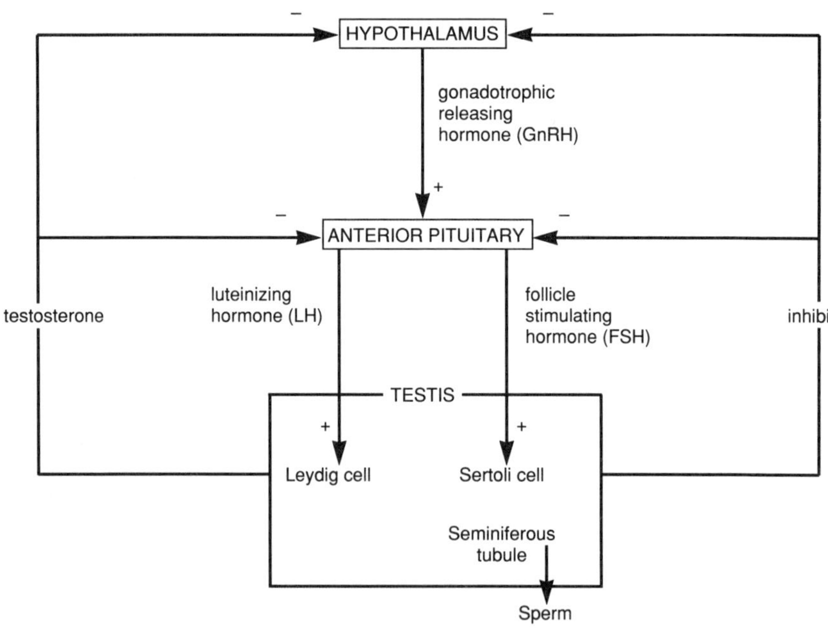

Figure 6.3: Hormonal regulation of testicular function

Phases of Germ Cell Development

Spermatogenesis is a complex process of cellular changes, which are divided into three groups. In animals, the changes take place in waves along the seminiferous tubules, but in man all types of cell may be seen in the same tubule and the process is more complex. The spermatogenic cycle in the testis is about 16 days in duration, but the total time from the commencement of spermatogenesis to expulsion of the spermatozoa in the semen during ejaculation is approximately 72 days.

The first (replication) phase of spermatogenesis involves spermatogonia, which undergo cell division to produce type A spermatogonia. These in turn produce intermediate and then type B spermatogonia. The recognition of these different spermatogonia is difficult with ordinary light microscopy. Spermatogonia divide in the second phase of spermatogenesis to produce spermatocytes, which undergo division with a halving of the number of chromosomes. The secondary spermatocytes divide in the final stage of spermatogenesis to produce spermatids and then spermatozoa. During spermiogenesis (third stage) the rounded spermatocytes become elongated and recognizable as sperms with an acrosomal cap on the sperm head, a midpiece, and a tail.

The Sertoli, or "supporting," cells play an essential role in testicular function and serve to capture hormones that nourish the germ cells. These cells rest on the basement membrane of the seminiferous tubules and send multiple cytoplasmic extensions into the lumen of the tubules between the germinal cells (Figure 6.4). The contents of a seminiferous tubule are "outside" the body, and special "tight-cell" junctions exist adjacent to the Sertoli cells. These allow the passage of fluid into the seminiferous tubule. The Sertoli cell is thought to contribute to the blood–testis barrier.

Assessment of Spermatogenesis

Spermatogenesis is assessed by performing a testicular biopsy, and it is important to avoid crushing the tissue while it is being obtained and to place it in a fixative solution that does not cause shrinkage of the seminiferous tubules. Bouin's, Cleland's, Stieve's, and a modified Zenker's solution are all satisfactory fixatives, but formalin (10% formaldehyde) is totally unsatisfactory. The specimen is fixed, sliced, and stained according to preference; some histopathologists prefer to use semithin sections. The histologic findings should be described, and there is much to recommend the additional use of a quantitative assessment. The widely used Johnsen (1970) technique counts the cells in the most advanced stage of spermatogenesis in 200 seminiferous tubules, and their average value is obtained (Table 6.2). The presence of Leydig cells is also noted. The

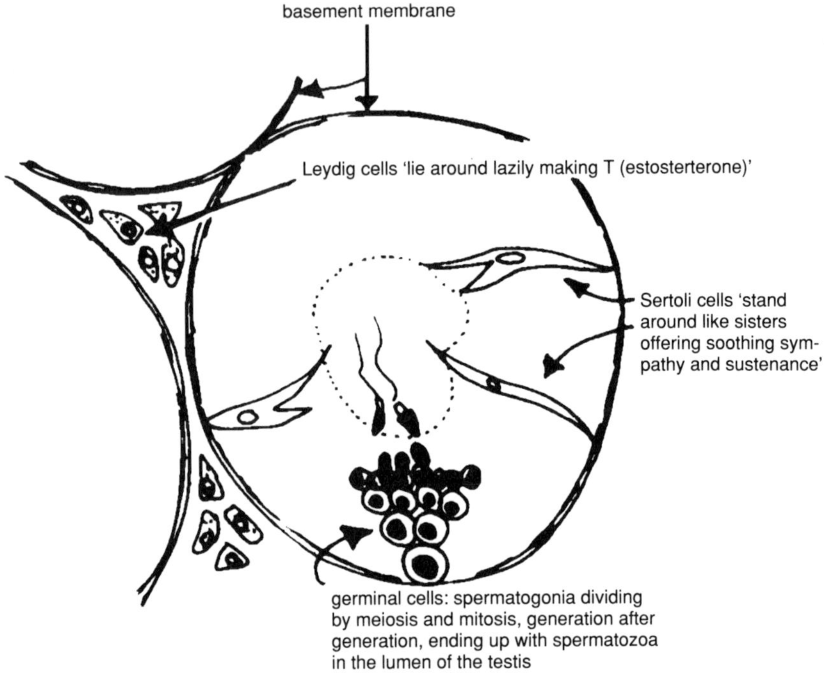

Figure 6.4: Histology of the testis. *Reproduced from Blandy J. Lecture Notes on Urology, 4th ed. Oxford: Blackwell Scientific Publications, 1991:292.*

ratio of the various components of the germ cells and Leydig cells in the testicular samples does not give a good indication of the expected semen quality or the likelihood of fertility.

Table 6.2: Correlation between Testicular Size and Spermatogenesis in Azoospermic Men

Testicular Size (ml)	*Biopsies number(%)*	*Mean Johnsen Score[a] (Number and %)* ≤2.0	2.1–7.9	≥8.0
2.5	11 (100)	11 (100)	—	—
7.5	71 (100)	36 (51)	34 (48)	1 (1)
15	118 (100)	39 (53)	35 (30)	44 (37)
25	198 (100)	11 (6)	35 (18)	152 (77)

[a]Johnsen (1970) described a method of scoring the stage (steps) of spermatogenesis in seminiferous tubules by the appearance of the cells: Sertoli cells, step 2; spermatogonia, step 3; spermatocytes, steps 4 and 5; spermatids, steps 6 and 7; spermatozoa, steps 8, 9, and 10

IMPAIRED SPERMATOGENESIS

Impaired spermatogenesis occurs for various reasons. Patients with primary testicular failure (either congenital or acquired) have elevated serum levels of FSH. In secondary testicular failure, a normal FSH level is seen, and the impaired spermatogenesis is the result of a hormonal deficiency.

Primary Testicular Failure

Primary testicular failure is characterized by azoospermia or severe oligozoospermia. Affected men have small testes and grossly elevated plasma FSH levels (Tables 6.2 and 6.3). Testicular exploration and biopsy are not required in the evaluation of these patients. The reported incidence of chromosomal abnormalities in infertile men varies from 2 to 20% of patients. The reported incidences depend on the populations studied, and some of the findings are of doubtful significance.

Klinefelter's syndrome (XXY), a common chromosomal abnormality, usually renders affected men infertile. The incidence of Klinefelter's syndrome is approximately 1 in 500 live births, 7% in infertile men, and as high as 25% in azoospermic men. The diagnosis is suspected on the clinical examination, which demonstrates small testes (99%), scant facial hair (77%), and a female hair distribution or gynecomastia (55%). The frequently associated hypospadias may already have been repaired during childhood, and men with a micropenis do not usually present to the infertility clinic. Azoospermia is found in 93% of men with Klinefelter's syndrome, and the testicular biopsy shows ghosting of the seminiferous tubules with very few testicular germ cells.

Testicular Maldescent

Argument persists as to whether failure of testicular descent is due to an intrinsic defect in the testis or to multiple external factors. There is no good evidence that an intra-abdominal testis will make sperm, and the

Table 6.3: Correlation between Plasma FSH Levels and Spermatogenesis in Azoospermic Men

FSH Level	*Biopsies Number (%)*	*Mean Johnsen Score (Number and %)* ≤2.0	2.1–7.9	≥8.0
Normal	114 (100)	4 (4)	26 (22)	84 (74)
Mild elevation	26 (100)	6 (23)	12 (46)	8 (31)
Gross elevation[a]	74 (100)	54 (73)	16 (22)	4 (5)

[a]FSH level greater than twice the upper limit of normal

occurrence of spermatogenesis following bilateral orchidopexy for truly undescended testes is uncertain. Such testes usually have normal numbers of Leydig cells but atrophy and/or fibrosis of the germinal epithelium. The incidence of carcinoma of the testis is increased in adults with undescended testes. Carcinoma was found in 25% of intra-abdominal testes compared to only 0.5 to 1% in men having a testicular biopsy as part of their evaluation for subfertility/infertility.

Sertoli-Cell–Only Syndrome

In Sertoli-cell–only syndrome, the seminiferous tubules have a uniform appearance and are lined by Sertoli cells. All germ cells are absent (germinal aplasia). The pattern is less uniform in some patients, in whom some seminiferous tubules show evidence of spermatogenesis. The patient is usually azoospermic and has elevated plasma FSH levels. This condition is medically and surgically untreatable.

Acquired Lesions

The germinal epithelium is sensitive to damage. Torsion of the testis may lead to the loss of germinal epithelium—sometimes patchy in distribution—and subsequent fibrosis, even if the blood supply is restored before the testis becomes fibrotic. It was previously thought that the ischemic testis was a source of antibody production that could lead to the later impairment of spermatogenesis. A careful recent study demonstrated that this is not the case. Biopsy of the contralateral testis at the time of the torsion revealed abnormalities, which account for the impaired fertility subsequently seen.

Mumps orchitis is characteristically associated with testicular atrophy and impaired spermatogenesis. Epididymo-orchitis may be associated with obstructive azoospermia. In severe cases, arterial thrombosis may occur, with subsequent loss of spermatogenesis and resultant infertility.

Radiotherapy and Chemotherapy

Exposure to radiation or chemotherapy damages the germinal epithelium. This effect is largely dependent on dosage. Testicular germ cells are highly radiosensitive. Spermatogenesis is impaired for up to 1 year by a radiation dose of 0.1 Gy, whereas sterility occurs for 2 to 3 years with dosages up to 2.5 Gy. Sterility is permanent with radioactive exposures of more than 4 to 6 Gy. Sertoli cells are relatively radioresistant, as are the Leydig cells in the testicular interstitium.

The actively dividing spermatogonia and the spermatocytes are particularly sensitive to the interference of cell division caused by chemotherapeutic drugs. The alkalinating agents and procarbazine, when administered as single-agent therapy, cause significant degrees of testicular damage. The damage is more difficult to ascertain when multidrug chemotherapy is utilized, for example, in Hodgkin's disease and germ cell testicular tumors. Spermatogenesis recovers in up to 50% of men with testicular cancer treated with multiagent therapy, although such recovery may take 1 to 2 years. Contralateral testicular abnormalities occur in nearly 1 in 5 men with testicular cancer.

Other environmental, occupational, and recreational (e.g., alcohol, caffeine, cigarette smoking) agents may play as yet undetermined gonadotoxic roles.

Secondary Testicular Failure

The problem in secondary testicular failure is usually a hormonal abnormality. This may follow pituitary ablation and give rise to "spermatogenic arrest," a term that is used frequently, is difficult to define, and implies that spermatogenesis proceeds to a certain stage and then stops. Secondary testicular failure classically occurs with a deficiency of gonadotrophic hormones (e.g., following hypophysectomy) at Johnsen steps 5 to 6. The cutoff in spermatogenesis is usually not confined to a single stage, and there is frequent spillover into adjacent stages. The term is so misused that it cannot be relied upon when a clinician assesses a testicular biopsy histological report issued by an unfamiliar pathologist. The various syndromes associated with endocrine abnormalities and infertility are shown in Table 6.4. It should be emphasized that such patients are an uncommon finding in an infertility clinic.

Hypogonadotrophic Hypogonadism

Patients with hypogonadotrophic hypogonadism usually present to the endocrinologist because of delayed puberty and the absence of develop-

Table 6.4: Hormonal Abnormalities and Infertility

		Effect on Hormone Levels			
Syndrome	*Hormone Deficiency*	*T*	*LH*	*FSH*	*Other*
Panhypopituitarism	Pituitary hormones	Low	Low	Low	Low
Hypogonadotrophic hypogonadism	GnRH, FSH, and LH	Low	Low	Low	Normal
Fertile Eunuch	LH	Low	Low	Normal	Normal
Isolated FSH	FSH	Normal	Normal	Low	Normal
Hyperprolactinemia	Excess Prolactin	Low	Low	Low	Prolactin high

ment of the secondary male sexual characteristics. The problem may be due to an isolated hypothalamic deficiency of gonadotrophic releasing hormone (GnRH). Kallman described this syndrome and noted its association with anosmia due to the agenesis of the olfactory bulbs. Other somatic abnormalities and birth defects may also occur, for example, cryptorchidism, cleft palate, harelip, cranial facial asymmetry, microphallus, and seizures. Two rare variants of hypothalamic GnRH release abnormality are the "fertile eunuch syndrome" and isolated follicle-stimulating hormone (FSH) deficiency. The former is due to an isolated luteinizing hormone (LH) deficiency in men with normal FSH levels. The man appears eunuchoid because of the relative deficiency of testosterone and failure of the full development of the secondary sex characteristics. Spermatogenesis is normal because there is sufficient FSH to stimulate spermatogenesis. The extremely rare syndrome of isolated FSH deficiency results in normal virilization with regard to body habitus but absent spermatogenesis.

Acquired hypogonadotrophic hypogonadism may be secondary to defects in the production of LH and FSH by the anterior pituitary as a result of adenomata, surgery, infarction, or infection. Extrinsic brain lesions may also impair pituitary function, and these deficiencies are associated with other abnormalities of pituitary function. Other manifestations of endocrine dysfunction and visual field defects are common.

Hyperprolactinemia

Increased production of prolactin by the anterior pituitary is characterized by the loss of libido, impotence, and infertility. Such patients are rarely seen in an infertility clinic. Minor elevations of serum prolactin levels (less than 1000 miu/L with a normal range of up to 200) are usually due to stress, exercise, or drugs; and extensive evaluations do not usually reveal pituitary adenomas (either micro- or macroadenomas). Other conditions that may cause elevated serum prolactin levels include liver cirrhosis, azotemia/uremia, a variety of neurotransmitters, and hypoglycemia.

SPERM MATURATION AND STORAGE

Spermatozoa pass from the rete testis into the long and tortuous epididymis, which serves as a storage reservoir for sperm (Figure 6.5). Testicular spermatozoa are immotile and have a low fertility potential, but during their passage through the epididymis they acquire motility and the ability to fertilize ova. These changes develop as a result of biochemical changes in the composition of both the epididymal fluid and sperm. The length of the epididymis is 3 to 4 meters, and it is highly coiled and convoluted. Anatomically and functionally, the human epi-

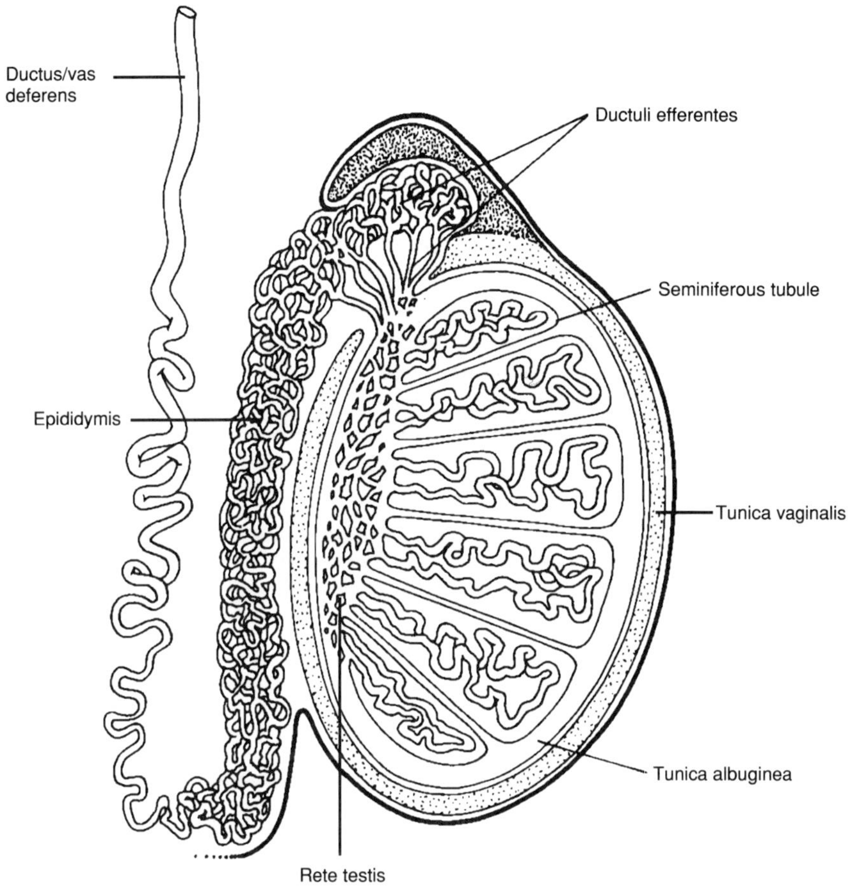

Figure 6.5: Human testis and epididymis. Note how the tubules are arranged in lobules, several tubules to each lobule, although for simplicity only one is shown. From the rete testis, the efferent ducts, or ductuli efferentes, open into the epididymal duct, where the sperm are stored until they are ejaculated through the ductus or vas deferens (After Dym). *Reproduced with permission from Webster G, Kirby K, King L, et al eds. Reconstructive Urology Vol 1. Boston: Blackwell Scientific Publications, 1993:79.*

didymis can be divided into segments: caput, corpus, and cauda epididymi. The lining of the epididymis is a pseudostratified epithelium, predominantly made up of tall columnar cells with prominent luminal microvilli, suggesting marked absorptive/secretory activity. Other epididymal cell types include apical cells (possible pinocytic function), basal cells, and lymphocytes. Ductal diameter increases from the caput toward the body and tail of the epididymis. They are under androgenic hormonal control (certainly testosterone) and may be temperature-dependent, which may be relevant in patients with varioceles.

The mechanisms whereby varioceles impair fertility are unknown. Many wives conceive even though their husbands have large, visible varioceles; yet others try unsuccessfully until small, subclinical varioceles are surgically treated. A bilateral variocele may cause spermatogenic arrest, and it is postulated that increased testicular temperature is the cause of this disturbance. An elevated temperature may also affect the epididymis and interfere with fertilization. In men, nearly 50% of the epididymal spermatozoa are in the cauda epididymis, suggesting some degree of storage in this segment. Sperm transport in the epididymis averages 2 to 12 days and is due to the contraction of the smooth muscle cells surrounding the epididymal tubules, rather than to innate sperm motility. Most of the observations on epididymal function are made on the basis of experimental work in animals and normal men. However, the findings are not negated by the results of microsurgical sperm acquisition in patients with obstructive male ductal lesions.

The important changes that occur in spermatozoa during their passage through the epididymis are discussed later with regard to capacitation and the acrosome reaction—two events that are important for fertilization. The functions of the epididymis, still poorly understood, are summarized in Table 6.5.

Table 6.5: Function of the Epididymis

- Sperm storage
  - Greatest in tail epididymis
- Sperm transport
  - Muscular contraction
  - Adrenergic innervation
- Sperm maturation/capacitance
  - Motility
  - Structural alteration in sperm tails (disulfide bonds)
  - Metabolic changes
  - Oocyte fertilization
  - Altered sperm morphology
    - Sperm head
    - Sperm tail
- Epididymal epithelial secretions
  - Proteins
  - Osmolarity
  - Electrolytes
  - Other chemicals

ACCESSORY GLAND SECRETIONS

Semen consists of the secretions of the seminal vesicles (65%), the prostate (30%), and the epididymis and testes (5%) (Table 6.6). These glands produce different chemical substances, and by getting men to produce a split ejaculate it is possible to study the order of emission. It is possible to split the ejaculate into six portions with care and a little practice! John Hunter (1786) was aware of the different components of human semen. The emission commences with clear fluid from Cowper's gland and then contains a sperm-rich portion from the ejaculatory duct and epididymis. The prostatic secretions, rich in citric acid, enter the ejaculate before the secretions of the seminal vesicles, rich in fructose. The accessory glands require testosterone for normal function. The precise roles of the individual chemical constituents of the secretions are uncertain (Table 6.7). Fructose was considered to be a form of energy for sperm, but this belief is no longer tenable. It may be that the main function of the accessory glands is the production of sufficient fluid volume to act as a buffer against the acidity of the vaginal secretions.

OBSTRUCTION TO THE SEMINAL TRACT

In some men, the total absence of spermatozoa in the ejaculate (azoospermia) is caused by a blockage of the sperm ducts. These men have normal-sized testes, no elevation of plasma FSH levels, and they require testicular exploration to determine the site of obstruction. The outcome in men who undergo testicular exploration is shown in Table 6.8. It should be noted that biochemical assessment of genital tract obstruction is only of value in patients with ejaculatory duct obstruction who have small-volume and acid semen that lacks fructose. Patients with congenital absence of the vasa have the same quality of semen but should be detected on clinical examination. Transrectal ultrasound may demonstrate distension and obstruction of the ejaculatory ducts as well as a dyskinetic conducting mechanism.

Table 6.6: Composition and Origin of Seminal Fluid

Volume	*Main Origin*	*Main Components*
65%	Seminal vesicle	Coagulation enzymes, fructose, prostaglandins
30%	Prostate	Liquefying enzymes, zinc, acid phosphatase, inositol, citric acid
5%	Epididymis	Carnitine, glycerophosphorylcholine

Table 6.7: Ejaculate Constituents

Constituents
Citric acid
Fructose
Polyamines
Prostaglandins
Cholesterol, lipids
Zinc
Dehydrogenase
Prostate specific antigen

Function
Coagulation
Liquefaction
Anti-infective
Promote fertility

The diagnosis of intratesticular obstruction is made when there is a normal testicular biopsy and no evidence of spermatozoa in the epididymis or of vasal obstruction by vasography. In some patients small cysts are observed in the junctional area between the testis and epididymis, and in others the epididymis may appear disconnected from the testis. These are congenital abnormalities. The epididyms may appear normal, and there is a round cell infiltrate in the testicular biopsy of some patients. Steroid therapy may be helpful in such patients.

Epididymal obstruction, particularly when situated at the junction of the caput and cauda, may be due to congenital causes. This may be associated with chronic respiratory disorders (Young's syndrome) or the use of mercury teething powders, which are fortunately no longer available.

Gonococcal infection classically causes an obstructive lesion in the tail of the epididymis, but more severe infections may be associated with

Table 6.8: Site of Obstruction in Obstructive Azoospermia

Intratesticular	47 (15%)
Epididymis	163 (51%)
Bilateral vasa aplasia	58 (18%)
Unilateral vasa aplasia and other obstruction	11 (3%)
Vasal	39 (12%)
Ejaculatory duct	3 (1%)

multiple extensive blockages of the genital tract and a less favorable clinical outcome regarding fertility and other functions.

Bilateral congenital absence of the vas deferens is associated with an absence of the corpus and cauda epididymis. Up to 80 to 90% of men with cystic fibrosis have absent vasa. It is now recognized that healthy men with vasal aplasia may have the gene deletion associated with cystic fibrosis carrier status (40%) or the gene deletion on both chromosomes (10%).

EJACULATION

Ejaculation occurs immediately after orgasm but is not essential for that process. It requires an intact sympathetic nervous system and is generally considered to consist of two phases: the emission of semen into the posterior urethra and its propulsion to the exterior.

Spermatozoa enter the epididymis from the testis passively as a result of fluid production in the seminiferous tubule. This movement is facilitated by the action of cilia in the caput epididymis. It should be noted that this segment of epididymis is present in men with vasal aplasia—a wolffian duct abnormality associated with the congenital absence of the remainder of the epididymis, vas deferens, and seminal vesicles—and is often the site of obstruction in men with congenital obstruction of the epididymis. A little fluid may pass along the epididymis and vas under normal circumstances, but most occurs at the time of ejaculation due to contraction of the vas. The simultaneous contraction of the seminal vesicles flushes the sperm from the ejaculatory ducts into the prostatic urethra.

The origin of ejaculation is from sensory stimuli arising mainly from the genital areas, and this stimulation must reach sufficient intensity to stimulate the ejaculation center, which is postulated to be in the hypothalamus. Nocturnal emissions are thought to occur as a result of stimuli arising from the cerebral cortex. Efferent stimuli descend in the anterolateral columns of the spinal cord and exit through the anterior roots between the ninth thoracic and second lumbar segments to join the sympathetic chains. The afferent fibers pass through the ganglia in the lumbar para-aortic region and then via sympathetics that accompany blood vessels to the pelvic organs. These fibers can be damaged during retroperitoneal node dissections for testis tumors or during vascular operations on the distal aorta and common iliac vessels. Every attempt should be made to perform a nerve-sparing operation in those situations. The sympathetic fibers can also be damaged during bowel operations in the pelvis; this is important in young men, particularly those requiring surgery for benign disease.

Surgical interference with the sympathetic fibers results in variable effects depending on the fibers that are damaged. Extensive and high damage (para-aortic region) may lead to a failure of emission of semen. More distal damage may prevent closure of the bladder neck and result in retrograde ejaculation. Some recovery occurs following surgical damage to the sympathetic fibers, but this may take up to 2 years. In some patients it may be possible to induce ejaculation with sympathomimetic drugs, for example, Desipramine (a drug that blocks the reuptake of sympathomimetic amines). Electroejaculation may be used to overcome ejaculatory failure and is performed either by the presacral implantation of electrodes or by stimulating the pelvic sympathetic fibers with a rectal probe (electroejaculation). Erections can be achieved with transrectal stimulation in most patients. However, ejaculation occurs in only about two-thirds of patients. Retrograde ejaculation can be due to mechanical abnormalities of the bladder neck, for example, following transurethral prostatic resection. Propulsion of semen along the urethra requires closure of the bladder neck to prevent retrograde ejaculation and rhythmic contractions of the bulbospongiosus muscles, which are innervated through the internal pudendal nerves.

SEMEN TESTING

Semen analysis is of great importance in the assessment of the fertility status of the man. However, the analysis can never prove that a man is fertile, no matter how much technology is available. Sperm quality, rather than quantity, is of paramount importance. Unfortunately, no definitive test of quality is widely available. After cleansing the glans penis, the semen sample should be produced by masturbation and the fluid collected into a sterile, wide-mouthed nontoxic container. It is preferable that the sample be produced in close proximity to the laboratory so that it can be examined fresh, usually within 1 to 2 hours. Semen quality varies greatly, and it is important not to place too much emphasis on the result of a single sample. In order to study any changes in the quality of the semen, it is important to ensure a fixed period of abstinence; in practical terms this is usually 2 or 3 days. The World Health Organization (WHO) has published a useful monograph on semen analysis and has done much to standardize the techniques used and the interpretation of results. The WHO criteria for semen normality are listed in Table 6.9.

A reduced semen volume is usually associated with a deficiency of seminal vesicular or prostatic secretions. This may occur with a congenital or acquired androgen deficiency or be associated with a congenital

Table 6.9: WHO Criteria for Normal Semen Parameters

Volume	>2.0 ml
pH	7.2–7.8
Sperm concentration	>20 × 10^6 spermatozoa/ml
Total sperm count	>40 × 10^6 spermatozoa
Motility	>50% with forward progression or >25% with rapid linear progression within 60 minutes of collection
Morphology	>50% with normal morphology
Viability	>50% live, i.e., excluding dye
White blood cells	<1 × 10^6/ml
Zinc (total)	>2.4 μmol per ejaculate
Citric acid (total)	>52 μmol (10 mg) per ejaculate
Mixed agglutination reaction test	<10% of spermatozoa with adherent particles
Immunobead test	<10% of spermatozoa with adherent beads
Fructose (total)	>13 μmol per ejaculate

absence of the seminal vesicles and vasa, or with ejaculatory duct obstruction, the causes of which are shown in Table 6.10.

Sperm concentration correlates poorly with fertility, and in many respects it is better to consider the total number of sperm in the ejaculate as this eliminates the variability of ejaculate volume. The number of sperm in the ejaculate varies, and the distribution appears to be on a log

Table 6.10: Causes of Ejaculatory Duct Obstruction (101 men)

Etiology	*Number*
Congenital	
Müllerian duct abnormality	17
Wolffian duct abnormality	19
Traumatic	15
Postinfective	
Tuberculous	8
Other	19
Adynamic	
Megavesicles	8
Ejaculatory dyskinesia	13
Neoplastic	2
Total	101

normal basis, as is found with other biological variables. It is useful to consider the significance of sperm concentration on fertility (Table 6.11). The association between the specificity and sensitivity of sperm numbers with regard to fertility is poor. In this respect it is useful to consider the prognostic significance of sperm numbers; that is, sperm counts of less than 2 million/ml are rarely associated with fertility.

Sperm Motility

Defects in motility are undoubtedly the cause of much male infertility. Estimation of the percentage of motile sperm with flagellar motion is not difficult, but of greater importance is the assessment of forward or progressive motility. This assessment may be carried out subjectively by trained technicians or objectively by computer analysis. The opinion of an experienced observer is more useful than the more expensive computer-generated printouts. It should be noted that the WHO classification of progressive motility tends to be replaced by a grading scale from 0 to 4 (0 = no motility; 4 = excellent straight-line motility). Computerized semen analysis may be quick, provide additional data, and add interest for the laboratory technician, but it is also expensive and does not provide a better assessment of fertility. This is because the critical assessment of the semen lies in the number of normal sperm with good progressive motility. Even in a normal sample, the number of sperm with good fertilizing capacity is probably only a small proportion of the total sperm ejaculated.

Defects in sperm motility may occur as a result of congenital abnormalities, for example, lack of dynein arms in the sperm tail (Kartagener's or the "immotile cilia" syndrome). In this condition, the affected man has immobile sperm and suffers from frequent respiratory tract infections and situs inversus. Genital tract infections (a more alkaline pH, increased number of white cells and organisms on culture) or sperm antibody production also results in impaired sperm motility. Although epidemiologic evidence suggests that genital tract infections (e.g., chlamydia, mycoplasma) are linked to infertility, direct evidence of this association is less than compelling. An association between antisperm antibody types and infertility is

Table 6.11: Significance of Sperm Concentration on Fertility

Total Number of Sperm in Ejaculate ($\times 10^6$)	*Interpretation*
Zero	Infertile
<1	Probably infertile
1–10	Some impairment of fertility
≥10	May be fertile

well known. Antibodies impair sperm transport through the cervical mucus, cause agglutination of spermatozoa, and may also prevent fertilization of the ovum. Antisperm antibodies can be assayed in the serum or more directly, on the spermatozoa themselves, using the Immunobead Assay. Infertile men with documented immunologically mediated infertility can be treated with corticosteroid immunosuppression.

It is important that the semen is not produced into a condom (which contains a spermicide) and that it is not chilled while being transported to the laboratory. When all the spermatozoa are immotile, it is important to perform a live/dead stain in order to assess sperm viability.

Sperm Morphology

The value of sperm morphology assessment in infertile men is debatable as it is the subject of significant observer bias. Round-headed sperm lacking acrosomal caps are incapable of fertilizing ova. The greater the proportion of abnormal sperm forms (amorphous, tapered, large- and small-headed), the greater the likelihood of impaired fertility. A normal ejaculate contains more than 60% of normal sperm forms. Electron microscopic examination occasionally demonstrates the cause for infertility (e.g., lack of dynein arm in the sperm tail) but is not otherwise of great value.

SPERM TRANSPORT IN THE FEMALE GENITAL TRACT AND FERTILIZATION

The deposition of sperm in the vagina is facilitated by normal potency (see Chapter 7) and ejaculation. Spermatozoa readily pass through the cervical canal and uterine cavity to fertilize the oocytes in the fallopian tube. The postcoital test is the single best test of cervical mucus–sperm interaction and fertility. The presence of many motile sperms (usually 10 to 20/hpf) is an excellent prognostic sign. A poor postcoital cervical mucus test—no sperm or absent motility—may be the result of failure of coital technique, suboptimal timing of the test, defective sperm motility, antisperm antibodies, or cervical mucus hostility. Bovine cervical mucus may allow better standardization of the sperm–mucus interaction and result in better reproducibility.

Antisperm Antibodies

Antisperm antibodies are probably nonspecific and impair fertility in a variety of ways. The testicular germ cells in the seminiferous tubules are separated from the rest of the body by the blood–testis barrier. Spermatozoa are not produced until puberty, by which time the body's immune system is mature. Spermatozoa are therefore recognized as "foreign," and if they enter the body, the immune system responds by producing antisperm antibodies. These antibodies may be agglutinating or spermicidal in nature. The specific nature of antisperm antibodies has not been completely elucidated. The presence of antisperm antibodies may be particularly suspected in couples with unexplained infertility or poor postcoital tests. The semen analysis may be poor and show sperm agglutination. The mixed agglutination reaction (MAR) test is rapid and useful for screening. However, it is of value only if the sperm have good motility. Tray agglutination tests remain the standard technique for measuring antisperm antibodies, and the correlation between these and the results of immunobead testing is uncertain. Antisperm antibodies contribute to reduced fertility in approximately 5 to 10% of infertile couples. Antisperm antibodies prevent sperm migration through the female genital tract and therefore interfere with fertilization. Bilateral vasectomy is associated with the formation of antisperm antibodies in about 50% of men. Antisperm antibodies may be produced in response to, for example, testicular torsion, ductal obstructions, or infections. However, the effect of antisperm antibodies on fertility after vasectomy reversal is uncertain and only of significance when they are present in the blood at high titers (1:512 or greater). These high serum concentrations are associated with significant titers in seminal plasma after vasectomy reversal. For these reasons, it is customary to ignore the possibility of antisperm antibodies after a vasectomy reversal until the couple have been trying to conceive for 1 year (less if the woman is more than 35 years old).

Varicocele

The pathogenetic role of varicoceles in fertility remains open to dispute. The current popularity of varicocele ligation is based on the finding of Tulloch that bilateral varicocele ligation in an azoospermic man improved fertility. The testicular biopsies at the time of the operation showed a spermatogenic arrest, and following treatment of the varicoceles sperm appeared in the ejaculate and the man fathered four children. He later returned for bilateral vasectomy, and the testicular biopsies showed normal spermatogenesis.

No one disputes that pregnancies occur following varicocele ligation, but controlled trials suggest that these may be no more than those expected from any new form of treatment. Our understanding has been hampered by the lack of a controlled trial—who would agree to have a placebo operation? Many pathophysiological explanations have been suggested; the most generally accepted is that there is an adverse effect on spermatogenesis as a result of the raised temperature of the scrotal contents (Table 6.12). It has been suggested that a varicocele—and size may

Table 6.12: Varicoceles and Infertility

Prevalence	*Etiology*	*Pathogenesis of Impaired Spermatogenesis*
15% in "normal" adult men 40% in infertile male population Usually left-sided Bilateral 5–10%	Valvular incompetence in spermatic vein "Nutcracker" phenomenon	Elevated scrotal temperature (bilateral) Toxic metabolites from kidney, adrenal Catecholamines Steroids Prostaglandins

not be important—may cause infertility by depressing spermatogenesis, impairing sperm motility, or by a more subtle interference with the sperm fertilizing function acting through the epididymis. None of these theories is proven, and it is important to maintain an open mind on the subject while awaiting scientific evidence.

Approximately 15% of normal, healthy adult men have a varicocele. Most varicoceles are left-sided, although bilateral varicoceles occur in between 5 and 10% of patients. However, in an infertile male population, varicoceles contribute to infertility in 40%. Although the anatomical defect is usually unilateral, the effect on spermatogenesis is frequently bilateral. Recent experience suggests that varicocele ligation in puberty can result in an increase in testicular size as well as improved spermatogenesis.

Fertilization and Unexplained Infertility

Fertilization is a complex process that occurs in the fallopian tube. To ensure their fertility potential, sperm need to undergo various changes after they are produced in the testes. Capacitation is essential in this regard, and this process is reversible. Capacitation reflects a stage of epididymal sperm maturation associated with changes in composition of the sperm and a more stable cell membrane. This process is reversed in the female genital tract at the time of the acrosome reaction prior to fertilization. During the acrosome reaction a complex series of changes occur in the sperm head which permit the passage of enzymes out of the sperm and the facilitation of sperm binding to the oocyte. Changes in sperm motility (increased hyperactivity) precede the acrosome reaction and are considered essential to the ability of the spermatozoa to penetrate the cumulus mass around the oocyte. Failure of spermatozoa to fertilize eggs was long suspected but only detected as a cause for infertility through use of the zona-free hamster egg penetration test. This investigated the ability of spermatozoa, after a suitable period of culture to allow sperm capacitation, to penetrate zona follucida free hamster eggs. This bioassay is unfortunately poorly standardized, although sperm penetration of 10 to 30% of ova is usually regarded as normal. There is no consensus on the usefulness or interpretation of the sperm penetration assay (SPA). The test is time-consuming, and it has been abandoned in favor of in vitro fertilization, where it is possible to study the fertilizing capacity of human sperm and ova.

ASSISTED CONCEPTION

In 1978, the first "test tube" baby was born in Oldham, England. Since then, thousands of babies have been born using this technique, and other, newer, techniques of assisted reproduction have been developed. The process depends on hyperstimulation of the female partner to produce eggs, which are then retrieved by laparoscopy or needle aspiration under ultrasound control. The eggs (usually no more than three) may be placed together with sperm, in the fallopian tube (gamete intrafallopian tube transfer (GIFT) or additional eggs cultured with sperm in-vitro (in vitro fertilization (IVF)). Individual oocytes are observed for 24 hours, and the developing embryos are transferred back into the uterus or fallopian tube at 48 to 72 hours. It is considered unethical to replace more than three or four embryos on each occasion, and spare embryos may be frozen and used for subsequent cycles should pregnancy not occur. The couple should have a realistic appreciation of the chances of having a child by assisted conception and realize that there is a 25% chance of miscarriage. There is little variation in the pregnancy rate when the concentration of motile sperms is in the range of 1 to 50 million/m. It is the number of sperm with good progressive motility that is important. Pregnancies usually do not occur unless there is progressive sperm motility. The quality of the sperm preparation is improved by removal of the seminal plasma using a layering technique with a Percoll gradient. This provides useful prognostic information in infertile couples. The overall pregnancy rates with assisted reproductive techniques are listed in Table 6.13.

Additional Techniques

Techniques for assisted conception have undergone steady refinement during the past decade (Table 6.14). In 1984, sperm obtained during open surgery in an azoospermic man resulted in fertilization of his wife. Techniques of sperm retrieval in azoospermic men are continually being refined. Up to 20% of women whose husbands have vasal aplasia can become pregnant as the result of microsurgical sperm aspiration and transfer.

Attempts to improve the fertilization rate for men with extreme

Table 6.13: Percentage Chance of a Live Birth (or Ongoing Pregnancy Nearing Delivery) in Women Undergoing a Cycle of Assisted Conception

Sperm Concentration (Number Motile × 10^6/ml)	*Number*	*Births (%)*
<1	32	4 (12.5)
1–4.9	75	16 (21)
5–9.9	83	20 (24)
10–19.9	193	55 (28.5)
20–49.9	551	162 (29)
≥50	149	55 (37)

oligozoospermia have been made by injecting the sperm directly into ova with altered zona pellucidas. These micromanipulation techniques will improve further over the next decade, and they have already rendered obsolete the technique of implanting sperm reservoirs.

Table 6.14: Assisted Conception Techniques

Sperm Manipulation In Vivo	*Sperm and Ova Manipulation In Vivo*	*Sperm and Ova Manipulation In Vitro*
Artificial insemination (AI) Intrauterine Cervical, vaginal Intraperitoneal	Gamete intrafallopian transfer (GIFT)	In-vitro fertilization with embryo transfer (IVF) Zygote intrafallopian transfer (ZIFT) Tubal embryo transfer (TEF) Micromanipulation techniques

SUGGESTED READINGS

Ford TF, Parkinson MC, Pryor JP. The undescended testis in adult life. Br J Urol 1985; 57:181.

A review of the incidence of carcinoma-in-situ and spermatogenesis in the adult undescended testis.

Johnsen SG. Testicular biopsy score count: a method for registration of spermatogenesis in the human testis: normal values and results in 335 hypogonadal males. Hormones 1970; 1:2.

Description of a useful technique to provide quantitative reports on testicular histology for the assessment of spermatogenesis.

Silber SS, Ord T, Balmaceda J, Patrizio T, Asch RH. Congenital absence of the vas deferens: the fertilizing capacity of human epididymal sperm. N Engl J Med 1990; 323:1788.

Demonstrates that a useful pregnancy rate can be achieved by microsurgical sperm retrieval from the epididymis.

Hellstrom WF, Overstreet JW, Samuels SJ, Lewis EL. The relationship of circulating antisperm antibodies to sperm surface antibodies in infertile men. J Urol 1988; 140:1039.

The immunobead test for antisperm antibodies is described and the potential role of antisperm antibodies in infertility discussed.

Smith RG, Johnson A, Lamb DJ, Lipshultz LI. Functional tests of spermatozoa: sperm penetration assay. Urol Clin North Am 1987; 14:451.

Concise review of the hamster oocyte penetration test. Technique, indications, and limitations are discussed. This test is probably the best in vitro test of sperm fertilizing capacity.

MacLeod J. Seminal cytology in the presence of varicocele. Fertil Steril 1965; 16:735.

Landmark study describing the "classic" semen abnormalities in varicocele—the so-called "stress pattern" of MacLeod.

Schoysman RJ, Bedford JM. The role of the human epididymis in sperm maturation and sperm storage as reflected in the consequences of epididymo-vasostomy. Fertil Steril 1986; 46:293.

Describes the outcome in a large group of patients undergoing reconstructive epididymal surgery. Particular emphasis on the acquisition of fertilizing capacity in the epididymis.

Liu DY, Baker HWG. Tests of sperm function and fertilization in vitro. Fertil Steril 1992; 58:465.

Comparison of the results of computer-assisted semen analysis, acrosome function, and sperm penetration of heterologous oocytes compared to in vitro fertilization rates.

Takihara H, Sakatoku J, Cockett ATK. The pathophysiology of varicocele in male infertility. Fertil Steril 1991; 55:861.

Discussion of the factors involved in the pathophysiology of varicocele-associated subfertility. Excellent synopsis of current hypotheses.

Howards SS. Subclinical varicocele. Fertil Steril 1992; 57:725–726.

Useful short review of the varicocele controversy presented from a more skeptical standpoint. Raises fundamental questions regarding the relationship of varicoceles to fertility.

Pryor JP, Hendry WF. Ejaculatory duct obstruction in subfertile males: analysis of 87 patients. Fertil Steril 56:735.

Review of this uncommon condition. The prevalence of genital-tract obstruction may well have been underestimated in the past. Diagnosis, evaluation, and treatment are all well discussed.

Hendry WF, Hughes L, Scamell G, Pryor JP, Hargreave TB. Comparison of prednisolone and placebo in subfertile men with antibodies to spermatozoa. Lancet 1990; 335:85.

Addresses the role of steroids in the treatment of subfertile men with antisperm antibodies.

CHAPTER 7

Penile Function

Michael P. O'Leary
Tom F. Lue

Penile erection and detumescence involve numerous, complex anatomic and physiologic processes. Knowledge of the normal anatomic, neurologic, and endocrine functions responsible for this aspect of male sexual function is essential to an understanding of the common urologic problem of erectile dysfunction. Over the last 10 years, there has been a remarkable explosion of knowledge pertaining to the pathophysiology of erection and impotence. These advances have led to a variety of new approaches to the diagnosis and treatment of erectile impotence.

Although the true prevalence of impotence is unknown, estimates place it at 10 million men in the United States. The incidence almost certainly increases with age, and the true prevalence may be closer to 30 million affected individuals. Patients with underlying conditions such as diabetes and peripheral vascular disease are at particular risk for the development of erectile dysfunction. An organic problem can now be identified in between 70 and 85% of men with impotence. Purely psychogenic impotence is now an uncommon diagnosis—a clear contradistinction to the situation 20 years ago, when organic impotence was infrequently diagnosed.

Impotence is the result of complex, interrelated pathophysiologies involving venous, arterial, sinusoidal, hormonal, biochemical, neurologic, social, and psychological factors. Risk factors for impotence include hypertension, diabetes mellitus, atherosclerosis, alcohol excess, smoking, and the use of such medications as antihypertensives and sedatives. Diabetes mellitus, the second most common cause of organic impotence, after vascular disease, in the United States, affects an estimated 2 million men. Erectile dysfunction affects between 35 and 75% of diabetic men, and it tends to be progressive with time.

ANATOMY OF THE PENIS

The penis is composed of three cylindrical structures surrounded by a thick fascial sheath known as Buck's fascia. These three cylinders are the paired corpora cavernosa and the corpus spongiosum (Figure 7.1). The corpus spongiosum, the "urethral body," has a similar histologic architecture to that of the paired corporal bodies, with smooth muscle arranged in sinusoids and lined by endothelium. The spongiosum, however, lacks a dynamic role in erection. The sinusoidal spaces of the spongiosum are larger and contain less smooth muscle than the sinusoidal spaces in the corpora cavernosa. The proximal ends of the corpora cavernosa, the crura, arise as two separate structures from the undersurface of the puboischial rami but then merge at the undersurface of the pubic arch and remain attached distally up to the glans penis. Surrounding the corpus cavernosum is a thick envelope, the tunica albuginea, composed of layers of wavy collagen and elastic fibers. These allow a considerable degree of

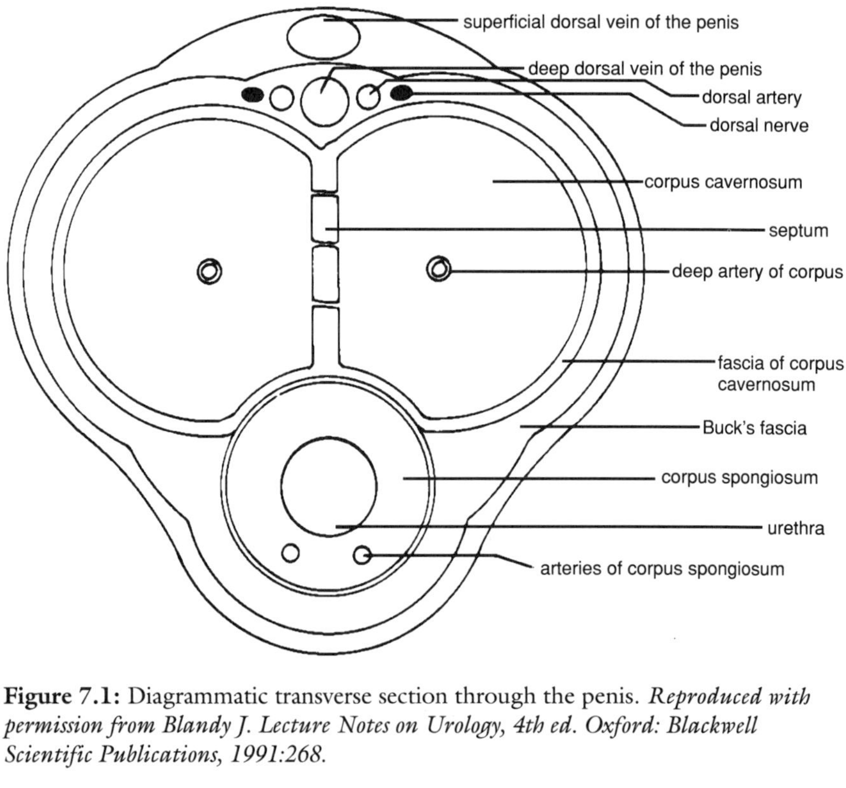

Figure 7.1: Diagrammatic transverse section through the penis. *Reproduced with permission from Blandy J. Lecture Notes on Urology, 4th ed. Oxford: Blackwell Scientific Publications, 1991:268.*

elongation and expansion during erection and maintain the structural integrity of the penis. The tunical covering is complete except where pierced by arteries and nerves, which are surrounded by a sheath of loose areolar tissue that protects them from compression during tumescence.

The emissary veins from the corpora are in direct contact with the tunica albuginea and thus can be easily occluded by the shearing action of the tunical layers during erection. The tunica encases the erectile cavernosal tissue, whose spongelike pattern is composed of multiple interconnected lacunar (or sinusoidal) spaces lined by vascular endothelium. These lacunar walls are formed by the trabeculae, which are thick bundles of smooth muscle admixed with collagen, elastin, and fibroblasts.

The urethra lies in a ventral groove formed by the paired corpora cavernosa and is surrounded by the corpus spongiosum. Distally the corpus spongiosum forms the cone-shaped glans penis. The sinusoids of the corpus spongiosum are larger in diameter with a thinner tunica, which is altogether absent where spongiosum becomes the glans penis.

PENILE ARTERIAL SUPPLY

The internal pudendal arteries are the main blood supply to the penis. Occasionally, accessory arteries arising from the external iliac or obturator vessels may become the dominant arterial supply to the corpus cavernosum. The internal pudendal artery becomes the penile artery after giving off a branch to the perineum. The three branches of the penile artery are the dorsal, bulbourethral (or spongiosal), and cavernosal arteries. The cavernosal artery enters the corpus cavernosum at the hilum of the penis where the crura merge. At the penile base, the cavernous artery is close to the septum, while in the middle and distal penis it becomes centrally located. Multiple helicine arteries supplying the trabecular tissue and sinusoids arise along its course. These arteries are contracted and quite tortuous in the flaccid state but become dilated and straight during erection. The helicine arteries (diameter 150 to 350 μm) branch off the cavernosal artery as multiple, muscular, corkscrew-shaped vessels that then open directly into the lacunar spaces and function as "resistors" to control the inflow of blood into the penis. The helicine arteries play a crucial role in the regulation of penile rigidity and flaccidity. The dorsal artery accompanies the deep dorsal vein between the tunica albuginea and Buck's fascia. It joins the spongiosal artery at the glans.

The entire corpus cavernosum is a conglomeration of sinusoids among the interwoven trabeculae of smooth muscles and supporting connective tissue that harbor the terminal cavernous nerves and helicine arterioles. The sinusoids are larger toward the center than at the periphery. In the flaccid state blood diffuses slowly from the central to the peripheral sinusoids with oxygen levels similar to that of venous blood. However, during erection the rapid entry of arterial blood to both the central and peripheral sinusoids alters this milieu.

PENILE VENOUS DRAINAGE

In the peripheral sinusoidal spaces immediately beneath the tunica albuginea, small subtunical venules drain the corpora. These venules travel in the trabeculae between the tunica and the peripheral sinusoids and form the subtunical venular plexus before coalescing into emissary veins that pierce the tunica albuginea. In the body of the penis the majority of these veins exit dorsally into the deep dorsal vein or laterally to the circumflex veins that then join the deep dorsal vein. Some exit ventrally to join the periurethral veins.

In the proximal corpora cavernosa and the crus of the penis, emissary veins follow an independent drainage pathway into the cavernosal veins. In the proximal crus, crural veins join the urethral veins and drain directly into the internal pudendal vein.

In the glans penis, because of the absence of a tunica, the sinusoids empty directly into a complex of veins forming the retrocorporal plexus. This is the origin of the deep dorsal vein. As it courses cephalad, the deep dorsal vein also receives a number of circumflex veins, and these eventually ascend behind the pubic bone and become the periprostatic plexus. The superficial dorsal veins are small vessels in the subcutaneous layer that drain the skin and generally empty into the saphenous vein. Each cavernosal vein originates at the penile hilum, courses through the penile crus, and then drains into the preprostatic venous plexus.

Thus, the deep dorsal and cavernosal venous drainage systems are independent, although they occasionally communicate via small connecting branches. Venous drainage from the cavernosal bodies is separate from that of the glans penis and corpus spongiosum.

NEUROANATOMY AND NEUROPHYSIOLOGY OF THE PENIS

Both psychogenic and reflexogenic mechanisms control penile erection. A "reflex" erection is mediated by a spinal reflex pathway. The efferent limb arises in the sacral parasympathetic center and proceeds via the pelvic nerves into the erectile tissue. The afferent limb comprises sensory penile/glandular receptors that join the pudendal nerve to reach the sacral spinal cord. Psychogenic erection results from the effects of psychogenic (visual, tactile, auditory) stimuli on the brain. These stimuli are integrated in the hypothalamus and control neural penile outflow via the thoracolumbar sympathetic and sacral parasympathetic spinal cord centers. A sensory stimulus from the penis travels along the paired dorsal nerves through the genitourinary diaphragm and joins the perineal nerve, which forms the pudendal nerve. This nerve joins the branches of S2, S3, and S4 and enters the dorsal roots of the spinal segments. These pudendal afferent fibers terminate in the medial dorsal horn and dorsal commissure of the sacral spinal cord. Information then passes through the spinal thalamic tract to the thalamus and sensory cortex for sensory perception. The supraspinal area presumed to be responsible for erection is the medial preoptic area. Efferent pathways from this area enter the medial forebrain bundle in the midbrain tegmental region. Pathological processes in these regions of the brain, such as Parkinson's disease or cerebral vascular accident, are often associated with impotence.

The parasympathetic nerve fibers to the penis arise from neurons in the intermediolateral cell columns of the second, third, and fourth sacral spinal cord segments. The preganglionic pelvic nerves (nervi erigentes) join the pelvic plexus, where they are joined by sympathetic nerves from the hypogastric plexus. The cavernous nerves containing parasympathetic and sympathetic fibers are branches of the pelvic plexus that innervate the penis. They course posterolateral to the apex of the prostate at the 5 and 7 o'clock positions and then become lateral to the membranous urethra at the 3 and 9 o'clock positions. Distally, at the level of the bulbar urethra, the nerves course anteriorly at 1 and 11 o'clock positions, where they finally enter the hilum of the penis. A clear understanding of the path of these nerves is essential to the prevention of iatrogenic impotence during prostatic and urethral surgery.

The sympathetic nerves originate from the eleventh thoracic to the second lumbar spinal segment and descend through the preaortic plexus and abdominal chains to the superior and inferior hypogastric plexuses. Branches from these communicate with parasympathetic nerve fibers to form the cavernous nerves. In animal models, stimulation of the pelvic plexus and the cavernous nerves induces erection, while stimulation of the hypogastric nerve or the sympathetic trunk causes detumescence. Thus, the sacral parasympathetic input is responsible for erection, and the thoracolumbar sympathetic pathway controls detumescence.

Tactile stimulation of the penis produces an erection in normal men and in patients with suprasacral spinal cord lesions but not in patients with sacral injury. These reflexogenic erections result from impulses that reach the spinal erection center (S2 to S4 and T10 to L2). Some impulses then follow the ascending tract and result in sensory perception, while others activate the autonomic nuclei to send messages via the cavernous nerves to the penis to induce an erection. This type of erection is preserved in patients with upper spinal cord injury. On the other hand, psychogenic erections may be provoked by audiovisual stimuli or cognitive thought. Signals descend from the brain to the spinal erection center to activate the erectile process. This type of erection is preserved in only a small percentage of patients with complete sacral cord lesions, suggesting that the sacral erection center is the main locus of erectile nuclei. The mechanisms for nocturnal erections occurring during rapid eye movement (REM) sleep are not clear.

HEMODYNAMIC MECHANISMS OF ERECTION

The hemodynamic changes during penile erection, detumescence, and flaccidity have recently been elucidated. During erection, the penis functions as a volume capacitor that accumulates blood under pressure.

The flaccid penis is in a moderate state of contraction and is under the dominant influence of the sympathetic nervous system. Flaccidity is characterized by contraction of the terminal arterioles and sinusoidal smooth muscles. The minimal blood flow through the sinusoidal spaces—approximately 2.5 to 8.0 ml/min/100 g of tissue—is only enough to serve the nutritional needs of the penile corporal tissues. In the flaccid state, the contracted penile smooth muscle provides maximal resistance to arterial blood inflow (Figure 7.2). Smooth muscle contraction in the flaccid penis is tonically mediated by alpha-adrenergic nerves (Table 7.1). Although both alpha$_1$- and alpha$_2$-adrenergic receptor subtypes have been identified in the corpus cavernosum, alpha$_1$-adrenergic stimulation appears to be the predominant mechanism for trabecular and arteriolar smooth-muscle contraction in the flaccid penis. During detumescence, increased sympathetic input causes a reduction in arterial blood inflow, collapse of the lacunar spaces, decompression of the subtunical venules, and increased drainage of the corporal bodies (Table 7.1).

For erection to occur, the penile arteries and the cavernosal trabecular smooth muscle must relax. Smooth muscle relaxation is regulated by

Table 7.1: Penile Detumescence Mechanism

Smooth muscle contraction
Alpha$_1$-adrenergic receptors
Increased venous blood egress
Reduced penile arterial inflow

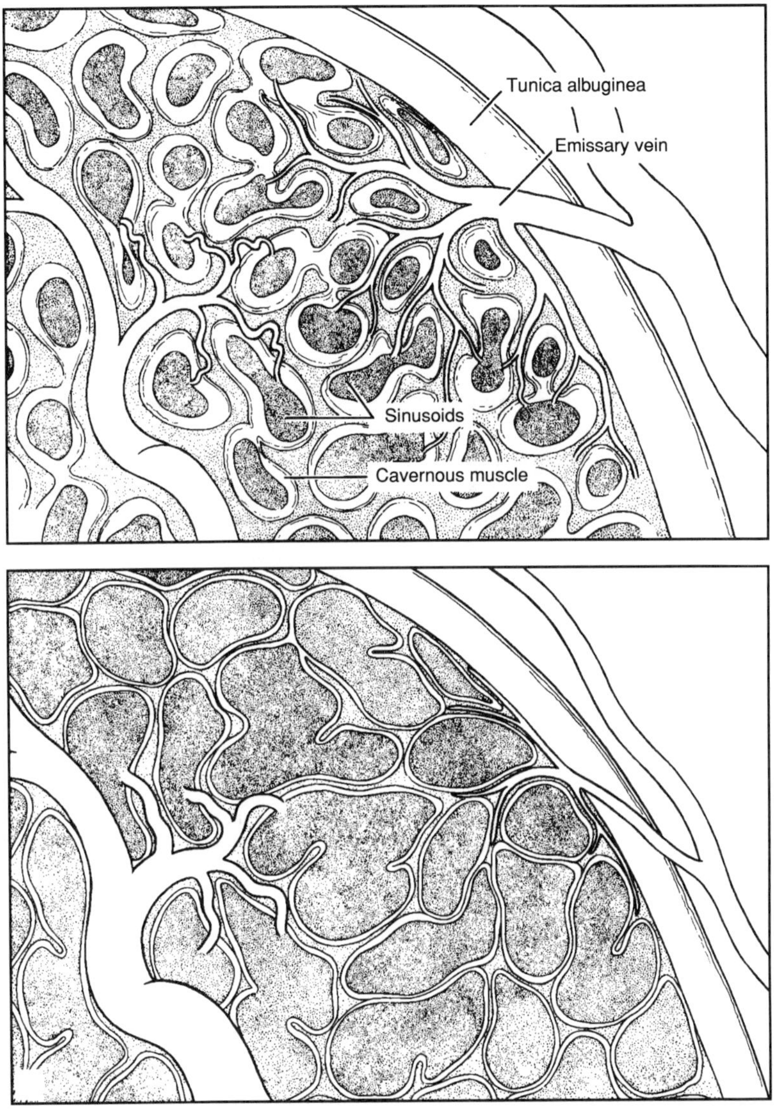

Figure 7.2: Mechanism of penile erection. In the flaccid state (a), the arteries, arterioles, and sinusoids are contracted. The intersinusoidal and subtunical venules are open with free flow to the emissary veins. During erection (b), the muscles of the sinusoidal wall and the arterioles relax, allowing maximal flow to fill the now compliant sinusoidal spaces. The small venules are compressed between sinusoids. The larger intermediary venules are sandwiched and compressed between the distended sinusoidal wall and the noncompliant tunica albuginea thus restricts the venous flow to a minimum. (After Lue). *Reproduced with permission from Webster G, Kirby K, King L, et al eds. Reconstructive Urology Vol 1. Boston: Blackwell Scientific Publications, 1993:75.*

a number of neuroeffector mechanisms. This increases the compliance of the sinusoids, causes dilatation of the helicine arteries, and results in increased arterial flow into the penis. Dilation of the penile arterioles is probably the first physiologic event leading to an erection. This results in reduced arterial resistance and increased penile blood flow and pressure. This decreased vascular resistance is mediated predominantly via cholinergic nerves. Erection is initiated by the sacral parasympathetic nerves in which the preganglionic neurotransmitter is acetylcholine. However, a number of experiments have demonstrated that the postganglionic neurotransmitter that mediates erection is a nonadrenergic, noncholinergic (NANC) neurotransmitter.

Cholinergic nerve endings are present in the corpus cavernosum. However, they do not mediate relaxation of trabecular smooth muscle by means of postjunctional receptors. Instead, the may contribute to relaxation of penile cavernosal smooth muscle via endothelium-dependent mechanisms. This event is mediated by one or more neurotransmitters.

Unlike other vascular organs, the penis requires arterial inflow and perfusion in addition to venous outflow obstruction for proper function, i.e., erection (Table 7.2). A key to understanding penile outflow resistance is the corporal veno-occlusive mechanism. Empirical observations and recent experimental studies have confirmed the critical roles of smooth muscle in the regulation of erectile function. The smooth muscles of the cavernosal/helicine arteries control penile blood inflow, whereas the smooth muscle of the trabeculae controls veno-occlusion. Furthermore, the endothelium lining the lacunar spaces contributes to trabecular smooth muscle tone.

Table 7.2: Penile Erection Mechanisms

Smooth muscle relaxation	
	Trabeculae
	Penile, helicine arteries
Veno-occlusion	
	Subtunical venules
	Emissary veins
Increased penile blood inflow	
	Dilation of lacunar spaces
	Cavernosal arterial inflow
Appropriate psychologic, hormonal milieu	
	Prolactin, testosterone
	Libido
	Stimuli

In the flaccid penis, the arterioles and sinusoids are contracted while the subtunical venules drain freely into the emissary veins. During erection, arterial and trabecular smooth muscles relax and result in decreased arteriolar resistance and an increase in arterial inflow and corporal perfusion. The systemic blood pressure is now directly transmitted through the cavernosal and helicine arteries to the lacunar spaces, which become engorged with blood. The expanded lacunar spaces then compress the subtunical venules against the relatively noncompressible tunica albuginea, resulting in venous outflow resistance and corporal veno-occlusion. With further engorgement, the uneven stretching of the layers of the tunical albuginea further closes off most of the emissary veins in the pendulous portion of the penis.

Dysfunction of the corporal veno-occlusive hemodynamic mechanism may contribute to or cause erectile impotence. Such dysfunction is due to insufficient trabecular smooth muscle relaxation and decreased tissue compliance as a result of alterations in the fibroelastic components of the trabeculae, for example, secondary to vascular risk factors, smoking, or diabetes. Veno-occlusive dysfunction from ineffective compression of the subtunical venules causes reduced venous outflow resistance, increased venous egress from the corporeal bodies, and failure to maintain a rigid erection. Restriction to venous outflow is a passive phenomenon mediated via compression of the venular plexus against the rigid tunica albuginea. Neurogenically mediated, direct venoconstriction, although postulated as a further mechanism of venous outflow restriction, has not been demonstrated.

Trabecular smooth muscle tone is an important regulatory mechanism of corporal veno-occlusion. Dilator autonomic nerves and an endothelium-derived relaxing factor (EDRF) control the relaxation of the trabecular smooth muscles of the corpora cavernosa. Chemical stimulation (e.g., acetylcholine, bradykinin) or physical shear stresses causes release of EDRF from the vascular endothelium. This local paracrine hormone diffuses to underlying smooth muscle and causes relaxation. There is now convincing evidence that EDRF from corporal tissue is nitric oxide (NO). NO can be synthesized in endothelial cells from L-arginine under the influence of nitric oxide synthase released from nonadrenergic, noncholinergic nerves or produced in the endothelium by neurotransmitter (e.g., acetylcholine, substance P) stimulation. Human cavernosal tissue relaxation is abolished by blockade of nitric oxide synthase, and this inhibition is reversible by administration of excess L-arginine. Immunohistochemical studies have shown a wide distribution of nitric oxide synthase (NOS) in the genitourinary tract—the penis, bladder neck, pelvic nerve ganglia, and membranous urethra. Nitric oxide may well be the crucial neurotransmitter involved in erection (Table 7.3). Nitric oxide relaxes smooth muscle by stimulating the formation of cyclic 3',5' guanosine monophosphate (cGMP) via the activation of guanylyl cyclase. This in turn stimulates protein phosphorylation by cGMP-dependent protein kinase, which results in reduction of cytosolic free calcium (Ca^{++}) and muscle relaxation.

The 28 amino-acid vasoactive intestinal polypeptide (VIP) has been proposed as a mediator of NANC neurotransmission and trabecular smooth muscle relaxation (Table 7.4). VIP may be a direct dilator or may function via stimulation of endothelial cell nitric oxide synthesis. In the penis, VIP and NO may function as cotransmitters. However, it appears that VIP is not the principal neurotransmitter in penile erection. Other chemical neurotransmitters function as modulators of corporal contraction, flaccidity, and detumescence (Table 7.4). Endothelin-1, a potent vasoconstrictor peptide synthesized by the endothelium of the human corpus cavernosum, causes sustained contraction of corporal smooth muscle. The endothelins may help to maintain penile flaccidity by providing sustained tone to the trabecular smooth muscle.

The human corpus cavernosum synthesizes a variety of prostaglandins including PGH_{2F}, PGE_2, PGI_2, and thromboxane. PGE_2 may promote relaxation of trabecular smooth muscle, whereas the other endogenous prostaglandins may cause constriction or have no effect on smooth muscle tone. The antiplatelet-aggregating property of PGI_2 released by the endothelium may be important in preventing coagulation during erection.

Various phases of penile erection have been characterized (Figure 7.3). The flaccid state is characterized by minimal blood flow in the cavernosum; that is, the cavernosal arterial diameter is 0.05 cm with a peak flow velocity of 15 cm/sec. Blood flow is highest in the latent (filling) phase—artery diameter 0.1 cm, peak flow velocity of 30 cm/sec with penile elongation and increased blood flow in the pudendal artery. The

Table 7.3: Nitric Oxide Neurotransmitter

Formed from L-arginine
Synthesis controlled by nitric oxide synthase (NOS)
NO released by endothelium, dilator nerves
NO is key mediator of penile smooth muscle relaxation
Endothelial release NO (EDRF)
Chemical stimulation
Physical forces
NOS widely distributed in penile vascular endothelium and adventitial nerves of penile arteries

Table 7.4: Penile Smooth Muscle Contractility

Neuroeffector systems
Adrenergic
Cholinergic
Nonadrenergic, noncholinergic (NANC)
Endothelium-derived vasoactivators
Nitric oxide
Endothelin
Prostaglandins
$PGE_{2\alpha}$, $TBXA_2$
Smooth muscle relaxation
Nonadrenergic, noncholinergic (NANC) neurotransmitter
Nitric oxide (previously EDRF) released by nerves, vascular endothelium
Vasoactive intestinal polypeptide (VIP)
? cotransmitter
Cholinergic innervation of endothelium leads to release of nitric oxide
Prostaglandins
Smooth muscle contraction
$Alpha_1$-adrenergic neurotransmitter
Endothelin-1

intracorporeal pressure increases during the tumescence phase, in which the penis expands and maximally elongates. Further increases, up to 90% of systolic pressure, in corporal pressure characterize the full erection phase with a rigid, straight penis. Blood is then trapped by the expanding sinusoids, which continue to elongate and expand. The subtunical venular plexuses become compressed against the tunica albuginea, reducing venous outflow. Once the tunica albuginea is stretched to its maximum, the emissary veins between the tunical layers are further compressed, maximally decreasing venous outflow. Intracavernous pressure is thus maintained at approximately 100 mm Hg.

Penile thrusting or stimulation of the glans penis triggers the bulbocavernosus reflex with contraction of the striated, ischiocavernosus muscles at the base of the penile shaft. This results in further restriction of venous outflow and an increased intracorporeal pressure well above systolic pressure. There is no inflow of blood during this rigid erection phase. Skeletal muscle fatigue limits the duration of this phase and prevents tissue ischemia and damage. Thus erection involves sinusoidal relaxation, arterial dilatation, and venous compression. During detumescence, tonic sympathetic discharges contract trabecular smooth muscle, reopen the venous outflow channels, and constrict the arterioles to

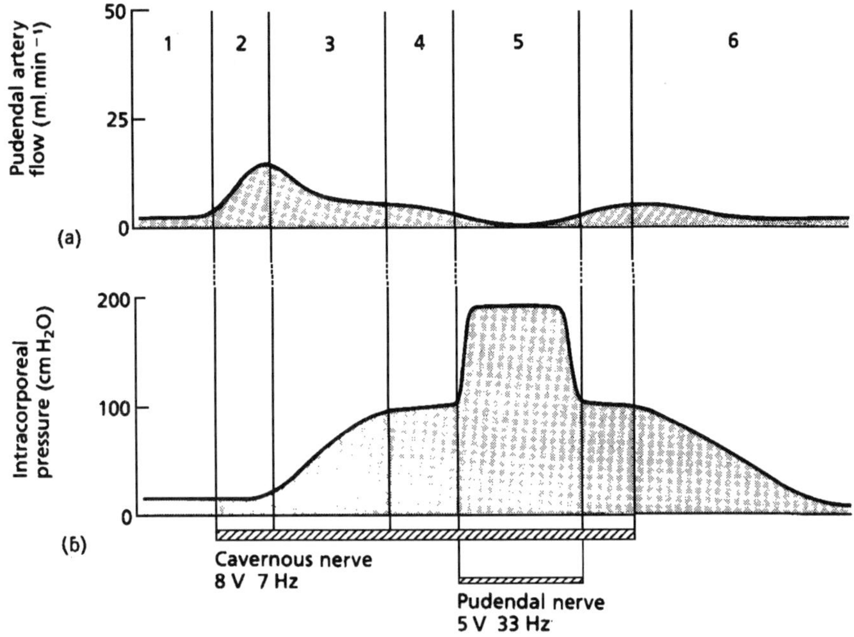

Figure 7.3: Phases of penile erection. (a) Intracavernous pressure; (b) flow within the internal pudendal artery (After Lue). *Reproduced with permission from Webster G, Kirby K, King L, et al eds. Reconstructive Urology Vol 1. Boston: Blackwell Scientific Publications, 1993:75.*

reduce blood flow to flaccid levels. The resulting increased compliance of the sinusoids and arteriolar walls lowers the resistance to blood flow.

PHARMACOLOGY OF ERECTION

While the precise neurotransmitter or transmitters and the chain of events they initiate leading to erection are still under investigation, most researchers agree that erection results from relaxation of smooth muscles of the arterioles and the cavernous trabeculae. Detumescence is the result of the contraction of these muscles.

Direct injection of vasoactive drugs to induce erection or detumescence was first described by Virag. A number of pharmacologic agents have been injected intracavernosally to produce erections (Table 7.5). High, local concentrations of these agents cause maximal and long-lasting relaxation of smooth muscle, which maximizes arterial inflow. The most commonly used drug has been papaverine, an opium alkaloid and a potent, nonspecific smooth-muscle relaxant that works by direct phos-

Table 7.5: Agents Inducing Erection or Detumescence

Erection	*Detumescence*
Alpha-adrenergics	Epinephrine
Phentolamine	Norepinephrine
Phenoxybenzamine	Phenylephrine
Yohimbine	Dopamine
Thymoxamine	Metaraminol
Smooth muscle relaxants	Terbutaline
Papaverine	Ephedrine
Nitroglycerine	
Theophylline	
Imipramine	
Calcium channel blockers	
Verapamil	
Prostaglandins	
Prostaglandin E_1	
Others	
Vasoactive intestinal polypeptide (VIP)	
Trazodone	

phodiesterase inhibition. This drug has been combined with phentolamine, an alpha-adrenergic blocker that induces vascular smooth muscle relaxation by its action on cell membrane receptors. More recently, prostaglandin E_1 (PGE_1) has been used for intracavernous injection. PGE_1 is a smooth muscle relaxant that acts as an alpha$_2$-antiadrenergic agent and potent vasodilator. It appears less likely to cause fibrosis of the corpora with repeated injection. All of these intracavernosally injected agents have the potential to cause prolonged erection, and they should be used with caution. Furthermore, none is currently approved by the Food and Drug Administration (although PGE_1 is in clinical trials). The alpha antagonist, thymoxamine (moxisylyte), has recently been used, although full rigid erections are rarely achieved. Careful, informed patient consent is required prior to using drugs for intracavernosal pharmacotherapy. Agents such as L-dopa, yohimbine, and amphetamine, which act on the central adrenergic receptors, may enhance sexual drive and improve erectile function, while drugs that act on the central serotoninergic receptors may suppress sexual behavior and potency (Table 7.6).

Pharmacologic agents are used for diagnosis as well as treatment of erectile impotence. Intracavernosal pharmacologic testing is now an integral step in the evaluation of the impotent man. Drugs are used singly or in combination. If a full erection is achieved within 10 minutes of intra-

Table 7.6: Centrally Active Agents and Potency

L-dopa: increased libido
Yohimbine: increased libido
Amphetamine: increased libido
Serotonin: decreased libido

cavernosal injection and sustained for 30 minutes, major vasculogenic impotence can be reliably excluded. In such patients, further evaluation to exclude neurogenic or psychogenic impotence may be indicated. If response (partial or no response) to the injection is inadequate, further testing for arteriogenic or venogenic impotence is required.

Pharmacologic injection therapy with one or a combination of the three most popular agents is widely employed in the treatment of impotence. Papaverine and PGE_1 are the mainstays of treatment. Phentolamine (alpha-blocker), which promotes tumescence but not rigidity, is always used in combination with other agents. The major complications associated with papaverine include hypotension, tachycardia, and reversible abnormalities in liver function tests. Papaverine has been largely replaced by prostaglandin E_1 or combination therapy. PGE_1 has virtually no systemic side effects and a low risk of prolonged erection because it is metabolized within the corpora as well as by the lungs and kidneys. The overall incidence of priapism with intracavernosal pharmacotherapy is 3 to 10%, and this risk is lower with PGE_1. In animal studies, long-term papaverine injection results in corporal fibrosis, whereas PGE_1 leads to smooth muscle hypertrophy. PGE_1 causes a dull penile ache in about 10 to 20% of patients; this effect is dose-related.

DRUGS RELATED TO IMPOTENCE

A multitude of drugs have been implicated in causing impotence (Table 7.7). A recent review reported that drugs can be responsible for impotence in up to 25% of patients. The effects may be manifested by a change in libido, diminished erectile function, or inability to ejaculate. Drug agents may act centrally or locally. However, it is often difficult to identify the offending agent because many older patients take multiple drugs.

Data on drug-induced impotence are usually uncontrolled, and the mechanism of action of most drugs causing impotence is unknown. Nevertheless, the antihypertensive and antidepressant classes of therapeutic drugs are probably the most common prescription drugs implicated in contributing to impotence. Among the antihypertensives, diuretics

Table 7.7: Major Drug Classes Causing Impotence

Drug Class	*Example*
Major Tranquilizers	
Phenothiazine	Chlorpromazine
Butyrophenones	Haloperidol
Thioxanthenes	Thiothixene
Antidepressants	
Tricyclics	Imipramine
MAO inhibitors	Tranylcypromine
Antianxiety Agents	
Benzodiazepines	Diazepam
Mephenesin-like compounds	Meprobamate
Anticholinergic Drugs	
Belladonna alkaloids	Atropine
Antispasmodics	Propantheline bromide
Antiparkinsonians	Benztropine
Antihistamines	Dimenhydrinate
Muscle relaxants	Diphenhydramine
Antiarrhythmics	Disopyramide
Antihypertensives	
Diuretics	Spironolactone
Central sympatholytics	Methyldopa
Neurotransmitter depletion	Guanethidine
Alpha-adrenergic blockers	Phenoxybenzamine
Beta-adrenergic blockers	Propranolol
Miscellaneous	
Cimetidine	
Clofibrate	
Digoxin	

alone rarely cause sexual dysfunction, except for spironolactone, which may cause gynecomastia, decreased libido, and erectile failure. The sympatholytics, methyldopa and clonidine, contribute to erectile failure by a central mechanism. The psychotropic agents contribute to erectile dysfunction by decreasing libido, inducing sedation, and interfering with anticholinergic activity.

Alcohol also contributes to impotence. Excessive alcohol intake causes central sedation and decreased libido. Chronic alcoholism may result in liver dysfunction with decreased testosterone and increased estrogen levels. Alcoholic polyneuropathy can affect penile nerves. A number of drugs have been associated with elevation of serum prolactin in erectile dysfunction. These include the phenothiazines, tricyclic antidepressants, haloperidol, amphetamine, and opiates. Digoxin may cause a decrease in serum testosterone and an increase in estrogen owing in all likelihood to its similarity in chemical structure to the sex steroids. Central neurotransmitter pathways (noradrenergic, dopaminergic, hydroxytryptaminergic) may be affected by antipsychotics, antidepressants, and centrally acting antihypertensives. Cimetidine, a histamine (H_2) receptor antagonist, has been associated with antiandrogenic effects and impotence.

PATHOPHYSIOLOGY OF ERECTILE DYSFUNCTION

Psychogenic Impotence

A psychological stimulus such as a visual image or fantasy can produce an erection or enhance an erection already induced by genital stimulation. This occurs because impulses from the brain send both facilitatory and inhibitory messages to the spinal erection centers, which in turn control the erectile response via the spinal nerves. Other stimuli such as anxiety, depression, or guilt may also send strong messages from the brain to the spinal erection center to inhibit or terminate an erection.

The exact mechanism of psychogenic inhibition is unclear. However, it may result from direct brain inhibition of the spinal centers or from increased peripheral catecholamine levels that render the cavernous smooth muscles less responsive to neurotransmitters. Whatever the mechanism, psychogenic causes of impotence should be explored using a careful patient history regarding performance anxiety, relationship conflict, sexual preference conflict, guilt feelings, fear of sexually transmitted disease, and so on. Psychogenic impotence can be distinguished from organic impotence by nocturnal penile tumescence monitoring. Men with psychogenic erectile dysfunction retain their normal nocturnal erectile activity associated with rapid eye movement (REM) sleep.

Neurogenic Impotence

Erection is a neurovascular phenomenon. Thus, neurologic dysfunction extending from the brain all the way to the receptors of the terminal arteriolar and cavernous smooth muscles may cause impotence. Among these, spinal disorders are probably the most common cause of impotence. It has been reported that nearly 95% of patients with complete upper cord lesions are capable of attaining an erection (reflexogenic erection), while only 25% of those with complete lower cord lesions are able to attain erection (psychogenic erection). The thoracolumbar sympathetic pathway carries impulses for psychogenic erection, and because only 25% of patients are able to achieve an erection through the sympathetic pathway, the sacral parasympathetic neurons appear to be the most important erectile center.

Central lesions such as strokes, Parkinsonism, Alzheimer's disease, or severe head injury probably cause erectile dysfunction through a derangement of the hypothalamic center or increased inhibition of the spinal erection center. Dysfunction at the spinal level, such as in multiple sclerosis, may affect either the afferent or efferent nerve pathways. Neuropathies associated with alcoholism, vitamin deficiencies, or diabetes may affect the cavernous nerve terminals and result in a deficiency of neurotransmitters. Indeed, the high prevalence of impotence among diabetics results, in part, from autonomic and peripheral neuropathies.

Arteriogenic Impotence

A marked increase of arterial flow into the cavernous arteries is required for initiation of erection. Disruption of flow in the terminal aorta, or hypogastric, pudendal, or penile arteries may therefore result in erectile failure. Although trauma or a vascular anomaly may cause arterial insufficiency, the majority of cases of arteriogenic impotence result from generalized atherosclerosis. Diabetes, hypertension, hypercholesterolemia, and cigarette smoking contribute to the formation of atherosclerotic plaques and may lead to impotence. Patients with arteriogenic impotence have delayed initiation of erections, require increased stimulation to produce a response, and suffer early detumescence. As arterial luminal diameter and resultant blood flow decrease, partial to complete erectile failure results. Factors such as obesity, cigarette smoking, and psychic overlay frequent aggravate the erectile failure of arteriogenic impotence.

Duplex ultrasonography and color Doppler sonography in conjunction with intracavernosal injection of vasoactive agents can assess blood flow, cavernosal arterial diameter, cavernous erectile tissue, and venous outflow. This relatively noninvasive technique has largely replaced selective pudendal arteriography, which is now reserved for the relatively rare patient who is a candidate for arterial revascularization (e.g., post-traumatic impotence).

Venogenic Impotence

Some impotent patients have adequate arterial inflow to the penis but excessive venous outflow as a result of dysfunction of the corporal veno-occlusive mechanism. However, the precise role of venous incompetence in impotence is still under active investigation. Certainly any tunical abnormality that leads to the inability to compress the subtunical venules may result in early detumescence—a characteristic of venogenic impotence. Abnormal venous channels or ectopic drainage of the corpora via large superficial dorsal veins or abnormally large cavernous and corporal veins may also lead to early detumescence.

Typically, a patient with venogenic impotence is able to achieve an adequate erection but loses it rapidly. Diagnosis is confirmed by dynamic cavernosometry and cavernosography performed after the veno-occlusive mechanism is activated by intracavernous injection of vasodilators, visual sexual stimulation, or passive saline infusion (Figure 7.4). Elevated infusion flow rates or rapid decrease in intracavernosal pressure coupled with radiographic evidence of venous drainage characterize low venous-outflow

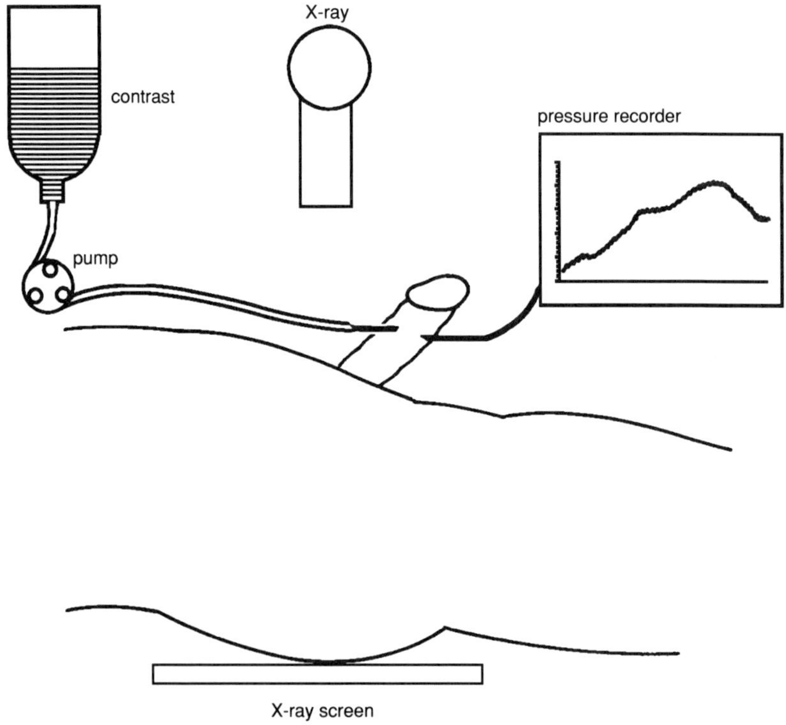

Figure 7.4: Dynamic cavernosography. Contrast is pumped at a constant rate into the corpus cavernosum while the pressure is measured and venous drainage monitored radiographically. *Reproduced with permission from Webster G, Kirby K, King L, et al eds. Reconstructive Urology Vol 1. Boston: Blackwell Scientific Publications, 1993:273.*

resistance and corporal veno-occlusive dysfunction. Venous ligation surgery is of some benefit in these patients, but its role is still incompletely defined. However, a simple treatment for venous impotence uses pliable constrictive bands that effectively restrict outflow when placed at the base of the penis.

Endocrinologic Impotence

Although diabetes is the most common endocrine disorder associated with impotence, the impairment results from vascular, neurologic and psychologic causes rather than a hormonal deficiency. Diabetics suffer from decreased tactile sensation, peripheral neuropathies with autonomic dysfunction, and alterations of cavernous erectile tissue as well as a variety of vascular abnormalities.

Thyroid abnormalities, including both hyperthyroidism and hypothyroidism, also affect sexual function through the inhibition of sexual drive. Hyperprolactinemia caused by a pituitary adenoma, chronic renal failure, or medication may inhibit the hypothalamic center and results in low testosterone levels and decreased libido.

The effects of androgens on libido and sexual behavior are well established. Androgens are essential for male sexual maturation. In the castrated adult, libido is decreased, seminal emission impaired, and the magnitude and frequency of erections decreased. However, it has been demonstrated that androgens are not essential for erectile activity, although they enhance penile tumescence. In spite of the progressive decline in serum testosterone levels after the seventh decade of life, as the result of testicular or hypothalamic-pituitary dysfunction, many elderly men are able to retain the ability to achieve adequate erections. Androgen replacement is therefore indicated only in the truly hypogonadal patient.

Iatrogenic Impotence

Erectile dysfunction may result from pelvic irradiation used to treat prostatic, bladder, or colonic cancers. Impotence following external beam radiation for clinically localized prostatic cancer reportedly occurs in approximately 30 to 40% of patients.

Interference with the penile vascular supply results from any decrease in the hypogastric blood flow such as occurs during reconstructive vascular surgery, for example, aortoiliac surgery or renal transplantation. During surgery for rectal or colonic carcinoma, injury to the pelvic parasympathetic nerves in the pararectal space can result in erectile dysfunction. Neurosurgical procedures in the lower spine may lead to impotence. Such surgical procedures as radical cystectomy, radical prostatectomy, retroperitoneal lymph node dissection are associated with the risk of vascular and/or neural injury in the pelvis or retroperitoneum and resultant impotence. Blunt or penetrating trauma to the pelvis or penis may disrupt the arterioles supplying the penis and lead to poor arterial inflow and erectile impotence.

DIAGNOSTIC EVALUATION OF THE IMPOTENT MALE

A utilitarian, goal-directed evaluation is recommended in all men with impotence. The invasiveness of the diagnostic tests and the available treatments need to be balanced against the patient's expectations and his mental and physical state (Table 7.8).

A careful history and physical exam are of paramount importance in all men with sexual dysfunction and should not be bypassed in favor of sophisticated or invasive testing. A variety of invasive and noninvasive studies may be considered later in the workup to try to discern the precise etiology of the impotence. A detailed history is obtained, including the time sequence of the impotence, assessment of risk factors (e.g., alcohol, cigarette smoking, hypertension, vascular disease, diabetes), psychosexual questioning (e.g., libido, relationships, stresses), and concurrent drug use.

Neuroendocrine Evaluation

The value of routine blood sampling for serum testosterone is debatable, since it is normal in most men with impotence. Nevertheless, it is important to document normal levels. Persistently low levels on at least two separate occasions raise the possibility of hypogonadism, and the serum luteinizing hormone (LH) level should be checked. Serum glucose and thyroid function studies are obtained on the basis of the patient's history. Serum prolactin screening is also recommended. In hyperprolactinemia,

Table 7.8: Impotence Evaluation—A Synthesis

Focused history and physical examination
Routine blood tests
Glucose, cholesterol
Testosterone, prolactin
Specific testing
Neurologic
Vascular
Psychologic
Hormonal

low serum testosterone levels result from suppression of gonado-trophin-releasing hormone. If serum prolactin and testosterone levels are normal, there is no need to check the luteinizing (LH) or follicle-stimulating (FSH) hormone levels (Table 7.9).

Nocturnal Penile Tumescence (NPT) Monitoring

Patients suspected of having psychogenic impotence should undergo testing to record penile tumescence and rigidity (Table 7.9). Rapid eye movement (REM) sleep and nocturnal erections are related. Erections normally occur during REM sleep. Lack of these normal nocturnal erections suggests organic rather than psychogenic causes of impotence. Reliable screening can be achieved using a penile snap-gauge consisting of a self-fastening ring with three bands that break with successive

Table 7.9: Tests for Impotence

Nocturnal Penile Tumescence (NPT)
Tumescence, rigidity testing
NPT monitor
Penile snap gauge
Penile Blood Flow
Penile blood pressure recording
Arteriography
Intracavernosal vasodilators
Duplex ultrasound
Cavernosal artery diameter
Blood-flow velocity
Venous outflow
Dynamic cavernosography, cavernosometry
Endocrine Evaluation
If prolactin, testosterone abnormal
Follicle-stimulating hormone (FSH)
Luteinizing hormone (LH)
Neurologic evaluation
Bulbocavernous reflex
Perianal, perineal sensations
Specialized
Biothesiometry
Reflex latency time
Dorsal nerve conduction velocity

increases in force. Testing of tumescence and rigidity is best performed at home, but occasionally a sleep laboratory test is indicated. A normal erection is characterized by an increase in penile base circumference of over 3 cm, increase in tip circumference of over 2 cm, and increase in rigidity of over 70%.

Vasculogenic Testing

The Penile Brachial Index (PBI) is obtained by determining the ratio between penile systolic blood pressure and brachial systolic blood pressure. The normal PBI is considered to be 0.75 or higher. Values of less than 0.6 suggest arterial insufficiency. This test is useful for screening, although it can be used in conjunction with other tests (Table 7.9).

Arteriography was previously the mainstay for the investigation of penile blood and vascular integrity. Because of the potential complications and costs of arteriography, it is currently reserved for patients considering penile reconstructive arterial surgery (Table 7.10). The nephrotoxicity of the high osmolarity contrast agents, painful intracorporeal injections, and risk of ionizing radiation limit the applications of penile arteriography. Arteriography has been largely supplanted by the intracavernous injections of vasoactive substances alone or in combination with duplex ultrasonography. This provides a functional evaluation of the penile arterial supply and is currently the best screening tool for vasculogenic impotence. The test is normal if a firm erection occurs within 10 minutes of injection and is sustained. A full erection following intracavernosal vasodilator injection in a neurologically normal man with impotence effectively excludes a vasculogenic (arterial or venous) etiology.

Real-time ultrasonography combined with pulsed Doppler scanning after injection of vasoactive agents is now an effective test of the functionality of the cavernosal arteries (Table 7.10). Blood flow in the dilated cavernosal arteries is identified and quantitated by color-coded Doppler flow analysis. A peak systolic velocity of less than 25 cm/sec suggests arterial insufficiency, whereas an end-diastolic flow of over 5 cm/sec is typical of corporal veno-occlusive dysfunction. The advantages of this test are its sensitivity and noninvasiveness, although the equipment is somewhat expensive. Patient anxiety may result in a false-positive test because of the increased sympathetic activity that restricts smooth-muscle relaxation and arterial dilatation.

Excessive venous outflow should be suspected in impotent men with partial erections and early loss of rigidity. Excessive venous outflow from the penile corporal bodies is the cause of impotence in a significant number of men. Dynamic cavernosometry and dynamic pharmacocavernosography are useful in evaluating patients with suspected "venous-leak" impotence

Table 7.10: Diagnostic Imaging in Impotence

Duplex Ultrasonography

May be combined with pharmacologic erection to evaluate vascular integrity
Advantages:
  Minimally invasive
  No radiation exposure
Disadvantage:
  Equipment cost

Dynamic Cavernosometry/Cavernosography

Highly accurate in the evaluation of suspected venous incompetence
Advantage:
  Diagnostic accuracy
Disadvantages:
  Invasive
  Radiation exposure
  Contrast media

Pudendal Arteriography

Reserved for candidates for arterial reconstruction
  (primarily young males, post pelvic trauma)
Advantage:
  Diagnostic accuracy
Disadvantages:
  Highly invasive
  Radiation exposure
  Contrast media

(Table 7.10). After injection of a vasoactive substance, a controlled infusion of saline is monitored while intracorporeal pressure measurements are obtained. Venous leak is suspected if more than 50 ml/min of flow is required to maintain an erection. This can be confirmed by controlled infusion of dilute contrast material with radiographic studies to detect the presence, location, and severity of excessive venous outflow. The information obtained with dynamic cavernosography is helpful in identifying patients who may benefit from venous ligation surgery. It not only confirms venous-leak impotence, but it also locates the leak and helps to tailor the surgical approach to treatment.

Neurologic Testing

Neurophysiologic testing is generally reserved for impotent men with a history of neurologic disease, for example, multiple sclerosis, or spinal cord lesions. Patients with suspected diabetic, alcoholic, or autonomic peripheral neuropathy may require careful neurologic evaluation. Dorsal nerve somatosensory evoked-potential testing assesses peripheral and central afferent pudendal pathways. Other more involved tests include sacral evoked-potential testing to identify suprasacral lesions and bulbocavernosus electromyography to test peripheral neurologic integrity. These tests are sophisticated and require expensive equipment and significant expertise, and they are not routinely performed.

Penile biothesiometry, which measures penile vibratory proprioception, is a simple screening test for afferent, somatosensory penile function. Assessment of the perianal sensation and the bulbocavernous (BC) reflex can be easily accomplished during the physical examination and can provide a gross assessment of the integrity of the S2 to S4 spinal segments (Table 7.9).

PRIAPISM

Priapism has been defined as a sustained, painful erection unassociated with sexual activity. Blood inflow into the corpora is controlled by the arterial resistance and outflow by the trabecular smooth muscle. Interference with constriction of the trabecular muscle leads to priapism. Veno-occlusive priapism results from persistent obstruction of venous outflow from the lacunar spaces (Table 7.11). The obstruction may be due to extravascular compression of the subtunical veins as a result of persistent corporal smooth muscle relaxation. This occurs with oral psychotropic drugs, for example, trazodone, or after intracorporeal injection of vasodilator agents. Less commonly, the obstruction is intravascular as a result of hematologic disorders, such as sickle cell hemoglobinopathy, leukemia, multiple myeloma, or reticuloendothelial malignancies.

Table 7.11: Priapism—Selected Aspects

Causes	*Pharmacologic Treatment*
Veno-occlusive	Alpha-adrenergic intracavernosal injection
Intracavernosal injection	Phenylephrine 200 μg q 5 minutes
Psychotropic drugs, e.g., trazodone	Epinephrine 10–20 μg q 5 minutes
Intravascular obstruction	
Sickle cell disease, leukemia	
"High-flow" priapism	
Lacerated perineal or pelvic artery	

The lack of blood outflow in priapism impedes arterial inflow and results in ischemia, acidosis, and pain with eventual corporal fibrosis if left untreated. Hypoxia and acidosis depress trabecular smooth muscle contractility and reduce the contractile response to norepinephrine, the endogenous adrenergic agonist that controls detumescence. Whatever the cause of priapism, the penile shaft is rigid and the glans is soft because blood is trapped under high pressure within the corpora but not the spongiosum. Pain results from tissue anoxia.

The most common cause of low-flow, veno-occlusive priapism is the diagnostic or therapeutic injection of intracavernosal vasodilators, such as papaverine or PGE_1. These drugs cause marked relaxation of intracorporeal smooth muscle with persistent veno-occlusion. An uncommon cause of priapism occurs after perineal or pelvic trauma resulting in lacerations of the main cavernosal artery or its branches. The vessel bleeds into the lacunar spaces, bypassing the arterial resistance bed of the helicine arteries. Treatment is tailored to stopping the unregulated arterial inflow, for example, by selective arterial embolization.

Underlying causes of priapism should be aggressively treated with transfusion in the case of sickle cell disease, or chemotherapy or radiation therapy in the case of hematologic or reticuloendothelial malignancy. As the mechanism of erection has become better understood, pharmacologic approaches have been applied to the treatment of priapism (Table 7.11). Needle aspiration of trapped corporal blood followed by instillation of dilute solutions of phenylephrine or epinephrine have resulted in vasoconstriction and detumescence. It is also theoretically possible that inhibition of nitric oxide synthase could be beneficial in the treatment of priapism.

SUMMARY

Increased arterial inflow, corporal smooth muscle relaxation, and decreased venous outflow are the anatomic and physiologic essentials of penile erection. Corporal smooth muscle tone can now be manipulated by pharmacologic agents, and this opens new pathways for the diagnosis and therapy of impotent men. Continued scientific and clinical research may allow even more precise manipulation of this event, providing more reliable and safer therapeutic options for the millions of men who suffer from impotence.

SUGGESTED READINGS

Krane RJ, Goldstein I, Saenz de Tejada I. Impotence. N Engl J Med 1989; 321:1648.

Excellent overview of impotence with an extended bibliography. The pathophysiologic rationale for the various tests of impotence are clearly described and treatment options discussed.

Walsh PC, Donker PJ. Impotence following radical prostatectomy: insight into etiology and prevention. J Urol 1982; 128:492.

Classic work describes the periprostatic nerves and their role in erectile function. Surgical implications pertaining to preservation and injury of the nerves are outlined.

Rajfer J, Aronson WJ, Burk PA, et al. Nitric oxide as a mediator of relaxation of the corpus cavernosum in response to nonadrenergic, noncholinergic neurotransmission. N Engl J Med 1992; 326:90.

Recent study that strongly suggests that nitric oxide is the principal neurotransmitter involved in penile erection.

Snyder SH. Nitric oxide: first in a new class of neurotransmitters? Science 1992; 257:494.

Excellent general review of nitric oxide and its neurotransmitter role in the penis, pelvic, and other organs.

Lue TF, Takamura T, Schmidt RA, Palubinskas AJ, Tanagho EA. Hemo-dynamics of erection in the monkey. J Urol 1983; 130:1237.

One of the earliest experimental studies describing the physiology of erection. The hemodynamics of erection in this animal model has clear parallels to human penile erection and flaccidity.

Virag R. Intravenous injection of Papaverine for erectile failure. (Letter to the editor.) Lancet 1982; 2:938.

One of the first descriptions of the use of vasoactive drugs to produce penile erections.

Aboseif SR, Breza J, Bosch RJLH, et al. Local and systemic effects of chronic intracavernous injection of papaverine, prostaglandin E_1, and saline in primates. J Urol 1989; 142:403.

Early study addressing the effects of the two main intracavernosal vasoactive agents used to produce pharmacologically induced erections.

Slag MF, Morley JE, Elson MK, et al. Impotence in medical outpatients. JAMA 1983; 24:1736.

Outstanding reference guide to the various drugs that contribute to erectile dysfunction in men.

Karacan I, Aslan C, Hirschkowitz M. Erectile mechanism in man. Science 1983; 220:1080.

Classic study demonstrating the presence of nocturnal erections in men. The relationship of REM sleep to nocturnal erections is described.

Forsberg L, Hojerback T, Olsson AM, Rosen I. Etiologic aspects of impotence in diabetics. Scand J Urol Nephrol 1989; 23:173.

Comprehensive discussion of a common sequela of diabetes mellitus, with particular emphasis on the pathophysiology of "diabetic impotence."

Kwan M, Greenleaf WJ, Mann J, Crapo L, Davidson JM. The nature of androgen action on male sexuality: a combined laboratory and self-report study in hypogonadal men. J Clin Endocrinol Metab 1983; 57:557.

Interesting discussion of the role of testosterone and androgens in male erectile function and dysfunction.

Meulman EJH, Bemelmans BLH, VanAsten WNJC, et al. Assessment of penile blood flow by duplex ultrasonography in 44 men with normal erectile potency in different phases of erection. J Urol 1992; 147:51.

Intracavernous injection of papaverine and duplex ultrasound was studied. The specific patterns of the Doppler spectrum during different phases of erection are presented and reference values defined.

Lewis RW. Venous ligation surgery for venous leakage. Int J Impotence Res 1990; 2:1.

Overview of the diagnostic, clinical, and treatment aspects of venous-leak impotence. Techniques and limitations of cavernosography/cavernosometry are discussed.

Saenz de Tejada I, Goldstein I, Krane RJ. Local control of penile erection: nerves, smooth muscle and endothelium. Urol Clin North Am 1988; 145:9.

Synopsis of the various neurotransmitters and neuromodulators involved in penile flaccidity and erection. Strong emphasis on basic biochemistry and pathophysiology.

CHAPTER 8

Basic Immunology

Stuart M. Flechner

The immune system, a highly complex and interactive system, is essential for human growth and development and the maintenance of normal health. The functions of the immune system include, but are not limited to, resistance to infectious and neoplastic disease, elimination of organic and inorganic substances, and rejection of transplanted organs and tissues. The immune system also contributes to autoimmune diseases, in which the host is pathologically triggered against itself.

The presence of an immune system was known long before its component parts were identified. Jenner observed that individuals who had contracted the more benign cowpox infection were protected from future exposure to smallpox. It was later observed that convalescing individuals develop serum "protective factors" that could be transferred to newly infected individuals to prevent or eradicate illness. These factors were eventually identified as gamma globulin proteins.

Early skin graft experimentation vividly defined the relationship between the immune system and the fate of tissue grafts. Inbred strains of animals would uniformly accept skin grafts from each other, whereas members of different strains would keep the grafts for only 10 to 14 days before necrosis and sloughing developed. These observations helped to define some of the basic elements of the immune response: the recognition of *self* and *nonself* inherent within a strain, *specificity* to respond to a unique product, *memory* to recall a previous challenge, and *amplification* to accelerate the response to a previously encountered challenge.

THE IMMUNE RESPONSE

The immune response is mediated by specific populations of cells and their products. A substance capable of inducing an immune response is termed an immunogen or more commonly, an antigen. Antigens can be parts of or whole microorganisms, chemicals, foods, drugs, pollen, or benign or neoplastic cells.

The immune system also includes an essential nonspecific barrier to "foreign" material termed innate immunity, which is available at short notice to protect the individual. These barriers include the skin, mucous membranes, the cough reflex, and surface chemicals such as fatty acids, enzymes, and pH differences. In addition, nonspecific cellular elements such as granulocytes, macrophages, microglial cells, and cellular products (interferons, pyrogens, lysins, and kinins) form an internal host defense network.

During the development of acquired immunity, the host produces two interactive populations of lymphocytes: one responsible for secretion of specific antibody (humoral immunity), the other for creation of antigen-specific cellular populations (cellular immunity). Classically, this response is divided into three phases, or limbs. The *afferent* limb includes the recognition of foreign antigen and its presentation to immune-competent cells. The *central* limb describes the processing of this information by immune-competent cells to acquire memory and specificity. The *efferent* limb constitutes the effector mechanism(s), humoral and cellular, of the immune response.

Cells of the Immune Response

Lymphocytes, the central components of the immune system, represent about 20% of the circulating leukocyte population. The interaction of lymphocytes with other immune-competent cells and molecules triggers the immune response. Lymphocytes vary from one another and have different functions at various stages of maturation. These differences are defined by the expression of various cell surface receptors or molecules, termed cluster designations (CD) (Table 8.1). There are two major classes of mature lymphocytes: the bursa-derived B cells, associated with humoral immunity, and the thymus-derived T cells, associated with cellular immunity.

B Lymphocytes

B cells develop from a common progenitor bone marrow stem cell and are distinguished by the presence of surface immunoglobulin (antibody) molecules. The antibodies (primarily IgD) are imbedded in the cell surface with their exposed antigen-binding regions acting as receptors. Each antibody molecule on the cell, or its progeny (clone), bears the same antigen-binding specificity.

B cells migrate throughout the body, populate the spleen and lymph nodes, and comprise 10 to 15% of circulating lymphocytes in healthy adults. With antigen binding, B-cells become activated and differentiate into mature plasma cells, which secrete antibody molecules with the same

Table 8.1: Commonly Defined Cell Surface Markers

Cluster Designation	*Other Designation*	*Description*
CD1	T6, leu6	Thymocyte differentiation marker
CD2	T11	E rosette receptor
CD3	T3, leu4	Molecular complex T-cell receptor
CD4	T4, leu3a	Helper/inducer subset
CD5	T1, leu1	T-cell marker
CD7	leu9	T cell and NK-cell marker
CD8	T8, leu2	Suppressor/cytotoxic subset
CD10	Calla	Common acute leukemia antigen
CD15	leu M1	Monocyte and granulocyte marker
CD16	leu11	Fc receptor on NK cells and PMNs
CD19	leu12	Mature B cells
CD20	B1	Mature B and dendritic cells
CD25	Tac	The IL-2 receptor
	leu19	NK cells

antigen specificity as that encountered by the original B-cell. B-cells express other cell surface markers, such as class II major histocompatibility complex (MHC) antigens and receptors for certain complement components.

T Lymphocytes

T cells also arise from bone marrow precursors but differentiate differently as they migrate through the thymus gland. In fact, an absent or abnormal thymus gland at birth results in a severely impaired adult immune system. T cells comprise about 80% of circulating lymphocytes and are classified into various functional subsets (Table 8.2): cytotoxic T cells (Tc), which specifically kill other target cells to which they are sensitized; helper T cells (Th), which expand populations of precursor T cells once they become sensitized to antigen, or help B cells mature into antibody-producing plasma cells; suppressor T cells (Ts), which retard the immune response; and T cells that mediate delayed type hypersensitivity (Td).

About 60% of circulating T cells in healthy individuals bear the CD4 surface marker and function as helper-inducer cells (Th). About 30% of circulating T cells express the CD8 marker and function as either cytotoxic (Tc) or suppressor (Ts) cells. There is some functional overlap, with one or more clones sharing these and other surface markers at different times during differentiation. Commercially available monoclonal antibodies for identifying T-cell subsets are prepared by the Ortho Co. and bear the descriptor OKT or T, and by the Becton-Dickinson Co. with

Table 8.2: Distribution of Cells in Peripheral Blood of Healthy Individuals (per microliter)

Differential	*%*	*Absolute Numbers*
White blood cells	100	5000–10,000
Granulocytes	60	3000–6000
Monocytes (leu M3)	10	100–500
Lymphocytes	25–35	1500–2500
T (CD3)	75–85	1200–1800
B (CD20)	10–15	150–500
Null	3–5	50–150
T-cell subsets		
Total T (CD3)	75–85	1200–1800
Helper/inducer (CD4)	40–60	600–1200
% total T	50–75	
Suppressor/cytotoxic (CD8)	20–40	350–600
% total T	25–40	
Helper (CD4)/suppressor (CD8) ratio		2.0

the descriptor Leu (Table 8.1).

The ratio of Th to Ts (CD4 to CD8) cells is a crude indicator of overall immune activity (Table 8.2). The normal ratio of about 2 rises two to three-fold during immune activity such as allograft rejection. An inverted ratio, often below 0.5, may occur with viral illness. This ratio may even approach zero in individuals infected by the human immunodeficiency virus (HIV), which obliterates the CD4-bearing helper-cell population.

Antigen-Presenting Cells

The early phases of the afferent immune response require antigen presentation in a form that can be recognized by immune-competent lymphocytes. Cells that can present antigen in an immunogenic form, antigen-presenting cells (APC), are the macrophages, monocytes, certain B cells, some endothelial cells, and dendritic interstitial cells. Antigen is internalized, processed, and then re-expressed on the surface of these cells in a form capable of triggering resting lymphocytes. In addition to APC, this process may require the presence of class II MHC antigen on the surface of these cells as well as the local secretion of cytokines (see Chapter 9).

Killer Cells

Animal experiments reveal that tumor masses implanted under the skin of certain recipients can be eliminated in a few days. This phenomenon is due to a distinct population of large granular lymphocytes, natural killer

(NK) cells, with spontaneous cytotoxic activity. These cells lyse target cells such as malignant tumors, virally infected cells, antibody-coated cells, and chemically transformed cells. NK cells lack the usual cell surface markers found on T and B lymphocytes, or macrophages, but do express the CD2 and CD16 markers. Activation of NK activity does not produce the memory, specificity, or amplification observed in a normal immune response. NK cells are activated prior to the T-cell response and may be important in the early stages of tumor growth. The NK response can be augmented by certain interferons, tumor cells, and viral particles and inhibited by prostaglandin E.

Another lymphocyte population with cytotoxic potential is the killer, or K, cell, with surface receptors for the Fc portion of antibodies. K cells recognize targets coated with specific antibody, which binds to the Fc receptors. K cells do not recognize targets without bound antibody, and this mechanism is therefore termed antibody-dependent, cellular cytotoxicity (ADCC).

Phagocytic Cells

Phagocytosis, a significant component of innate immunity, is especially important during inflammation. Phagocytic cells ingest and destroy invading foreign particles, such as bacteria, and include polymorphonuclear leukocytes (PMN), macrophages, monocytes, and cells of the reticuloendothelial system, such as liver Kupffer cells. The foreign material is entrapped in vacuoles, into which lysosomes or other granules release hydrolytic enzymes that digest the invader. Phagocytosis is enhanced by factors (opsonins) such as antibodies and components of the complement system. Phagocytes usually express receptors for the Fc portion of antibody molecules and various activated complement components like C3b and C3d.

NONCELLULAR ELEMENTS OF THE IMMUNE RESPONSE

The cellular elements of the immune response intercommunicate via the secretion of chemical messengers termed cytokines. These small proteins, peptides, and glycoproteins are of low molecular weight (under 50 KD) and are soluble in plasma. Products secreted by lymphocytes are called lymphokines, and their functions range from expansion of sensitized cell populations to the recruitment of unsensitized precursor cells. The CD4+ T-helper is a potent source of lymphokine and a central actor in the repertoire of T-cell function. The finely integrated interactions between the immune cellular elements also depend on antibody production, regulation by inherited MHC gene products, and the triggering of the T-cell antigen receptor.

Lymphokines

Lymphokines are essential for the induction, maintenance, and control of the immune response (Table 8.3). Interleukins 1 and 2 (IL-1, IL-2) are the best characterized. Initially called lymphocyte activation factor, IL-1 is produced by many cells, including activated macrophages and some T cells in the presence of class II MHC-associated antigen. IL-1 is a potent pyrogen and causes the release of acute phase proteins from the liver (haptoglobin, complement, fibrinogen, etc.). It stimulates proliferation of helper T cells by inducing IL-2 release and expression of IL-2 cell surface receptors. IL-1 also stimulates endothelial cell procoagulant activity and the release of vascular mediators such as prostaglandin E_2.

IL-2 stimulates T-cell proliferation after activation by contact with antigen and IL-1. IL-2 is secreted by T helper cells and binds to specific receptors on the surface of activated T cells. In turn, IL-2 induces the expression of these IL-2 receptors (CD25), which results in further expansion of sensitized clones. The receptor for IL-2 has been identified on the surface of activated B cells and some monocytes and macrophages. The IL-2 receptor, a cell surface glycoprotein of molecular weight 55 KD, referred to as Tac, is a unique indicator of T-cell activation.

Interleukin 3 (IL-3), a small glycoprotein secreted by T lymphocytes, supports the growth and differentiation of a number of blood cell lines. It is referred to as a colony-stimulating factor for erythrocytes, granulocytes, megakaryocytes, and macrophages. Initially described as b cell stimulating factor, IL-4 has been shown to induce the expression of class II MHC molecules on the surface of B cells and macrophages and

Table 8.3: Interleukins and the Immune Response

Molecule	*Source*	*Major Actions*
IL-1, alpha, beta	Macrophages, endothelial cells	Activates resting T cells, mediates inflammation, induces fever
IL-2	T cells	Growth factor for activated T cells, activates cytotoxic T cells
IL-3	T cells	Growth factor for bone marrow, stem cells, mast cells
IL-4	T cells, mast cells	Growth factor for activated B cells, class II expression on B cells
IL-5, IL-6	T cells, monocytes, epithelial cells	Differentiation of B cells into plasma cells, T-cell activation, eosinophil growth factor

to help in the activation of resting B cells. IL-5 is another B-cell growth factor required for maturation. IL-6, once thought to be involved in only the late stages of B-cell maturation, now appears to have functions related to IL-1. In fact, IL-6 can be induced by IL-1.

Interferons

The interferons (IFNs) are a class of cytokines first identified in the supernatant of virally infected cell cultures. These small glycoproteins and polypeptides "interfere" with viral infection and protect other cells of the same species from attack by viruses. IFNs are a multigene family divided into three main groups: alpha, beta, and gamma. The IFN proteins consist of 165 to 187 amino acids with a molecular weight of 17 to 25 KD. The production of interferons using recombinant DNA technology has permitted the study of these molecules and their clinical use (Table 8.4).

Alpha IFN is most efficiently induced in peripheral blood mononuclear cells and beta IFN from fibroblasts and epithelial cells. Stimuli for IFN production are viruses, bacteria, and double-stranded RNA. Cytokines also induce IFN secretion, for example, tumor necrosis factor, colony stimulating factors, and IL-1 and IL-2. The IFNs bind to specific receptors and then either up-regulate or down-regulate other cellular genes. IFNs induce enzymes, a synthetase and a protein kinase, that inhibit cellular protein translation and interrupt the viral life cycle. Alpha and beta IFNs are also potent inhibitors of normal and malignant cell growth. They act as negative growth regulators by arresting the G_1 phase of the cell cycle.

Table 8.4: Cytokines and the Immune Response

Molecule	*Source*	*Major Actions*
Interferon gamma (MAF)	T cells, NK cells	Activates macrophages, augments NK, antiviral activity, induces class I and class II expression
Interferon alpha, beta	Leukocytes, fibroblasts	Induces fever, antiviral activity, antiproliferative, class I expression
Tumor necrosis factor Alpha—cachectin Beta—lymphotoxin	T cells	Cytotoxic to some tumors, acute phase response, mediates inflammation, induces catabolism
Colony stimulating factor	T-cells	Stimulates neutrophilic, macrophage, and eosinophilic bone marrow colonies

Gamma IFN is produced by activated T-cells, both helper CD4+ and suppressor CD8+, after stimulation by mitogens or antigens. CD16+NK cells also produce gamma IFN. This interferon, also termed macrophage-activation factor, causes increased size, lysosomal content, phagocytosis, and enhanced ability to kill ingested organisms. While class I MHC genes are up-regulated by all types of IFN, gamma IFN can also induce surface class II MHC molecules on macrophages and other non-immune cells. For example, the tubular epithelium of a rejecting renal allograft will express class II molecules in the presence of gamma IFN. Gamma IFN may therefore play a critical role as a positive feedback loop in the immune response.

Tumor Necrosis Factor

One of the most important recent advances in immunology is the recognition that activated immune cells secrete cytokines that mediate the inflammatory response to infection and injury. The most potent of these mediators are two soluble proteins, tumor necrosis factors, with antitumor and catabolic properties.

The tumor necrosis factors are TNF alpha (cachectin) and TNF beta (lymphotoxin) (Table 8.4). The genes for these TNFs are tightly linked to each other and reside on chromosome 6 in humans, within the major histocompatibility complex. Human TNF alpha is a 233 amino acid prohormone, which is processed to a 157 amino acid active molecule with a molecular weight of 17 KD. Human TNF beta shares about 30% homology with TNF alpha, but has a similar biological activity and competes for common receptors in normal tissues (liver, muscle, lung, bowel, kidney). The TNF alpha is made principally by macrophages and cells of the reticuloendothelial system. Most TNF beta is produced by T lymphocytes and perhaps by B cells.

The stimuli for TNF biosynthesis include bacterial endotoxin/lipopolysaccharide, toxic shock syndrome toxin, viruses, complement components, fungal and parasitic antigens, IL-1, and mycobacteria. Corticosteroids inhibit TNF biosynthesis, whereas gamma IFN promotes it. The active 17-KD molecule interacts with high-affinity cell surface receptors in normal tissues, and this receptor–ligand complex is then internalized. Details of further intracellular responses are currently being elucidated.

TNF is a potent pyrogen that induces IL-1 synthesis, enhances chemotaxis of macrophages and neutrophils, and increases their phagocytic and cytotoxic activity. TNF plays a role in abscess formation and the early walling-off of infections. After the intravenous administration of bacterial endotoxin, TNF levels peak coincident with fever, myalgias, rigors, headache, and nausea. Sterile injections of recombinant TNF can induce lethal shock syndrome and tissue injury similar to clinical septic shock. Interestingly, septic shock and death are preventable in a primate model by the simultaneous administration of anti-TNF antibody.

Persistent animal exposure to TNF leads to cachexia, anorexia, weight loss, and the depletion of protein and lipid body stores. In culture, adipocytes and myocytes become catabolic. Elevated serum TNF levels have been reported in patients with chronic illness or wasting disorders. Paradoxically, the biological properties of TNF also include some tissue remodeling. TNF can act as a growth factor for fibroblasts and mesenchymal cells in wounds. These functions may contribute to the coordinated removal and replacement of senescent tissues after inflammation or injury.

The discovery that TNF promotes tumor lysis in endotoxic mice created great anticipation of its role as an antineoplastic agent. However, animal and early phase I clinical studies have shown poor efficacy at doses with tolerable toxicity. Pronounced systemic and organ-specific toxicity has been observed including fever, rigors, hypotension, and hepatotoxicity. Trials of TNF in conjunction with other cytokines are in progress, but it remains to be established whether TNF toxicity can be reduced. Future manipulations of the TNF molecule or further understanding of some of its intermediaries may permit selective enhancement of its ability to kill tumor cells.

The T-Cell Antigen Receptor

The T-cell antigen surface receptor is composed of two polypeptide chains, alpha and beta, linked by disulfide bonds. Each chain is about 40 to 50 KD in size and contains both constant and variable regions. Analogous to the immunoglobulin molecule, the constant regions contribute primarily to the structure of the molecule and its surface associations, while the variable regions provide for diversity of specific antigen recognition. A second receptor structure, composed of gamma and delta chains, has been identified, but its function is currently unknown.

The alpha and beta chain genes of the T-cell receptor undergo genetic rearrangement of the germline sequences similar to those of immunoglobulin genes. These include sequences for variable, joining, diversity, and constant regions. During T-cell differentiation inversions or deletions of these sequences may occur, which can give rise to as many as 10^{12} combinations of alpha and beta chains. Such genetic rearrangement, which occurs as the T-cell migrates through the thymus gland, explains the tremendous antigenic diversity recognizable by T cells. T-cell receptor expression occurs at an earlier stage of T-cell maturation than the expression of either the CD4 or the CD8 antigen.

Intimately associated with the alpha and beta chains of the T-cell receptor are a group of invariant proteins that form the CD3 molecule. These CD3 polypeptides are produced intracellularly and then packaged with the alpha and beta chains for transport to the T-cell surface. Both the alpha and beta chains, as well as the CD3 molecule, are required for T-cell activation. Receptor activation by antigen causes an influx of calcium into the cell with stimulation of the phosphatidylinositol pathway and release of lymphokines and other factors that stimulate cellular differentiation and proliferation. The immunosuppressive efficacy of the monoclonal antibody OKT3, an anti-CD3, is due to its blocking or masking of the interaction between the T-cell receptor and CD3.

Other Cell Surface Molecules

The interactions of immune-competent cells with other cellular or soluble antigens are not limited to those of the T-cell receptor and human leukocyte antigen (HLA) molecules. Additional molecules on the surface of lymphocytes play a role in immune activation via cell adhesion, activation (signal transduction), and certain effector functions. They can interact as receptor–ligand pairs, and promote adhesion or binding between cells. One identified couple is termed leucocyte function associated antigen (LFA-1) and its ligands, intercellular adhesion molecules (ICAM 1 and 2). The sheep erythrocyte receptor on T cells (CD2) and its ligand LFA-3 promote cell-to-cell interaction. Other receptor–ligand pairs may be involved with homing, the recruitment of circulating lymphocytes to sites of inflammation.

The initial descriptions of the CD4 (helper/inducer) and the CD8 (suppressor/cytotoxic) molecules as markers for T-cell subset function have been expanded. It has been conclusively demonstrated that CD4 binds MHC class II molecules and CD8 binds MHC class I molecules. This binding may allow preferential interaction between certain immune-competent cells and certain targets, as well as regulation of binding avidity between different cell populations. The CD4 molecule is the receptor for the human immunodeficiency virus (HIV 1) that selectively invades cells expressing this molecule.

THE MAJOR HISTOCOMPATIBILITY COMPLEX

The products from a region of closely linked genes on the 6th chromosome in humans are critically involved in the immune response. This gene region, the major histocompatibility complex (MHC), encodes for cell surface glycoproteins that are potent antigenic triggers of the immune response.

HLA class I antigens consist of two polypeptide chains with carbohydrate moieties attached in different regions (Figure 8.1). The heavy, or alpha, chain has a molecular weight of 45 KD and is inserted into the plasma membrane at its carboxyterminus. A light, or beta chain with a molecular weight of 12 KD is noncovalently bound to the alpha chain on the cell surface. The alpha chain is encoded by an HLA gene; the beta chain (beta$_2$-microglobulin) is common to all class I antigens. The HLA class I alpha chain is divided into three external domains (alpha$_1$, alpha$_2$, and alpha$_3$) caused by folding and disulfide bridging. The alpha$_3$ domain of the molecule is closest to the cell surface and considered to be the constant region since its amino acid sequence is homologous for most class I antigens. The alpha$_1$ (the aminoterminus) and alpha$_2$ domains represent the variable regions of the molecule, and their amino acid sequences provide for the polymorphism of the class I antigens.

HLA class II antigens consist of two polypeptide chains: a heavy (alpha) chain with a molecular weight of 34 KD and the light (beta) chain with a molecular weight of 29 KD. Each chain is inserted into the plasma membrane at its carboxyterminus, has an extracellular aminoterminus, has carbohydrate side groups, and is contoured into domains by disulfide bridges (alpha$_1$, alpha$_2$, and beta$_1$, beta$_2$). Both chains are encoded by genes of the MHC, and antigenic diversity is accounted for by the variable amino acid sequences of the aminoterminus alpha$_1$ and beta$_1$ domains.

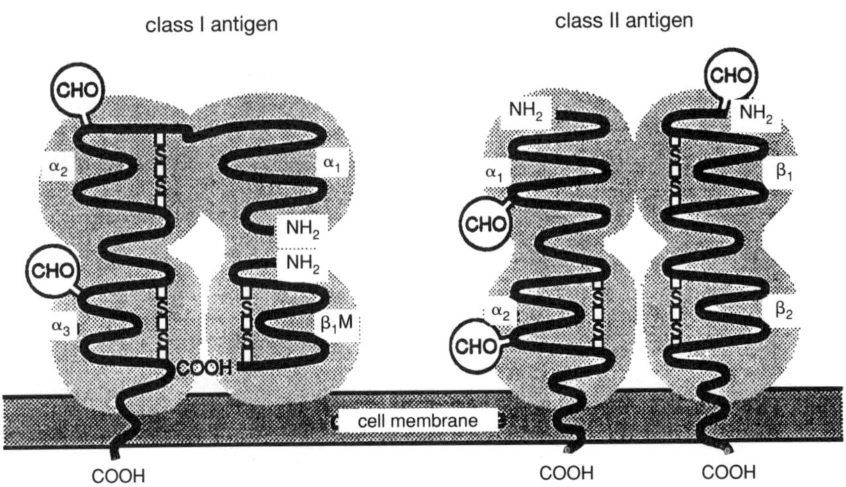

Figure 8.1: Structure of the HLA class I and class II surface antigens. Class I antigen with three domains (alpha$_1$, alpha$_2$, alpha$_3$) formed from the heavier alpha chain and linked noncovalently to the beta$_2$-microglobulin unit that is similar for every class I molecule. Class II molecule with two chains (alpha and beta), each with two domains.

Three genetic loci or regions (A, B, and C) code for the HLA class I antigens, and three regions code for the HLA class II specificities: DR, DP, and DQ. At each locus there are many potential alleles or forms of genes that code for the different antigens. An individual inherits one allele from each parent at each locus. Each individual inherits two 6 chromosomes and therefore two HLA-A, -B, -C and -DR, -DP, -DQ genes. A complete HLA match between two siblings consists of 12 antigenic determinants. The genetic distribution of chromosome 6 follows a mendelian inheritance pattern and is codominant (whatever is inherited will be expressed). Thus, one out of four siblings from the same parents will be HLA identical.

Serological typing is the main technique for identification of HLA antigens. This method relies on the availability of known antisera with reactivity against specific HLA antigens on the surface of lymphocytes. Peripheral blood lymphocytes or fractionated T cells are used to identify class I specificities, and an enriched pool of B cells is used to define class II specificities. After the cells are incubated with the known antisera long enough to coat their surfaces, rabbit complement is added to the cell culture. If the complement is activated by the presence of a specific HLA antigen and antibody binding, it will lyse the cell and permit entry of a vital dye such as eosin. The cells can then be counted using a phase contrast microscope and the HLA type established.

A uniform nomenclature of human HLA antigens has been recognized by the World Health Organization. The letters correspond to the genetic loci that code for the specificities, and the numbers represent the approximate order of identification of the various antigens. An HLA type is usually reported using the serologically defined HLA-A, -B, and -DR antigens. Newer methods of typing using molecular DNA probes are currently under investigation. The ability to type by precise gene sequences may provide identification of single amino acid alterations in a specific HLA antigen.

The 19 known HLA-D specificities can be identified only by proliferative responses in the 5-day mixed lymphocyte culture (MLC). The D region represents the cumulative response to the DR, DP, and DQ specificities. MLC typing is useful in establishing HLA identity among family members.

The products of the MHC play a strategic role in the regulation of the immune response. In order for a specific immune response to occur, T cells must recognize foreign antigen in combination with self class I or class II molecules. For example, a foreign antigen must be presented with a self class II molecule in order for a resting T helper cell to become activated and produce lymphokines. If the same antigen is presented on cells with different class II specificities, the immune response is not initiated. This function is called genetic restriction of the immune response. Restriction is also evident in the effector arm of the immune response. Cytotoxic T-cells will destroy target cells with only certain specificities. The lysis of target cells expressing the foreign antigen will not occur unless the target cells also express self class I antigens.

CELLULAR INTERACTION, RESTRICTION, AND REGULATION

The activation of resting B and T lymphocytes by antigen is the core of normal and abnormal immune function (Figure 8.2). The humoral immune response to a specific antigen describes a process by which resting B cells proliferate, differentiate into mature plasma cells, and produce antibodies. This requires the presence of both antigen-presenting cells (APC) and T cells of the helper subset (expressing CD4). These CD4+ T cells recognize antigen on the surface of APCs by their T-cell receptor in combination with self-MHC class II molecules. This cell surface interaction coupled with the presence of macrophage-derived IL-1 leads to further differentiation of T-helper cells. The CD4+ T helper cells produce IL-2 and express the receptor for IL-2 (CD25).

B-cell activation and differentiation requires IL-2, other interleukins, growth factors, and interferons produced by activated T helper cells. These factors act as second signals or modulators of B-cell activation to augment the primary signal of B-cell surface antibody binding to specific antigen. This sequence of events is referred to as T-cell-dependent antibody formation and results in durable immunity characterized by specificity, memory, and amplification. The responses are usually polyclonal with IgG antibody production. Certain very large and repetitive antigens such as bacterial lipopolysaccharides activate B cells directly. These are referred to as T-cell-independent antigens and work by crosslinking various cell surface receptors. Such responses are less durable, produce IgM antibody, and often exhibit less antigen binding avidity.

The CD4+ T cell plays a central role in the cellular immune response. In events similar to B-cell activation, the APCs present antigen in combination with self-MHC class II molecules in the presence of macrophage-derived IL-1 in order to activate the CD4+ T helper populations. These activated T cells produce interleukins (principally IL-2), which act as second signals to expand populations of cytotoxic T cells primed against specific antigen. The primary signal for this subset of resting CD8+ T cells is the recognition of antigen on APCs in combination with self-MHC class I molecules. Further exposure of the CD8+ T cells to IL-2 induces proliferation

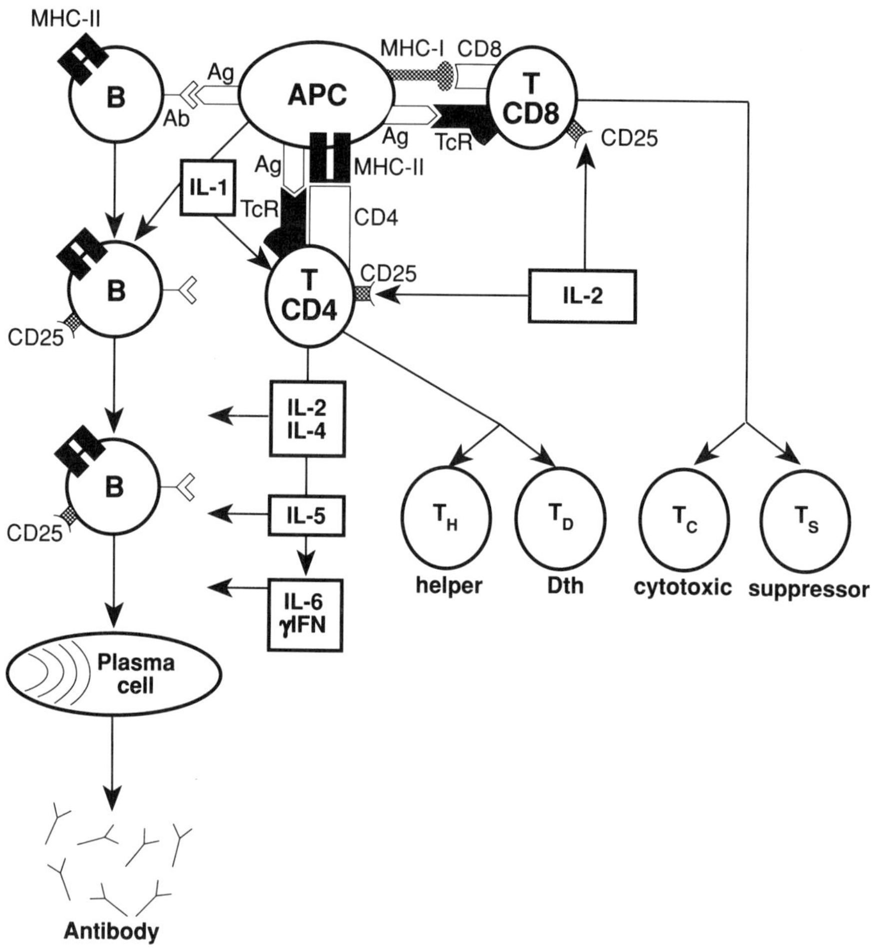

Figure 8.2: Lymphocyte activation pathways. MHC, major histocompatibility antigens; IL, interleukin; IFN, interferon; B, B lymphocyte; T, T lymphocyte; APC, antigen presenting cell.

and differentiation of specifically sensitized clones of cytotoxic T cells.

The two chains of the T cell surface receptor carry the specificity for both antigen and MHC recognition. Cells with receptors for CD4 appear to be MHC class II restricted, and those with receptors for CD8 are MHC class I restricted. Such a control mechanism may be advantageous in focusing sensitized immune cells on certain targets, for example, directing cytotoxic T cells to self-cellular targets infected with viral organisms rather than to infectious particles themselves. Such restriction may also help in the recognition of neoantigens or embryonic antigens on developing tumors. The recognition of altered self may promote the early elimination of these cells prior to dedifferentiation and metastasis. The recognition of small changes in MHC structure among organ and tissue allograft recipients also explains why these differences are a strong stimulus for rejection.

The immune system does not discharge to a predetermined end point once antigen is encountered. There are numerous regulatory stop signals. Indeed, the absence of these regulatory mechanisms can cause autoimmune diseases. A simple method of negative feedback exists by the elimination of the foreign antigen, which reduces the ongoing stimulation of the immune response. An excess of specific antibody also diminishes ongoing humoral immune responses. A potent stop signal to a specific immune response is produced by a T-cell subset that usually bears the CD8 molecule. These T suppressor cells are specifically activated and expanded by many of the cellular and cytokine signals that trigger effector functions. These cells produce cytokines (suppressor factors) that retard further expansion of the specific immune response.

MONOCLONAL ANTIBODIES

During evolution, the immune response attained the flexibility to act as an umbrella against numerous pathogens. One aspect of this protective role is the production of different antibodies during the humoral immune response to a specific antigen. This diversity strengthens the host response but complicates the use of antibodies as diagnostic reagents or therapeutic agents because immune sera usually contain a mixture of antibodies that differ from each other in affinity and specificity. When an apparently pure antigen is used for immunization in either animals or humans, large amounts of antibody are also produced against minor immunogenic contaminants. The most potent or specific antisera contain antibodies with different affinities for antigen, including different classes and subclasses with varying abilities to fix complement, agglutinate, precipitate, or cross react. Each pool of antiserum is a unique serological reagent with properties that may differ from another batch, even from the same individual. This antibody diversity is due to the fact that an immune response against a specific antigen is polyclonal due to different clones of antibody-producing plasma cells.

Antibodies have a major role as laboratory tools for disease diagnosis, detection of drug levels in body fluids, and quantification of tumor antigens and viral and bacterial products. Unfortunately, several factors limit the consistency of preparations and thus the quality control of many assays. In addition to the previously described heterogeneity, a major barrier in generating human antibodies is the ethical and practical limitation of immunizing and bleeding patients. Even in animals, the quantity of antibody cannot always be predicted and certain antigens are weak immunogens.

Cell biologists are able to fuse different animal cells in culture to produce hybrids with genetic material from both cell lines. Kohler and Milstein (later to receive the Nobel Prize) demonstrated that mouse myeloma cells could be fused to normal spleen cells after the animals were immunized with sheep red blood cells. Some of these hybrids produced large amounts of homogeneous antibody against the immunizing sheep red blood cells, could grow continuously in culture, and could be frozen or recovered. This process could be repeated for any number of antigens. These findings were truly revolutionary because it was not only possible to generate homogeneous antibody but also the production was immortalized with a virtually unlimited capacity for product. In addition, impure antigens or weak antigens could be enriched as the antibody-forming hybrids would result from the fusion of a single cell producing only one antibody type. Thus, although the immunizing event was polyclonal, the antibody eventually recovered came from a single hybrid and was monoclonal.

Hybridoma technology has been most frequently employed in the murine system. Animals are repeatedly immunized with an antigen in order to generate a secondary response (Figure 8.3). The spleen is removed 2 to 4 days later and a cell suspension made. The splenocytes are fused with an established murine myeloma cell line using polyethylene glycol, a surface-active agent that promotes fusion of cell membranes. Only one out of 2×10^5 spleen cells actually forms a viable hybrid, and it is therefore necessary to eliminate the unfused spleen and myeloma cells by isolating the hybrids in selective growth medium. Mouse myeloma cells lacking the enzyme hypoxanthine phosphoribosyl transferase (HPRT) are used as the myeloma parent and hypoxanthine, aminopterin, and thymidine are added to the culture medium. The cells with only the myeloma genetic material lack HPRT and cannot use exogenous hypoxanthine to synthesize purines. Aminopterin blocks their endogenous synthesis of purines and pyrimidines, and therefore the myeloma cells die. However, the hybrids possess the essential transferase enzyme provided by the normal spleen cells, and can utilize the exogenous hypoxanthine and thymidine to survive. The hybrids double every 24 to 48 hours and rapidly outgrow the few nondividing unfused spleen cells.

The spleen of a well immunized animal contains about 10^8 nucleated cells and generates about 300 to 500 hybrids. About 2 to 4 weeks after fusion the hybrids become visible on culture plates, and their supernatants are screened for specific antibody. About half of the hybrids produce some antibody, and anywhere from 1 to 10% produce antibody

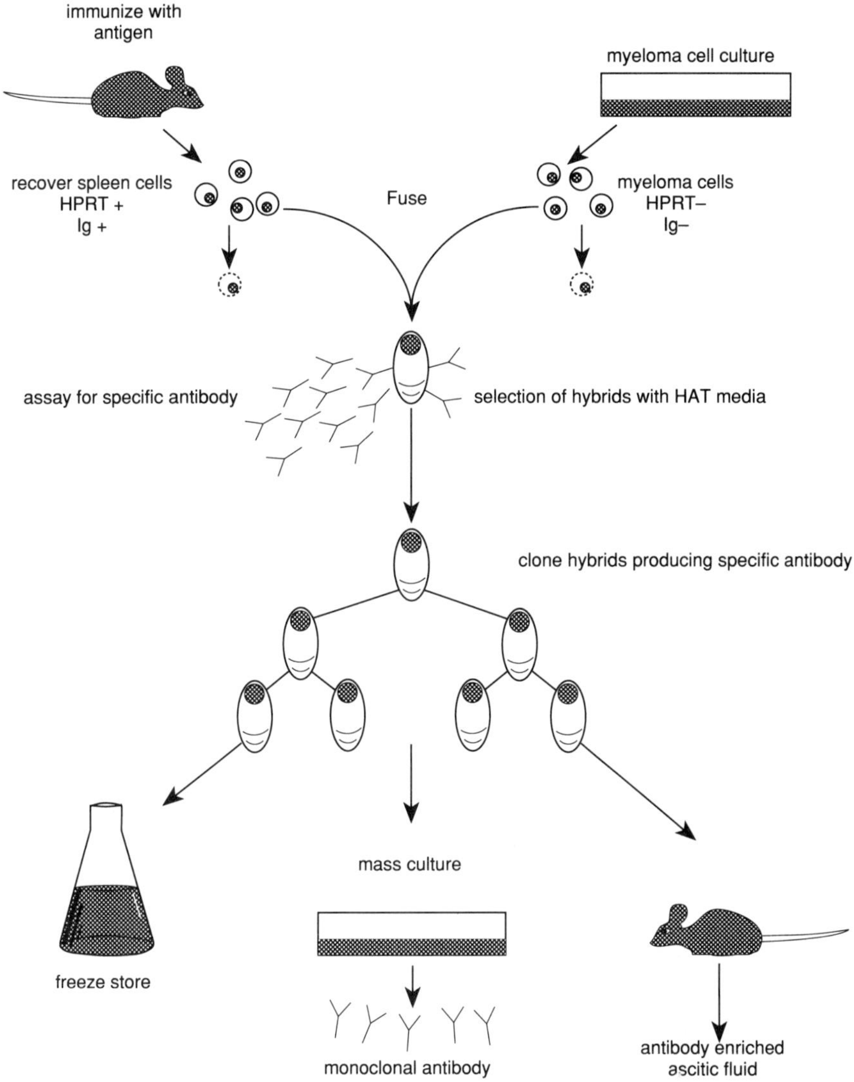

Figure 8.3: Hybridization schema for production monoclonal antibody. HPRT, hypoxanthine phosphoribosyl transferase; Ig, antibody; HAT media, Hypoxanthine, Aminopterin, Thymidine.

that reacts with the immunizing antigen. Enzyme linked or radioimmunoassays are used to screen for a desired antibody, and once identified, selected hybrids are cloned to ensure homogeneity of the selected antibody. The selected cell lines can be frozen for later use, placed in mass culture for antibody collection, or injected intraperitoneally into mice to produce antibody-enriched ascites. Hybridomas secrete between 10 and 100 μg/ml of monoclonal antibody in tissue culture medium. When injected into the mouse peritoneum, the ascitic fluid can contain 1 to 10 mg of antibody per milliliter of fluid. Since each mouse produces about 10 ml of ascitic fluid, it is clear that hundreds of milligrams of antibody can be quickly generated.

While monoclonal antibodies are continually being developed for diagnostic assays and as therapeutic agents, they are also used as probes to dissect the mechanisms of immune activation and effector function (Table 8.5). The use of monoclonal antibodies has inherent drawbacks. Since the majority of monoclonal antibodies are derived from murine cell lines, the antibodies are themselves immunogenic in other species and can be eliminated through a host response. Indeed, the potent anti-CD3 monoclonal antibody (OKT3) use in human immunosuppression is neutralized by this process after one or two administrations.

The limitations in immunizing humans and the inability to harvest human spleen routinely are drawbacks to the production of human monoclonals. Human peripheral blood cells are not as potent partners for fusion as other sources of lymphocytes, and human myeloma cell lines are limited and do not fuse as well as their murine counterparts. The creation of so called "designer antibodies" may expand the horizons of current hybridoma technology. Designer antibodies are immunoglobulins that have been genetically engineered so that specific regions of an antibody gene can be altered or connected to portions of a different immunoglobulin gene. For example, a rodent or murine variable region (which contains the antigen binding site) is combined with human constant

Table 8.5: Applications of Monoclonal Antibodies

Current Uses
Routine serology, hormone and drug levels
Tissue and blood typing
Diagnosis of infectious disease
Identification of differentiation antigens—lymphocyte subsets
Identification of tumor antigens—characterize leukemias and lymphomas
Future Uses
Manipulation and/or amplification of immune response
Location of tumor cells and tumor immunotherapy
Identification of autoantibodies—therapy of autoimmune disease

regions. This markedly reduces the antigenicity of the antibody in humans and takes advantage of murine hybridoma techniques to select the desired antigen binding sited. Designer antibodies have been generated that can select for certain effector functions by selecting for the desired Fc portion of the antibody or making certain antibody–toxin conjugates. "Humanizing" antibodies from other species would seem to offer some hope for the therapeutic use of monoclonal antibodies in humans.

TUMOR IMMUNOLOGY

Immune Surveillance

The concept of immune surveillance arose from observations of the growth of specific transplantable tumors in animals. The theory is based on the fact that during its life a normal organism is subjected to a continuous barrage of somatic mutations that may induce the expression of non–self surface markers or antigens early in the course of malignant transformation. Proponents of the immune surveillance theory suggest that the immune response has evolved as an early defense against potentially lethal tumors while they are still small. The mechanisms responsible for organ or tissue allograft rejection (primarily cell mediated immunity) target neoplastic cells as nonself. Perhaps the best support for immune surveillance in humans comes by inference. Recipients of organ or tissue allografts who receive immunosuppression have an increased incidence of cancer following transplantation (see Chapter 9). Tissues with a naturally high turnover rate, such as lymphoid elements, skin, and cervical epithelium, are especially susceptible.

However, there is doubt regarding the existence of immune surveillance, and the relationship of the immune system to neoplastic transformation may be coincidental. Indeed the athymic "nude mouse" (lacking mature T lymphocytes) does not exhibit increased spontaneous tumor formation. Furthermore, many tumors possess weakly immunogenic surface antigens and do not necessarily flourish in the host. Many observations about tumor regression caused by immunologic mechanisms have been nonspecific, and are related to natural killer (NK) cell function. Interestingly, the athymic mouse has a significantly increased number of NK cells. Thus, the theory of immune surveillance, although attractive, remains controversial and unconfirmed.

Immune surveillance aside, there is no doubt that an immune response (in vivo and in vitro) can be induced against tumors. Why do malignant tumors escape from immune control? The answer may lie in the physical relationship of the tumor to the host, and in the ability of the immune system truly to recognize nonself in tumor tissue. Rapidly growing tumors may outstrip the host's capacity to deliver sensitized effector cells precisely. Each tumor and host may have a critical mass, after which the immune response is ineffective. Certain areas in the body have poor penetration by immune-competent cells. These "privileged" immunological sites include the anterior chamber of the eye, parts of the central nervous system, the tunica albuginea of the testes, and capsules of several visceral organs. Tumor cells, as they dedifferentiate, may shed previously expressed surface antigenic determinants and form a nonhomogeneous tumor cell population. Immune clearance of certain tumor cells expressing one set of antigens may enhance the growth of other tumor clones within the same tissue.

Induction of suppressor networks accompanying the normal immune response can predominate in a tumor–host relationship and dampen a potentially lethal antitumor response. Certain soluble antigens, antibodies, antigen–antibody complexes, or other immune mediators may unintentionally block or mask newly expressed tumor antigens. Local release of immune-expanding cytokines may have a positive effect on tumor cell growth in certain settings. The control of tumor cell growth by immunologic mechanisms is subject to an array of factors that may limit antitumor effector function. Further understanding of this relationship should permit manipulation of the response so as to maximize the beneficial interactions for the host.

Tumor Antigens

Tumor cells may have surface antigens that allow the immune system to differentiate them from normal cells. Such antigens induce cellular and humoral immune responses and are of two types: unique tumor-specific antigens and tumor-associated antigens found on tumor cells as well as some normal cell populations. Qualitative and quantitative differences in tumor-associated antigen expression may provide useful markers for tumor cell identification. Expression of these tumor antigens reflects a heritable change in the genetic material of the cell undergoing malignant transformation.

Spontaneous and experimentally induced (carcinogens, radiation, etc.) tumors express tumor antigens. The latter arise from molecular alterations within the cell and are expressed on the cell surface or secreted into the extracellular space. Molecular mechanisms responsible for new tumor antigen formation include alteration of existing molecular structure, uncovering of normally protected molecules, de-novo synthesis of a new molecule, and expression of molecules normally restricted to the fetal stages of development. These mechanisms are activated by environmentally induced genetic mutations or the incorporation of new genetic material as occurs with oncogenic viruses. Tumor-associated antigens are increasingly being identified using monoclonal antibody technology. The best characterized tumor-associated antigens are the oncofetal antigens found in fetal tissues. They disappear during adult life but are re-expressed on certain tumor tissues.

Tumor Markers

Tumor markers, when present, are useful tools for the diagnosis, treatment, and monitoring of cancer patients. An ideal tumor marker would be produced only by cancer cells, correlate with tumor size, be readily retrievable from body tissues and fluids, be accurately measured by uniform testing, be detectable when tumor burden is small (therefore curable), and correlate with various forms of therapy. Although there are no tumor markers that fulfill all these criteria, several are clinically useful. The tumor markers that currently enjoy the most widespread use are those associated with urologic malignancies (Table 8.6).

Testicular Cancer

The alpha fetoprotein (AFP) and human chorionic gonadotropin (HCG) markers are essential for the accurate staging and management of patients with testicular germ cell tumors. Up to 50 to 90% of patients with active disease have detectable levels of one or both markers in the serum.

Table 8.6: Common Urologic Tumor Markers

- Alpha fetoprotein (AFP)
  - Glycoprotein
  - Molecular weight = 70 KD
  - Half-life of 5 days
  - Absent in pure choriocarcinoma, seminoma
- Human chorionic gonadotrophin (beta-HCG)
  - Glycoprotein
  - Molecular weight = 38 KD
  - Two chains—alpha, beta
  - Half-life 24–36 hours
  - Present in 5–10% pure seminomas
- Prostate specific antigen (PSA)
  - Glycoprotein
  - Molecular weight = 34 KD
  - Produced by prostatic epithelial cells
  - Increased in BPH, prostate cancer
  - Half-life 2–3 days

The HCG molecule is a glycoprotein of molecular weight 38 KD normally secreted by the placenta during gestation. It has two chains, alpha and beta, and closely resembles the pituitary hormones TSH, LH, and FSH. It differs primarily in the carboxy terminal of the beta chain subunit, which can be measured separately by radioimmunoassay. HCG is secreted by syncytiotrophoblast cells found in germ cell tumors, and to a lesser extent by some other solid organ cancers (liver, pancreas, stomach, lung, breast, etc.). The HCG molecule has an elimination half-life (T1/2) of 24 to 36 hours, although each subunit is cleared much faster (20 to 60 minutes). Virtually all patients with choriocarcinoma, 50 to 60% with embryonal cell carcinoma, and 5 to 10% with pure seminoma have detectable serum levels of beta HCG. The giant synctial cells sometimes present in seminomas is the source of HCG in those tumors.

The AFP molecule is a single chain glycoprotein of molecular weight 70 KD and is the major serum binding protein in the fetal circulation. It is produced by the fetal yolk sac, liver, and the GI tract and falls to low adult levels by 1 year of life. The elimination half-life (T1/2) of AFP is about 5 days. Elevated levels occur with embryonal cell carcinoma, teratocarcinoma, yolk sac tumor, and "mixed" tumors. Pure choriocarcinomas and seminomas do not produce AFP.

HCG and AFP levels correlate with tumor burden, although 10 to 15% of patients with high-stage nonseminomatous germ cell tumors have normal levels. Following curative surgery both markers are expected to reach normal levels (after about five T1/2 periods). Persistently elevated markers usually herald residual disease. In general, changes in markers parallel the course of therapy (surgery, radiation, or chemotherapy). However, testicular malignancies are notorious for changes in the predominant cell type after therapy, and marker analysis alone may be less than ideal in individual patients. Testicular tumor markers such as placental alkaline phosphatase, lactate dehydrogenase, carcinoembryonic antigen, and human placental lactogen have also been reported to be useful in monitoring patients. However, they are less specific and not widely used.

Bladder Cancer

Because bladder cancer is well visualized by cystoscopy and amenable to repeated biopsy, the development of tumor markers has focused on the identification of lesions with a propensity for muscle invasion. The availability of sloughed bladder cells in the urine provides a ready source of tissue for observation of changes in cell structure. The most promising results have been reported using differences in chromosome banding, DNA content, and loss of blood group surface antigens. Invasiveness seems to be associated with a progressive increase in the modal chromosome number and in certain banding patterns on autosomes. Flow cytometry can assess the ploidy of cell populations in the urine. The blood group antigens A, B, and H are lost when the urothelium undergoes malignant transformation. Much of the technology required for these evaluations is cumbersome and not widely available.

Kidney Cancer

Several reports have described associations between renal cell carcinoma and some normally occurring serum products (e.g., erythropoietin, renin, prostaglandins, cholesterol, ACTH, and parathormone). However, none has achieved reliable clinical utility. Preliminary reports have described monoclonal antibody preparations that can identify epitopes specific to renal cell carcinoma. This promising area of investigation awaits further advances.

Prostate Cancer

Prostate specific antigen (PSA) comes as close as any known endogenous substance to fulfilling the criteria for an ideal tumor marker. PSA was initially discovered in seminal plasma by two independent labs (Hara et al. in Japan and Li and Beling) in the early 1970s. By 1979, it was established that PSA originates from and is specific for prostatic tissue. Further investigations confirmed that the same substance could be isolated from prostatic tissue, seminal plasma, and human serum; and by the 1980s, PSA could be reliably measured in the serum using enzyme-linked assays. The two most common diseases of the prostate, benign prostatic hyperplasia (BPH) and prostate adenocarcinoma, cause PSA elevations. During the latter part of the 1980s the role of PSA determinations in the diagnosis and management of patients with prostatic disease had been established, and current investigations seek to incorporate serum PSA measurement into the evaluation of the aging adult male.

PSA is a glycoprotein monomer of 240 amino acids and 4 carbohydrate side chains with a molecular weight of 34 KD. The gene encoding PSA has been sequenced and resides on chromosome 19 in humans. Functionally, PSA is a serine protease produced only by the epithelial cells lining the ducts and acini of the prostate gland. PSA is detectable in the epithelial cells of BPH tissue, primary prostate cancer, and in metastatic deposits of prostate cancer. The enzymatic action of PSA is similar to the proteases of the kallikrein family, to which it bears significant genetic homology. PSA is normally secreted into the lumina of the prostatic ducts, and it has a significant role in the liquefaction of the seminal coagulum formed during ejaculation. The seminal coagulum contains a structural protein of high molecular weight that is cleaved by PSA into several protein fragments of lower molecular weight, promoting liquefaction.

The average concentration of PSA in seminal plasma is about 2 mg/ml.

PSA is measured in patient sera using one of two commercially available assays. Over 90% of centers use the Tandem-R PSA (Hybritech, Inc.) method, and much of the clinical literature is based on this assay. Although absolute numbers differ, the trends and relationships observed in prostate disease have been similar in both assay systems. The Tandem-R assay is a solid phase immunoradiometric assay that uses two murine monoclonal antibodies specific for different epitopes on the PSA molecule. Female sera are used as the media for dilution standards. Studies have failed to establish a circadian pattern to PSA levels in the serum, but did demonstrate up to a 20% fall in PSA levels when patients are hospitalized and put to bed rest. In addition, various reports of manipulations of the prostate, such as digital rectal exam, transrectal ultrasound, several modes of biopsy, cystoscopy, and transurethral procedures, can falsely elevate serum levels. Therefore, the most appropriate time to measure serum PSA in an ambulatory patient may be prior to prostatic examination or instrumentation.

The disappearance of PSA from the serum after total prostatectomy follows first-order kinetics. The elimination half-life of PSA in the serum is between 2 and 3 days. This is important in patients after radical prostatectomy, as nearly 3 weeks must elapse after prostate removal before serum PSA levels fall to zero.

It has been observed that 100% of healthy men under age 40 and 97% of healthy men over age 40 have values between 0.0 and 4.0 ng/ml. The majority of those healthy men with PSA levels over 4.0 ng/ml had levels less than 10 ng/ml. Healthy females have a range of 0.0 to 0.2 ng/ml. The assay curve is linear over the working range of 0.0 to 100 ng/ml. Some authors have reported that BPH raises the serum PSA about 0.3 to 0.5 ng/ml per gram of tissue, and that prostate adenocarcinoma raises it about 3 to 4 ng/ml per gram of cancer. However, since both BPH and prostate cancer elevate the PSA level, and both are detected with greater frequency with increasing age, significant overlap prevents precise tissue diagnosis by PSA level, at least in the early stages of disease. In addition, since PSA is prostate-tissue rather than prostate-cancer specific, not all prostate cancers will cause a detectable increase in PSA. While these limitations may limit the role of PSA as a cancer screening tool, its usefulness in screening high-risk groups or for serial determinations in the same patient are the subject of ongoing investigation.

Pretreatment serum PSA values in patients with clinically localized prostate cancer have been correlated with the pathologic step-sectioning of radical prostatectomy specimens. PSA correlates with increasing stage and cancer volume in a particular gland, but there is considerable overlap.

As previously discussed, the amount of coexistent BPH tissue also influences these findings. Thus, no single PSA value defines local extension or capsular penetration of prostate cancer. Certain ranges of values may be clinically useful. One large study reported that a cancer is unlikely to be organ-confined if the preoperative PSA exceeds 50 to 75 ng/ml. In addition, a large retrospective study found that among 306 patients with pretreatment PSA levels under 20 ng/ml, only one had a positive bone scan. Therefore, the PSA value may help refine clinical staging prior to therapy.

The clinical utility and impact of PSA is perhaps best demonstrated in the monitoring of patients with prostate cancer. After total removal of the prostate, PSA should fall to undetectable levels, generally considered less than 0.5 ng/ml. Higher levels or increasing levels over time represent residual cancer. PSA is also a useful marker of disease activity in patients treated with radiotherapy or antiandrogen therapy. In over 80% of patients with early tumor control or remission, the PSA levels fall dramatically, often up to 10-fold. Rising PSA levels correlate with biopsy-confirmed disease progression and clinical symptoms. Longer follow-up of existing patient cohorts and future studies may further define high-risk groups who would benefit from adjuvant therapies. The use of PSA may prove to be even more essential in the future as newer anticancer agents and biological preparations are developed and tested against prostate cancer.

IMMUNOTHERAPY

The spontaneous regression or disappearance of cancer is extremely rare, occurring in less than 0.1% of cancer patients. Nevertheless, such events suggest that the immune system is capable of attacking and eliminating cancer cells. Anecdotal reports of patients who live for many years with a stable and measured tumor burden exist, further supporting the notion that the immune system is capable of controlling tumor growth.

Although the host immune system is often unable to control tumor growth in-vivo, continued investigation into the tumor–host relationship holds promise that future manipulations can amplify the response to promote tumor eradication. These immunotherapy approaches are appealing because healthy cells are spared. Recent technological advances have stimulated enthusiasm for successful tumor immunotherapy. These advances include the ability to separate distinct lymphocyte subpopulations, the retrieval of lymphocytes that infiltrate tumors, the identification and purification of newer tumor-specific and tumor-associated antigens, the production of large quantities of cytokines using recombinant DNA technology, and the production of antibody–toxin conjugates with specific tumor-killing activity. These advances have contributed to a variety of immunotherapeutic approaches (Table 8.7).

Table 8.7: Cancer Immunotherapy

Rationale
Theory of immune surveillance
Tumor-specific and tumor-associated antigens
Spontaneous tumor regression
Augment immune response to tumors
Approaches
Direct immunization with tumor cells
Adoptive cellular immunity
Lymphokine activated killer (LAK) cells
Interleukins (ILs)
Tumor infiltrating lymphocytes (TILs)
Interferons (alpha, beta, gamma)
Specific monoclonal antibodies

Immunization with Tumor Cells or Antigens

Direct immunization of tumor-bearing hosts with fresh tumor cells or purified tumor antigens has generally not led to primary tumor regression. This is due to the presence of billions of cells in tumors over 1 cm^3 in volume and the triggering of Ts (suppressor cells) networks that inhibit antitumor responses. Appropriate tumor sensitization requires a diminished tumor burden and depletion of the Ts cell population, but this may not be practical. The main limiting factor in tumor immunization is the intrinsically weak immunogenic nature of the tumor antigens. Several techniques have been used to modify the antigens so as to augment the immune response, for example, attempts to alter or uncover hidden surface markers using neuraminidase or binding haptens such as trinitrophenol to surface structures. Thus far, this has resulted in limited success in animal models. A more adventurous scheme would be to insert genes that encode known highly immunogenic tumor antigens into weakly immunogenic tumor cells using recombinant vectors such as viruses. These approaches, currently reserved for preclinical investigation, may become clinically useful in the future.

Adoptive Cellular Immunotherapy and Cytokines

The same reasoning that spawned attempts to immunize hosts against cancer cells led to trials of passive immunotherapy, whereby cancer patients were given transfusions of whole blood or serum from other patients who had successfully convalesced from cancer. These transfusions did not result in tumor regression, nor did transfusion from animals heavily immunized with human cancer cells. No doubt the host allograft and/or xenograft response against these cells blunted their antitumor activity. However, adoptive immunotherapy or cell transfer of tumor-specific immune cells to tumor-bearing hosts causes tumor regression in certain inbred strains of mice. Human experimentation is limited by the inability to raise sufficient numbers of tumor-specific human lymphocytes. In vivo sensitization to tumor antigens also induces populations of Ts cells, and those need to be eliminated prior to cell transfer in order to maximize antitumor potency.

The identification and purification of the T-cell growth factor, interleukin-2 (IL-2), opened the door to the generation of sufficient quantities of human tumor-specific lymphocytes. The availability of IL-2 and other cytokines allowed the cloning of specific lymphocytes in culture. Advances in recombinant DNA technology made the IL-2 itself abundant, so it could be used in experimental protocols. Animal studies clearly demonstrated that tumor-specific T cells could be extracted from tumor-immunized mice and grown in culture, and that the cultured cells would retain their antitumor properties when reinjected into tumor-bearing hosts. In addition, IL-2 enhances tumor regression if given with the transferred cells, presumably by locally expanding the cytotoxic cell population. Much of this work and the subsequent clinical trials was done by Rosenberg and his colleagues at the National Cancer Institute.

The isolation of T cells with antitumor activity is more difficult in humans. During experiments aimed at growing T-cells and tumor in culture with IL-2, Yron and Spiess noted that a new population of cells was induced by the cytokine, that is, cells with cytolytic activity against several different tumor types. Even human peripheral blood lymphocytes in culture would kill a variety of human cancer cells in-vitro when exposed to IL-2. These in-vitro activated cells were named lymphokine-activated killer (LAK) cells. When LAK cells were further characterized, they were found not to be cytotoxic T cells or B cells, but null lymphocytes similar to natural killer (NK) cells.

Since 1985, over 300 patients have been treated with LAK cells, IL-2, or a combination of both. The therapy is most effective in patients with metastatic renal cell carcinoma or melanoma. For kidney cancers, complete regressions occur in about 10% of patients, while 25% demonstrate a 50% reduction in tumor mass. Overall, the use of IL-2 and LAK cell adoptive immunotherapy is estimated to benefit about 20% of cancer patients who fail conventional forms of therapy. The toxicity of the therapy, primarily related to high doses of intravenous IL-2, is severe and requires hospitalization in intensive care units. Fever, chills, rigors, lethargy, GI symptoms, anemia, hypotension, azotemia, and a capillary leak syndrome causing pulmonary edema can occur. Fortunately, most side effects disappear with cessation of treatment.

The encouraging clinical trials using LAK cells and IL-2 stimulated the search for truly tumor-specific cell populations. It was reasoned that the likely source of these cells, already activated against the patient's cancer, was the tumor itself. Tumors were surgically removed, enzymatically digested, and cultured with IL-2 and other growth factors. Tumor cells and LAK cells generally stop proliferating by 1 to 2 weeks, leaving a residual population of lymphocytes with specific antitumor cytotoxicity. These cells were named tumor-infiltrating lymphocytes (TIL), and they are classic cytotoxic T cells. Early clinical trials of TIL and IL-2 therapy suggest that they are more potent than LAK and IL-2 therapy for patients with metastatic melanoma. Since the TILs have more specific antitumor activity, they require less IL-2, and this diminishes the toxic side effects of therapy. Trials with TILs await longer follow-up to establish the durability of responses and the justification of the high cost and complexity of administration.

Recent studies have confirmed that adoptively transferred TILs work at the site of the tumor in the host. This was conclusively determined using the first FDA-approved recombinant gene therapy in a human. In culture, the TILs had a foreign gene inserted to be used as a marker when they were reintroduced into the host. The foreign gene encoded for a protein that normally renders a bacteria resistant to neomycin. This protein was subsequently found in the tumor site after TILs were injected peripherally, thus establishing their path to the tumor.

Interferons

Interferons inhibit the growth of some transplantable tumors and the development of experimental metastases in animals. This is also observed when human tumor xenografts are transplanted to nude mice. Alpha IFN has induced significant responses in hematologic malignancies, including (in descending order) hairy cell leukemia, chronic myeloid leukemia, essential thrombocythemia, and lymphoma. The responses of solid tumors to alpha IFN are few, and the initial enthusiasm for alpha IFN in renal cell carcinoma has waned. The antitumor activity of the IFNs may be related to negative growth regulation rather than immunomodulation of the host anticancer response.

Gamma IFN is a more potent modulator of the immune response than either alpha or beta IFN. However, it does not have increased antitumor efficacy compared to alpha IFN. Advanced solid tumors are not sensitive to gamma IFN. One phase II study did report that 7 of 14 patients with advanced renal cell carcinoma did demonstrate significant responses, two of which were described as complete. In the future, the IFNs may have a place as adjuvant agents in urologic cancer therapy.

Specific Antibody Therapy

The ability to generate monoclonal antibodies ("designer antibodies") has increased the potential for antitumor antibody therapy. In the future, monoclonal antibodies themselves may be highly selective triggers for antibody-dependent cellular cytotoxicity (ADCC), which has been shown to be more potent than complement-dependent tumor cell killing in vitro. The ability to conjugate cytotoxic drugs, toxins, or radioisotopes to antibodies may generate true "magic bullets" for killing tumor cells. Tumor antigens that are endocytosed are particularly appealing targets for conjugates with toxins or cytotoxic drugs. It also may be possible to deliver ionizing radiation to regions of a tumor that express certain epitopes. The eventual applicability of these techniques will depend on the identification of true tumor-specific antigens, since the more common tumor-associated antigens are also present on some normal cell populations that would need to be protected from the antitumor therapies.

SUGGESTED READINGS

Balkwill FR. Interferons. Lancet 1989; 1:1060.

Comprehensive summary of the production of the various interferons and their clinical uses.

Kohler H, Milstein C. Continuous culture of fused cells secreting antibody of predefined specificity. Nature 1975; 256:495.

Seminal description of the theory and production of monoclonal antibodies.

Mayforth RD, Quintans J. Designer and catalytic antibodies. N Engl J Med 1990; 323:173.

Insightful analysis of the potential uses and actual creation of hybrid antibodies in the laboratory.

Nossal GJ. Basic concepts of the immune system. N Engl J Med 1987; 316: 1320.

Elegant overview of the basic principles of cellular and humoral immunity and regulation. Integration of the concepts with clinical diseases is also presented.

Oesterling JE. Prostate specific antigen: a critical assessment of the most useful tumor marker for prostate cancer. J Urol 1991; 145:907.

Detailed description of PSA including the integration of laboratory and clinical findings.

Rosenberg SA, Packard B, Aebersold P, et al. Use of tumor infiltrating lymphocytes and IL-2 in the immunotherapy of patients with metastatic melanoma. N Engl J Med 1988; 319:1676.

Documents the clinical results and complexity in the use of tumor-infiltrating lymphocytes and IL-2. Prior treatment results with LAK cells and IL-2 are refined.

Rosenberg SA, Lotze M, Yang J, et al. Experience with the use of high dose IL-2 in the treatment of 652 patients with cancer. Ann Surg 1989; 210:474.

Largest known compilation of the results of clinical immunotherapy for metastatic cancer. Emphasis on the complexity and toxicity of immunotherapeutic protocols.

Rosenberg SA, Aebersold P, Cornetta K, et al. Gene transfer into humans: immunotherapy of patients with advanced melanoma using tumor infiltrating lymphocytes modified by retroviral gene transduction. N Engl J Med 1990; 323:570.

Detailed report of the first approved and successful transfer of a gene from the laboratory to a human.

Tracy KJ, Vlassara H, Cerami A. Cachectin tumor necrosis factor. Lancet 1989; 1:1122.

Comprehensive review of the identification and possible clinical uses of tumor necrosis factors.

Wood MR, Cohen MJ. Monoclonal antibodies defining distinctive human T cell surface antigens. Science 1979; 206:347.

Significant study that demonstrated the use of monoclonal antibodies to identify lymphocyte populations by phenotype of cell-surface antigens.

CHAPTER 9

Renal Transplantation

Joseph M. Hayes
Andrew C. Novick

Renal transplantation is an established and, in most cases, the preferred treatment for advanced chronic renal failure. Perhaps the most striking development in renal transplantation over the last 15 years has been the steady decline in morbidity and mortality. Mortality within the first year, during which time most deaths occur, is less than 5% for living donor graft recipients and approximately 10% for cadaveric donor recipients. Comparisons of dialysis and transplantation as therapy for patients with chronic renal failure have revealed that patients treated by dialysis are subject to a rather constant yearly death rate, whereas the death rate following transplantation falls sharply after the first year. The success of clinical transplantation in the last three decades has been achieved primarily as a result of advances in immunobiology.

The experiments of Alexis Carrel in the early twentieth century noted the process of host allograft rejection of animal organs. In the early 1950s attempts at human transplantation in unmodified recipients were generally unsuccessful. In 1954, Merrill, Murray, and associates performed the first successful human renal transplant between monozygotic twins. This success and subsequent experience demonstrated the effectiveness of renal transplantation in restoring a normal physiologic state to uremic patients.

TRANSPLANTATION IMMUNOLOGY

The Major Histocompatibility Complex

The intensity of tissue transplant rejection is related to the degree of tissue or histocompatibility. Transplantation or histocompatibility antigens are surface glycoproteins encoded by a set of closely linked gene loci collectively known as the major histocompatibility complex (MHC), located on human chromosome 6. Transplantation antigens are termed human leukocyte antigens (HLA) (Table 9.1). The segment of each chromosome that encodes for the MHC products is referred to as a *haplotype.* MHC antigens are divided into class I, II, and III antigens (Figure 9.1). The class III gene products include complement components that, when activated, serve as biologically active mediators and aid the nonspecific inflammatory response via alterations in vascular permeability, regional blood flow, inflammatory cell infiltration, and wound repair.

The class I antigens, HLA-A, -B, and -C, are present in varying concentrations on the cell surface of nucleated human cells and platelets and serve as recognition molecules for antibody and cell-mediated reactions against transplanted tissue. The structures of these antigens are described in Chapter 8. The HLA system is complex, with over 60 HLA-A, HLA-B, and HLA-C specificities recognized. Since virtually any HLA-A antigen may be linked with any B, C, or class II D antigens, the number of haplotypes present in the human population is enormous. Each individual receives two different chromosomes (one from each parent) such that the number of possible genotypes is large.

Lymphocytes from different individuals, when mixed in tissue culture, undergo a proliferative response because of their immunogenetic disparity. The transplantation antigens that trigger this proliferative response are the class II antigens. These cell surface glycoproteins are coded for by the MHC region termed HLA-D and subdivided into DQ, DP, and DR subregions. Class II antigens differ from class I antigens in their limited tissue distribution. They reside on antigen-presenting cells, for example, monocyte/macrophages, endothelial cells, dendritic cells, B-lymphocytes, and activated T-lymphocytes.

Table 9.1: Human Leukocyte Antigens (HLAs)

Closely related genes on chromosome 6
Inherited in mendelian, codominant fashion
Each individual inherits two sets or haplotypes of HLA genes
Individual haplotypes
25% chance HLA identical
25% chance HLA dissimilar
50% chance single haplotype match
Recombinant frequency between HLA genes
Roughly 1%
1 in 100 persons have haplotype resulting from gene crossover between original parent chromosomes

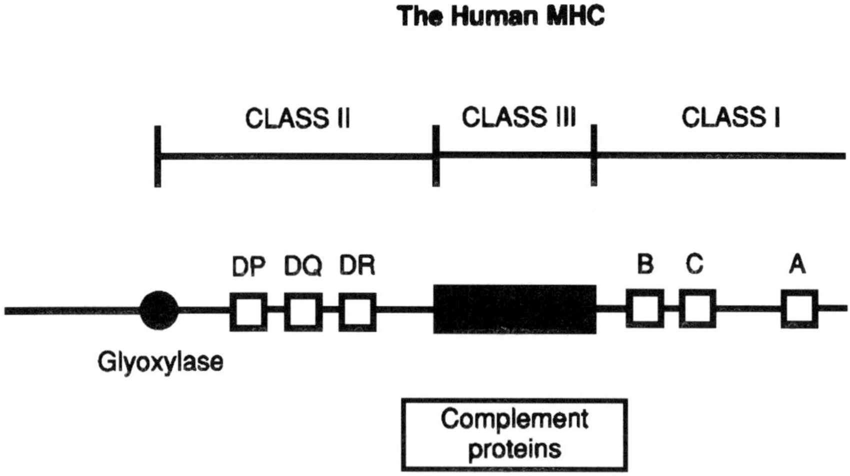

Figure 9.1: The major histocompatibility complex in humans. Located in the short arm of chromosome 6, genes are encoded for all three classes of immunologic activity and self-recognition.

Genetics of HLA Inheritance

The combination of closely linked alleles at each HLA locus on a single chromosome in inherited as a haplotype. Each individual inherits one chromosome 6 from each parent, resulting in two HLA haplotypes. Both alleles at a given HLA locus are usually expressed; that is, the expression is codominant and detectable on the cell surface—for example, an individual cell could express HLA-A1, -A2; -B8, -B12; -DR1, and -DR4. This is referred to as the HLA profile or phenotype. An individual may be homozygous for a given antigen when the same allele is present on both chromosomes. For example, an individual may be HLA-A1, -A1, while having different HLA-B and HLA-DR antigens.

Each parent has two haplotypes, and one is contributed to the inherited combination in the offspring. Four genotypic combinations are therefore possible, and the chance of two individual siblings sharing both haplotypes (haploidentical) is 25%, one haplotype 50%, and 0 haplotypes 25%. Due to recombination between HLA loci during meiosis, new haplotypes are occasionally seen (Table 9.1). Siblings may be haploidentical but ABO incompatible, because the antigens are encoded by genes on different chromosomes.

Histocompatibility Testing

The two techniques for histocompatibility testing (tissue typing) are serology and mixed lymphocyte reactions (MLR). The MLR is based on the fact that T cells are stimulated to proliferate in the presence of cells carrying foreign class II antigens. In practice, test cells are mixed with typing cells (usually B cells) that are homozygous for a particular specificity. The test T cells bearing for example, HLA-DR3,4, or HLA-DR1,2 antigens are cultured with B cells, pretreated by irradiation or mictomycin-C to prevent proliferation, and bear a homozygous antigen-HLA-DR3,3. In the case of HLA-DR3,4 no proliferation will occur. In the case of HLA-DR1,2, the test cells recognize the DR antigens on the typing cells as foreign and thus proliferate. After a 6-day culture, the proliferation of test lymphocytes is assessed by the incorporation of tritiated thymidine into DNA over a 12 to 24 hour period. In such a mixed lymphocyte culture (termed one way), the treated cells are designated as *stimulators* and the test population as *responders.*

In serological typing, antisera of a defined specificity, for example, anti-HLA-A2, is applied in a microtiter plate to the cells being tested (lymphocytes) in the presence of complement and a vital dye such as eosin. Cell death (uptake of dye) confirms the expression of that antigen (A2) on the cell surface. Serologic methods are also employed to detect class II antigens by use of immunofluorescence and enzyme-linked immunosorbent techniques. In clinical transplantation, tissue-typing techniques allow donor and recipient matching on the basis of HLA typing. In living related transplantation, HLA matching influences graft survival by as much as 10% at 3 years in patients with one and two haplotype matches.

Tissue typing is also used to screen potential recipient serum for cytotoxic antibodies, and to cross match potential donor cells with recipient serum. The transplant recipient's serum is periodically screened for preexisting cytotoxic anti-HLA antibodies by incubating the serum with a panel of cells obtained from various donors bearing well characterized HLA antigens. Complement-dependent cell lysis (CDC) is indicative of antidonor antibodies formed in response to previous antigen exposure during blood transfusions, pregnancy, or transplantation. The extent of the sensitization is measured by the percentage of the panel test cells lysed or the percent reactive antibody (PRA). A PRA of over 50% indicates a highly sensitized patient, for whom finding a compatible donor is difficult.

The technique of cross-matching, applied at the time of transplantation, refers to the incubation of a potential donor's cells with the recipient serum and the addition of complement. CDC is indicative of previous antigenic exposure and the presence of cytotoxic, anti-HLA antibodies (positive cross match).

In recent years new methodology has been applied to the identification of antidonor antibodies. Detection of host presensitization by the standard visual assessment of the CDC assay is insensitive. A modified complement-dependent assay technique, the antihuman immunoglobulin (Ig) technique, increases the assay sensitivity and detects subliminal antidonor Ig reactivity. The sensitivity of the cross-match assay has been further improved by flow cytometry, which uses an antihuman Ig conjugated to an immunofluorescent marker. There is controversy regarding the clinical relevance of very low levels of alloantibody detected by the antiglobulin or flow cytometry cross-match techniques in the face of a negative standard cross match.

Another new tissue-typing approach uses recombinant DNA technology to identify the DNA codes for HLA class II antigens. With this technique, HLA antigens have been found to be much more polymorphic at the gene level than at the serologic level. DNA fragments are isolated using restriction enzymes. Southern hybridization with class II DNA probes enables a comparison of the number of matched fragments between donor and recipient. The efficacy of DNA typing in renal transplantation is incompletely agreed upon, but refinement and practical applicability of these techniques hold promise for the future. A further refinement is the use of immunomagnetic beads to separate T and B cells for subsequent typing. Currently, the combination of flow cytometry and conventional cross match using immunomagnetically separated cells appears to offer the maximum characterization of a recipient–donor cross match.

Allograft Rejection Mechanisims

The immune response can be divided into the cellular and humoral components, although in the actual response to an allograft, a complex communicative interaction occurs between the two. The cells involved include lymphocytes, monocyte/macrophages, neutrophils, and antigen-presenting cells (APCs), such as endothelial cells and dendritic cells. The specificity of the immune response rests with the lymphocyte's ability to recognize and respond to foreign antigens. Lympocytes differ from one another by specific receptors and functional characteristics. A common precursor cell in bone marrow gives rise to two broad classes of lymphocytes: those that migrate to the thymus (T lymphocytes), and those that remain in the bone marrow and mature into B lymphocytes. These cells then migrate to lymphoid organs such as the spleen and lymph nodes. T cells have been further separated into various subpopulations on the basis of functional characteristics and cell surface receptors (see Chapter 8).

Cytokines

Cytokines, soluble protein and glycoprotein products made by various cells of the immune system, function in cell–cell communications, inflammatory responses, and immunoregulation. Cytokines stimulate cell proliferation (interleukins-2, -3, -4, -5, -7, and colony stimulating factors), attack foreign materials (interferons, tumor necrosis factor), mediate inflammatory cell mobilization and migration (migration inhibitory factor, interleukin-8, interleukin-1), stimulate adhesive interactions between cells (IL-1, TNF, or tumor necrosis factor, and interferon gamma), and activate cells for effector responses (IL-1, gamma interferon, IL-2, IL-6, and tumor necrosis factor) (see Chapter 8). The cytokines have broad cellular activity, and many cytokine actions are synergistic and overlapping. Many cytokines act as primers on various target cells, serving to enhance the response to other cytokines.

Accessory Cells

Most antigens are incapable of stimulating lymphocytes unless they are presented by the accessory immune cells in conjunction with class I or II antigen. Cells of the monocyte/macrophage lineage are the prime APCs in transplantation immunobiology. Macrophages take up foreign proteins, internalize and process them, and make them accessible to the immune system in a recognizable form. They also interact with lymphokines to become microbicidal and tumoricidal; affect T and B lymphocyte activity in many immunologic responses, and secrete complement proteins, growth factors (e.g., interleukins), bioactive lipids (e.g., prostaglandins), enzymes, tissue reorganization factors (e.g., angiogenesis factor), inflammatory enhancing proteins such as TNF and IL-1, and clotting factors. An important accessory cell is the dendritic cell. Dendritic cells are APCs that express MHC class II antigen and reside in lymph nodes, the spleen, and at low levels in blood. They are strong T-cell stimulators and activators of the allogeneic MLR. They may be present in many nonlymphoid organs. Dendritic cells in transplanted organs are referred to as passenger cells. Immunogenic dendritic cells may leave the graft after transplantation and enter draining lymph nodes, where they can potentially sensitize the host. The exact role of the neutrophil in allograft rejection remains uncertain. Neutrophils are among the first cells to infiltrate an allograft, and they may play a role in the attraction of other cells to enhance the nonspecific inflammatory and specific immune response. Neutrophils may also play a role in the preparation of the endothelium to infiltration by macrophages and lymphocytes.

The Immune Response

The immune response to an allograft can be divided into afferent and efferent arms (see Chapter 8). Allograft HLA antigens interact initially with host APCs that process antigen and present it to the T helper cell together with MHC class II antigens. Host lymphocyte recognition of alloantigen results in the proliferation and differentiation to specifically sensitized effector lymphocytes capable of target-cell lysis or antibody secretion. An elaborate amplification process takes place with graft antigen interacting with recipient T-cells and macrophages to produce lymphokines, which further stimulate clonal production of T cells and activation of B lymphocytes and macrophages.

The effector phase has specific and nonspecific components. The nonspecific activation of the complement and clotting mechanisms, the release of mediators such as leukotrienes or prostaglandins, and the accumulation of neutrophils or macrophages serve to amplify and concentrate the local immune response. Cytotoxic T cells respond to IL-2, differentiate, proliferate, and bind to target cells recognizing MHC class I products and antigens, and are thereby able to lyse specific allogeneic target cells. Binding is mediated by adhesion molecules (LFA-1 and ICAM-1) present on both the lymphocyte and target cell. Membrane permeability changes following binding, with resultant cell swelling, disruption, and allograft loss. Down-regulation of the immune response may occur via the action of CD8+ suppressor lymphocytes or suppressor products such as prostaglandins, which are secreted by T lymphocytes and accessory cells.

CLINICAL RENAL TRANSPLANTATION

Organ Donor Physiology, Selection, and Management

In the United States, over 20,000 patients currently appear on national waiting lists for solid organ transplants. It is estimated that greater than 25,000 potential organ donors die each year in the United States, for an overall loss of perhaps 100,000 transplantable organs. Despite what seems to be an adequate donor pool, only approximately 15% of potential donors become actual donors. Early donor recognition, rapid and accurate declaration of brain death, physiological maintenance, and coordination with local organ procurement agencies are important aspects of donor management.

Cadaveric Donor Selection

A thorough history and physical examination are vital in the initial assessment of donor suitability. The donor must be "brain-stem" dead and supported on a ventilator. The clinical diagnosis of brain death is based on the absence of brain-stem and cerebral function. Clinical tests of brain death include electrocerebral silence documented by electroencephalography as well as the absence of the following: cerebral responsiveness; motor activity; cough reflex with deep tracheal suctioning; corneal, pupillary, and oculocephalic/oculovestibular reflexes; an increase in heart rate in response to atropine; respiratory efforts on apnea testing with a $PaCO_2 > 60$ mm Hg. Hypothermia, metabolic encephalopathy, drug intoxication, and shock all must be excluded. The physician who makes the diagnosis of brain death should not be a member of the organ procurement or transplantation team, and the diagnosis should be made in strict accordance with local state laws.

Underlying conditions that generally exclude donors are advanced artherosclerosis, insulin-dependent diabetes, severe hypertension requiring multiple drug treatment, untreated systemic viral or bacterial infections, and extracranial malignant diseases. A history of cardiac arrest or prolonged hypotension is not an absolute contraindication for organ donation. Many centers have successfully used donors under 10 and even under 3 years of age. Other centers, however, are hesitant to use single kidneys from donors under 5 or 6 years of age. The upper limit of age is also controversial, and the shortage of kidneys for transplantation has persuaded some centers to extend their donor age limit beyond 50 to 55 years.

Donors with a history of chronic renal insufficiency are generally excluded. Donor laboratory evaluation includes tissue typing, a biochemical assessment of individual organ function or disease, and a microbiological/serological evaluation to prevent the transmission of infectious diseases such as viral hepatitis or encephalitis, acquired immunodeficiency syndrome, or venereal diseases to the potential recipient. Serological screen should also determine the presence or absence of cytomegalovirus (CMV) infection. An often-ignored aspect of organ donation is the need for continuing support of the donor's family. Frequently, second thoughts concerning the decision to permit organ removal, continuing worry about the patient, or the questions about the logistics of surgery require the availability of chaplains, social workers, physicians, nurses, and transplant coordinators to assist during the final stages of what is usually an unexpected injury or tragic illness.

Donor Management and the Physiology of Brain Death

Routine general care of the potential organ donor is of utmost importance. Maintenance of pulmonary care, nasogastric suction to prevent aspiration, lubrication and protection of the eyes, removal of all intravascular catheters placed before admission or during resuscitation, and maintenance of normothermia prevent infection and other complications that may render organs unsuitable for transplantation. Monitoring should include central venous and arterial pressure catheters and a Foley bladder catheter. The donor's temperature should be monitored with a probe calibrated to record temperatures below 35° C.

Deterioration of brain function and loss of central neurohumoral regulatory control results in severe systemic hypertension (Cushing's reflex) with elevated circulating catecholamines and sympathetic activity. Beta blockers can be used to protect the myocardium and antagonize the circulating catecholamines. Bradyarrhythmias may arise in association with hypertension. Atropine has little effect in the brain-dead patient. Brain herniation destroys the medullary and pontine vasomotor structures and causes hypotension and tachyarrhythmias. Adequate systemic organ perfusion is the most important factor in maintaining optimal organ viability. Maintenance of a minimum systolic pressure of 90 to 100 mm Hg is recommended. If vasopressors are required, Dopamine hydrochloride is the preferred vasopressor. A urine output of over 100 ml/hour is an important prognostic factor in determining renal allograft function.

The destruction of the hypothalamic–pituitary axis results in low levels of circulating antidiuretic hormone and "central" diabetes insipidus. Excessive free water loss leads to hypernatremia, hypokalemia, hypomagnesemia, hypocalcemia, and hypophosphatemia. Vasopressin administration may be needed to correct these fluid and electrolyte imbalances and maintain adequate urine outputs. An arterial oxygen saturation of at least 95% should be maintained, and antibiotics should be administered for documented or suspected infection. Aminoglycosides or other nephrotoxic drugs should be avoided.

Agents beneficial to post-transplant function include diuretics, alpha adrenergic blockers (phenoxybenzamine), and heparin. Pharmacologic agents of some benefit in the pretreatment of the brain-dead donor include lidocaine, calcium channel blockers, trifluoperazine, and drugs protecting against free radical injury. Experimental studies suggest that triiodothyronine, cortisol, and insulin can reverse cardiac and renal abnormalities.

ORGAN PROCUREMENT, RENAL ISCHEMIA, AND PRESERVATION

Procurement

Renal harvest is usually done in conjunction with procurement of other solid organs such as the liver, heart, or pancreas. The techniques for multiple organ harvest are well described. Following removal of the other intra-abdominal organs, the exposed kidneys are removed en-bloc while in-situ cold perfusion via an aortic cannula continues. In organ donors who are not candidates for liver or heart procurement, the current technique of harvest is en-bloc removal of both kidneys and ureter with a segment of abdominal aorta and vena cava (Figure 9.2). This technique is independent of renal vascular anatomy and avoids dissection in the renal

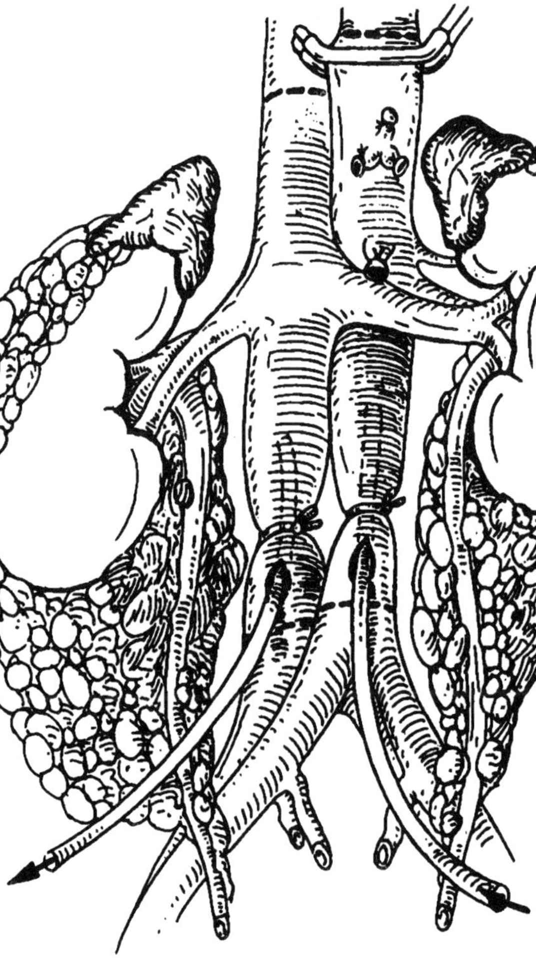

Figure 9.2: En bloc dissection for cadaveric kidney donation with cannulas in place for in-situ perfusion. Notice perihilar and periureteral fat are left in place. *Reproduced with permission from Webster G, Kirby R, King L, et al eds. Reconstructive Urology Vol 1. Boston: Blackwell Scientific Publications, 1993:202.*

hilum, which may compromise ureteral blood supply. Preservation of the aorta and vena cava allows the formation of Carrel patches, which are particularly useful if multiple vessels are present. After removal, the kidneys are placed in ice-slush solution; care is taken to protect the kidneys from direct contact with the ice.

Living-donor assessment consists of ascertaining that the donor will suffer no disadvantage from donor nephrectomy, or long-term loss of function secondary to being uninephric. Screening for renal or systemic disease requires a thorough history, physical examination, chest x-ray, electrocardiogram, 24-hour urine estimation of protein and creatinine, exclusion of urinary-tract infection, an intravenous pyelogram, and a renal arteriogram. Living-donor nephrectomy can be carried out through an eleventh rib flank incision to avoid entering the abdomen. The ureter and gonadal vessels are identified, and the vessels are ligated and divided distally. The ureter is dissected deeply in the pelvis; care is taken to maintain an adequate amount of periureteral tissue. Dissection proceeds to maintain a cone of tissue between the gonadal vessels, ureter, and the lower pole of the kidney. The gonadal vessels are followed to the renal vein. The renal vein and artery are then dissected with minimal manipulation to avoid spasm. After the vessels are mobilized, a brisk diuresis is induced with fluids and diuretics (e.g., Lasix, Mannitol) so that urine flows freely from the cut end of the ureter. The renal artery and vein are then ligated and divided. The kidney is removed and immersed in a cold preservation solution for flushing on a back-bench.

Renal Ischemia

Ischemic, hypoxic tissues lose the purine intermediate compounds used to make high energy ATP, but they recover and reconvert them if oxygen is restored. Cellular resynthesis pathways permit hypoxanthine and other compounds to be reconverted to ATP. Once these nucleotides are degraded beyond the xanthine level, however, they are irreversibly lost (Figure 9.3). The xanthine oxidase inhibitor allopurinol inhibits degradation of xanthine and was thought to be a possible renal protective agent for periods of warm ischemia of up to one hour. However, a randomized double blind study did not show a beneficial effect of allopurinol on the recovery of ischemically damaged human kidneys. Other agents effective

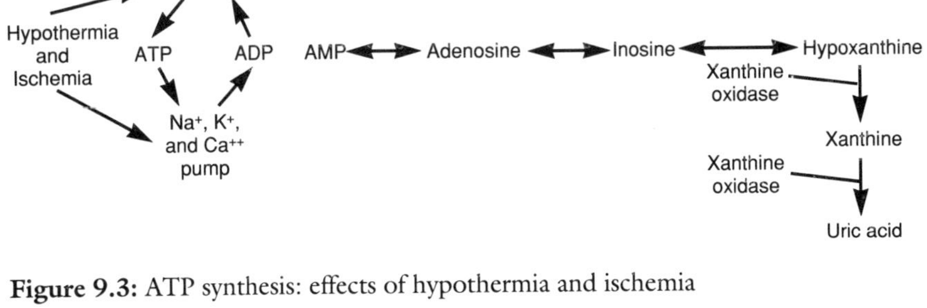

Figure 9.3: ATP synthesis: effects of hypothermia and ischemia

in the perioperative protection of ischemic and reperfusion injuries include captopril, trifluoperazine, and mannitol. Failure to perfuse and oxygenate the renal cortex is thought to be a key factor in the development of post-transplant, delayed graft function. Prolonged cold storage results in progressive deterioration in the integrity of renal cortical microcirculation. Failure of blood flow to return to all of the previously ischemic tissues, the *no-reflow phenomenon*, leads to reperfusion injury with cell necrosis and disruption.

Preservation

During the 1960s, the protective benefits of cold preservation in maintaining renal viability (for up to 72 hours) changed clinical renal transplantation. An effective preservation solution should prevent the reperfusion injury initiated by oxygen free radicals, provide adequate amounts of substrate for regenerating high-energy phosphate compounds (ATP) during reperfusion, prevent acidosis and interstitial space expansion, and minimize cell swelling due to sodium, chloride, and water influx that occurs during anaerobic, hypothermic ischemia.

The tendency of cells to accumulate water can be counteracted by substances known as *impermeants.* Solutions without substances that provide a colloidal osmotic pressure result in rapid diffusion of the solution into the interstitial space with tissue edema and capillary compression. The anaerobic metabolism that predominates during ischemia generates lactic acid and increased concentrations of hydrogen ions. Acidosis causes mitochondrial damage and activation of lysosomal enzymes with rupture and lysis of membranes. During reperfusion, ATP is needed for regeneration of several metabolic processes. The availability of ATP precursors during organ reperfusion is essential because ATP is rapidly degraded during hypothermic ischemia with loss of the end products, for example, hypoxanthine, inosine, and adenosine (Figure 9.3). Another important property for a preservation solution is protection from injury induced by reactive oxygen intermediates during reperfusion. Human livers and kidneys have high levels of endogenous superoxide dismutase, low levels of endogenous xanthine oxidase, and enhanced ability to scavenge superoxide anions compared to lung and intestine, which are sensitive to oxygen free radical damage.

The major prerequisites for successful organ preservation are hypothermia and suppression of cell swelling. Hypothermia reduces the demand for oxygen, conserves energy in the form of adenine nucleotides, and slows metabolism and catabolic enzyme activity. Rapid cooling suppresses "warm" ischemic injury; the optimal temperature appears to be 0 to 8° C. Simple hypothermic storage following an initial flush perfusion is the most widely used technique in the preservation of cadaveric renal allografts. The ionic composition of most preservation solutions mirrors that of intracellular fluid with low sodium and high potassium concentrations. Cold storage solutions include Eurocollins solution (EC), Sacks solution, hyperosmolar citrate solution (HC), University of Wisconsin–Lactobionate solution (UW), and phosphate-buffered sucrose (PBS). The compositions of these solutions are listed in Table 9.2.

The Collins solution and its Eurocollins derivative are the most widely used and contain high concentrations of potassium and magnesium. Phosphate and glucose act as impermeants to suppress hypothermically induced cell swelling; phosphate also acts as a hydrogen ion buffer. Glucose, the main impermeant, counteracts the osmotic force of intracellular anions and proteins. Collins solution is not an effective impermeant for the liver, which is able to better metabolize glucose than the kidney. Belzer and Southard developed the University of Wisconsin, or UW, solution which contains more effective impermeants—raffinose and lactobionate. UW solution improves preservation of the liver and pancreas and is now being increasingly used in renal transplantation.

Table 9.2: Composition of Kidney Preservation Solutions

Components (mM/liter)	*Collins*	*Eurocollins*	*Hyperosmolar Citrate*	*Buffered Sucrose*	*University of Wisconsin Lactobionate*
Sodium	10	10	80	120	20
Postassium	115	115	80	—	140
Magnesium	30	—	35	—	5
Sulfate	30	—	40	—	5
Phosphate	57.5	57.5	—	60	25
Chloride	15	15	—	—	—
Bicarbonate	10	10	—	—	—
Glucose	140	195	—	—	—
Citrate	—	—	55	—	—
Mannitol	—	—	185	—	—
Sucrose	—	—	—	140	—
Lactobionate	—	—	—	—	100
Raffinose	—	—	—	—	30
Adenosine	—	—	—	—	5
Glutathione	—	—	—	—	3
Allopurinol	—	—	—	—	1
Hydroxyethyl starch	—	—	—	—	50
Osmolality (mOsm/L)	360	375	400	310	320

HC contains mannitol, an effective kidney impermeant, and citrate as its main buffer. PBS uses sucrose as its osmotic agent. Sucrose, a larger molecule than mannitol or glucose, is more effective in preventing cell swelling, especially with preservation periods of over 48 hours. Phosphate is a superior buffer to citrate in the pH range of 6 to 7. An advantage of PBS is its simplicity (containing only three components) and low cost. Table 9.3 illustrates the roles of the various additives in cold-storage preservation solutions. It may well be unnecessary to mimic the intracellular ionic composition for effective preservation. Perhaps the more important factor is an osmotically active impermeant.

Table 9.3: Role of Additives in Organ Preservation Solutions

Additive	*Putative Role*
Buffers	Buffer lactic acid and hydrogen ion
Phosphate	
Citrate	
Impermeants	Suppress hypothermic induced cell swelling
Glucose	
Sucrose	
Mannitol	
Raffinose	
Lactobionate	
Colloids	Prevent expansion of interstitial space during flushing
Hydroxyethyl Starch	
Electrolytes	Cofactors in metabolism, maintain cell ultrastructure, osmotically active
Sodium	
Potassium	
Magnesium	
Metabolites	
Glutathione	Reduces cytotoxic agents such as peroxides and free radicals
Adenosine	Stimulates regeneration of energy products
Free radical inhibitors/scavengers	
Allopurinol	Inhibits free radical generation
Germanium	Free radical scavenger
Vasoactive substances/calcium	Interfere with calcium-dependent reactivation and stabilize renal microcirculation
Trifluoperazine	
Captopril	
Verapamil	

Simple cold-storage preservation is the method of choice at most transplant centers, although machine perfusion preservation may give slightly better organ preservation in terms of initial function. However, prospective, randomized studies have shown that this does not translate into long-term differences. Due to its simplicity and low cost, cold storage is preferred by most transplant centers. Hypothermic organ preservation extends organ preservation time for more than 72 hours, reduces the incidence of delayed graft function, and prevents immunologic alteration of organs.

Technique of Transplantation

The techniques of renal transplantation are essentially the same in both cadaveric and live donor transplantation. In adult recipients, the renal allograft is usually performed in the iliac fossa, whereas in children weighing less than 20 kg it is placed retrocecally with end-to-side anastomoses to the vena cava and either the aorta or common iliac artery. The standard techniques are well described. In male recipients the spermatic cord is mobilized, preserved, and retracted medially. Fatty tissue surrounding the kidney and the donor blood vessels is carefully dissected, and the hilum of the kidney is avoided. All divided tissue should be tied with fine sutures to prevent bleeding from vessels inadvertently damaged during the donor nephrectomy, to avoid the development of a lymphocele, and to enable the unhindered performance of the anastomoses.

In order to insure blood supply to the corpora cavernosa and reduce the risk of impotence, male recipients of second allografts who had their first transplant performed using the contralateral internal iliac artery, should have their second kidney graft anastomosed using the external or common iliac artery. Many centers prefer an extravesical ureteroneocystostomy because it is faster, better enables preservation of distal ureteral blood supply, and avoids the need for a separate cystostomy.

Allograft Rejection: Pathologic Types and Therapy

Rejection is the most frequent cause of allograft loss. Other causes of allograft dysfunction include acute tubular necrosis, technical complications, cytomegalovirus infection, cyclosporine toxicity, and the development of recurrent renal disease. Allograft rejection is classified on the basis of morphology and clinical presentation into hyperacute, acute, acute accelerated, and chronic rejection. Antidonor lymphocytotoxic antibody cross-matching has reduced the occurrence of hyperacute rejection to less than 1%. Hyperacute rejection occurs within minutes of revascularization but occasionally may not be apparent for hours after transplantation. The initially normal kidney (color and consistency) rapidly becomes swollen, mottled, and blue. Hyperacute rejection is caused by preformed anti-HLA or ABO antibodies. Histologically, IgG and complement deposits are seen in the glomeruli and peritubular capillary walls. Peritubular infiltrates of neutrophils, intrarenal glomerular capillary and arterial thrombosis, and extensive fibrin and platelet capillary aggregates are present. Cortical infarction and extensive tubular necrosis ensue.

Acute rejection is a common cause of renal allograft loss. Even with current immunosuppression regimens, more than 50% of allograft recipients will experience a rejection episode and 75% of these episodes are of acute rejection. Acute rejection, a major problem in the post-transplant management of recipients, can occur with HLA-identical matches. The kidney becomes swollen with microscopic interstitial edema and hemorrhage and a cellular infiltrate of small and large lymphocytes, macrophages, plasma cells, and occasionally, eosinophils, basophils, and neutrophils. Lymphocyte infiltration between tubular epithelial cells is common. Biopsy specimens obtained for diagnosis of acute rejection must include an adequate amount of cortex because the medulla is not predictably involved in acute cellular rejection. The T lymphocyte is generally regarded as the primary effector of acute cellular rejection. Most of the pathologic changes in acute rejection are reversible with antirejection therapy.

Acute accelerated rejection occurs within a few days to a week post-transplantation, with a clinical picture of the rapid onset of weight gain, edema, and deteriorating renal function with or without fevers. Proteinuria, frequently seen with acute rejection, is conspicuously absent. The microscopic features are consistent with vasculitis characterized by fibrin platelet deposits, thrombosis, cortical infarcts, and fibrinoid necrosis. Immunoglobulin and complement deposition within glomeruli are usually demonstrated. This form of rejection rarely responds to currently available immunosuppressive therapy; however, plasmapheresis may be successful. Some of the newer immunosuppressive agents (discussed in a later section) are successful in the treatment of acute accelerated rejection.

Chronic rejection is an increasingly important cause of renal allograft failure. Chronic low-grade rejection occurs in most renal allograft recipients and results in gradually decreasing renal function over months or years. Chronic rejection is the least understood of the immunologic processes resulting in graft loss. However, predisposing factors include multiple acute rejection episodes within the first 6 months post-transplant, acute rejection with vascular features, and longer ischemia times. Antibody-dependent lympocytotoxicity is also believed to play a role in chronic rejection. The main target in chronic rejection is the arterial endothelium. The pathologic findings are those of chronic vascular changes and interstitial fibrosis.

Although a number of radiologic techniques, including renal flow and function scan, Doppler ultrasound, and magnetic resonance imaging, are used to evaluate suspected acute rejection, the renal biopsy is the diagnostic gold standard. Acute rejection is characterized by increased lymphocytes and monocytes within the graft, with activated blast cells being an important component of the infiltrate. Immunofluorescent staining for class II antigen and glomerular infiltration by CD8+ lymphocytes both correlate with the intensity of acute rejection.

The primary therapy of acute allograft rejection is an increased dosage of corticosteroids. Polyclonal and monoclonal antilymphocyte globulins are used for refractory or recurrent acute rejection. Monoclonal antibodies have broadened the treatment options in acute rejection, and up to 90% of acute allograft rejection episodes can be reversed with these agents.

Immunosuppressive Therapy

Immunosuppressive drugs interfere with different portions of the allograft immune response (Table 9.4), and several immunosuppressive regimens are currently used. Cyclosporine (CsA) monotherapy is advocated by several European centers. The advantage of CsA monotherapy is the avoidance of complications caused by long-term corticosteroid therapy. With CsA monotherapy, steroids are withdrawn after 6 months to 1 year in patients considered immunologically stable.

A commonly used immunosuppressive regimen is double therapy with CsA and steroids (Table 9.5), which gives excellent short-term and long-term results. CsA and steroids are started at the time of transplantation regardless of the degree of renal function. Other centers have advocated triple immunosuppressive therapy consisting of CsA, corticosteroid (Cst) therapy, and azathioprine (AZA). The advantage of triple therapy is the ability to use lower doses of each agent and thus minimize toxicity. CsAs nephrotoxicity may result in a more prolonged period of delay graft function but does not impact significantly on overall allograft survival. In contrast, many centers employ prophylactic therapy with antilymphocyte globulin (ALG) or anti-CD3 during the periods of delayed graft function. This approach prevents the detrimental effects of CsA and renal ischemia. Prophylactic therapy is continued during the period of primary dysfunction with CsA started as allograft function improves, overlapping for several days with ALG or anti-CD3. Therapy is then continued with either CsA and prednisone alone or with CsA, AZA, and steroids. Regardless of the immunosuppressive regimen used, most centers report 1-year graft survival rates of 75 to 85% for cadaveric grafts and 90 to 95% for living related donors grafts with patient survival exceeding 90%. While these results are gratifying, long-term resolution of the patient's disease is the

Table 9.4: Common Immunosuppressive Drugs

Drug	*Mechanism of Activity*	*Side Effects*
Corticosteroids	Inhibition of cytokine release IL-2, IL-6, ?IL-2 Anti-inflammatory effects Blocks early lymphocyte activation cascade	Cushing's syndrome, obesity, hypertension, hyperlipidemia, mood and stress disorders, bone disease, peptic ulcers
Azathioprine	Antimetabolite Inhibition of cell division Blocks distal lymphocyte activation pathway	Bone marrow suppression, alopecia, cholestasis, risk of malignancy, interaction with xanthine oxidase inhibitors
Cyclosporine	Undecapeptide Blocks early segment of activation pathway Interferes with transcription IL-2 via binding to cyclophilin Inhibits T-cell lymphokine production Reduces T-, B-cell proliferation Variable dose: level relationships Lipophilic Variable metabolism Drug interaction	Nephrotoxicity, hyperkalemia, tremor
ALG/ATG (polyclonal antilymphocyte)	Block T-cell and other lymphocyte receptors	Chills, fever, arthralgias, urticaria, phlebitis, antibodies, leukopenia, thrombocytopenia, viral infection, rare serum sickness
OKT3 (monoclonal antilymphocyte antibody)	Blocks T-cell receptor CD3 antigen Activates nonimmune lymphocytes to release cytokines	"First-dose reaction": chills, fever, capillary leak, aseptic meningitis, pulmonary edema, viral infections, antibody with repeat dosing

ultimate goal. Unfortunately, available current data indicate that the incidence of late graft loss has changed little over the last 20 years.

Azathioprine

The purine analogue azathioprine (AZA) is a valuable immunosuppressive

Table 9.5: Immunosuppressive Drug Regimens

Cyclosporine induction therapy
Cyclosporine
Prednisone
± Azathioprine
Sequential induction therapy
T-cell antibody (polyclonal or monoclonal)
Prednisone (rapid taper)
Azathioprine
Add Cyclosporine, stop T-cell antibody (5 to 10 days)
Double-drug maintenance therapy
Prednisone + Cyclosporine
or
Cyclosporine + Azathioprine
Triple-drug maintenance therapy
Cyclosporine
Prednisone
Azathioprine

drug. AZA was synthesized in an attempt to increase the therapeutic efficacy of 6-mercaptopurine (6-MP) and has been used in clinical transplantation for nearly 30 years. It is metabolized in vivo to 6-MP and other metabolites. AZA and its metabolites are incorporated into cellular DNA and inhibit purine nucleotide synthesis and metabolism. The resultant alteration in RNA synthesis and function prevents mitosis and proliferation. Rapidly dividing cells such as T and B lymphoblasts are most susceptible to AZA. AZA has little effect on established immune responses and is used to prevent acute rejection rather than treat ongoing rejection.

Myelosuppression is the primary toxicity of AZA (Table 9.4). AZA is metabolized in the liver, and its metabolites are eliminated in the urine. While the dose is not automatically adjusted during periods of renal insufficiency, toxicity may occur from retention of metabolites and the apparent increased sensitivity noted in uremic patients. The issue of hepatic toxicity is controversial. Nevertheless, during periods of hepatocellular dysfunction, azathioprine can be discontinued in favor of the alkylating agent cyclophosphamide. Other chronic toxicities include anemia, alopecia, and an increased incidence of malignant disease in renal transplant recipients.

Corticosteroids

Corticosteroids (Csts) are potent immunosuppressive agents with diverse systemic effects. The primary immunologic effects of Csts are inhibition of IL-2 production and class II antigen receptor expression. Steroids suppress acute and chronic inflammatory responses as well as inhibiting extravascular extravasation of cells and fluid (via microvasoconstriction), thus preventing cellular migration and recruitment. Lymphocytes and monocytes are redistributed into lymphoid tissue with resulting decreased peripheral blood counts. While initially used in high doses to reverse acute allograft rejection, Csts are currently either administered at lower doses or removed altogether from the immunosuppressive regimen. The complications and side effects of Cst therapy are many (Table 9.4). These side effects usually subside with dose tapering. Other effects include infection, cataracts, osteoporosis (secondary to decreased calcium absorption and secondary hyperparathyroidism), Cushing's syndrome, proximal limb myopathy, and growth retardation (in prepubertal children). Hypercholesterolemia and hypertriglyceridemia, hypertension, weight gain, and diabetes contribute to the high incidence of cardiovascular disease in transplant patients. Serious bacterial, viral, and fungal infections also occur. There is no direct relationship between Csts and the development of malignancy in transplant recipients.

These complications have led to alterations in immunosuppressive regimens aimed at reducing or limiting steroid therapy. Newer immunosuppressive agents may eliminate steroid immunosuppression altogether. However, steroids are currently an important mainstay of therapy in many immunosuppression protocols.

Cyclosporine

CsA, a cyclic fungal metabolite, is a potent, primary, lymphocyte-specific immunosuppressive agent, and its use has had a profound effect on solid organ transplantation. CsA is believed to bind to the cytosolic protein (cyclophilin) to affect second messengers within the cytoplasm and cause an interruption of the signals necessary to activate protein kinases, cyclic nucleotides, and phospholipases. Such signals may be necessary for T-cell activation and are known to inhibit the transcription of the IL-2 molecule. CsA also inhibits the production of IL-3 and interferon gamma, although receptor expression for these lymphokines is unaffected.

CsA, rapidly absorbed after oral administration, achieves peak serum or whole blood concentrations in 2 to 4 hours. Concentration is measured either by high-performance liquid chromatography or by radioimmunoassay. CsA is metabolized in the liver, and drugs that stimulate the P-450 enzyme system will increase metabolism and decrease blood levels

(Table 9.6). Examples of such drugs include rifampin, phenobarbital, phenytoin, and norfloxacin. Drugs that inhibit or are metabolized via this system cause increased blood levels of CsA and may lead to toxicity. These drugs include aminoglycosides, ketoconazole, diltiazem, erythromycin, high-dose corticosteroids, and verapamil. Since CsA is absorbed primarily in the small intestine, gastric emptying affects its bioavailability. Drugs or diseases that affect gastric emptying (e.g., metoclopramide, diabetes) affect bioavailability and CsA blood levels.

CsA has had a major positive impact on clinical renal transplantation. However, CsA can be difficult to use and costly and has the potential for serious complications and side effects (Table 9.4). Toxic effects correlate poorly with blood CsA levels. CsA nephrotoxicity has been extensively studied. Increased renal vascular resistance, and reductions in renal blood flow, GFR, and urine output occur in a predictable manner with cyclosporine therapy. Most evidence suggests that renal vasoconstriction is at least partially mediated via release of the vasoconstrictor, thromboxane A_2. Renal ischemia has been noted to exacerbate these effects. Morphologic abnormalities associated with CsA include tubular atrophy and interstitial fibrosis. The use of CsA has also been associated with significant hypertension. While the mechanism for the altered renal hemodynamics and hypertension noted with CsA therapy is not known, current evidence suggests it is not renin–angiotensin mediated.

CsA therapy is associated with a decreased incidence of nonviral infections compared to AZA. Its effect on cytomegalovirus (CMV) infection is not completely known. An increased incidence of non-Hodgkin's and B cell lymphomas and Kaposi's sarcoma has been noted. This con-

Table 9.6: Cyclosporine Drug Interactions

Raised Drug Levels	*Reduced Drug Levels*
Diltiazem	Phenytoin
Verapamil	Phenobarbital
Cimetidine	Carbamazepine
Ranitidine	Norfloxacin
Metoclopramide	Isoniazid
Oral contraceptives	Rifampin
Ketoconazole	Ethambutol
Aminoglycosides	
Doxycycline	
Erythromycin	
High dose methylprednisone	

trasts sharply with conventional immunosuppression. CsA can cause hyperglycemia and hyperlipidemia.

Early clinical trials clearly established CsA as an important immunosuppressive agent, allowing improved graft survival, increased patient survival, and decreased morbidity. The effectiveness of this agent and its apparent synergy with other agents has resulted in the use of lower doses of all immunosuppressive agents and reduced post-transplant morbidity.

Polyclonal Antilymphocytic Antibodies

Injection of human lymphocytes, thymocytes, or splenocytes into goats, rabbits, or horses produces antilymphocyte serum from which the globulin fraction can be separated and purified. The commonly used antilymphoid globulin preparations are Minnesota antilymphocyte globulin (ALG) and antithymocyte globulin (ATG). Polyclonal antilymphocyte preparations have been used for prophylaxis and antirejection therapy and result in prevention and/or reversal of rejection and improved graft survival. ALG/ATG preparations are given intravenously (5 to 21 days) as a prophylactic adjunct, for antirejection therapy, or to protect against early post-transplant ischemic insults. With the exception of rabbit ATG, which may be given intramuscularly or intravenously, most preparations are administered via a large-bore central venous catheter or a high-flow arterial venous hemodialysis fistula. A dose of 10 to 30 mg/kg/day usually results in an acceptable level of immunosuppression, that is, T-cell fraction less than 10% of circulating lymphocytes. Administration takes place over 4 to 6 hours after a subcutaneous diluted test dose confirms the absence of prior sensitization to species-specific globulin. Pretreatment administration of an antihistamine, antipyretic, and steroids decreases the incidence and severity of side effects.

The long-term benefit of ALG/ATG therapy has not been established. Some studies have demonstrated significant survival benefit utilizing ALG as an immunosuppressive adjunct, but others have failed to show beneficial long-term effects. However, the effectiveness of ALG for acute rejection is well established. Toxic effects (flushing, chills, and fevers) occur in up to 25% of infusions (Table 9.4). Other side effects include erythematous rash, arthralgias, urticaria, myalgias, phlebitis, nausea, and vomiting. Extraneous antibodies can result in leukopenia and thrombocytopenia. Anaphylactoid reactions and serum sickness can develop, necessitating discontinuation of therapy. There is no increase of spontaneous malignancy in ALG treated patients compared to patients receiving conventional immunosuppression. CMV infections are a clinical toxicity of ALG/ATG therapy.

Monoclonal Antibodies

Unlike polyclonal antibody preparations, which contain antibodies to multiple antigens on many cell types (clones), monoclonal antibodies (MCAs) react with a single antigen (see Chapter 8). Their introduction in the 1980s began a new era of immunosuppression in organ transplantation. MCAs that target molecules on T-cells and their subsets are the most useful in clinical transplantation.

MCAs are used in similar fashion to polyclonal preparations, that is, as prophylactic therapy or for acute rejection. The most widely used MCA is the anti-CD3 OKT3 (Muromonab CD3, Ortho Pharmaceutical Corp.). OKT3 binds to the CD3 molecule on T cells and medullary thymocytes. The CD3 receptor is closely linked to the T-cell antigen receptor and plays an important role in T-cell function and activation. OKT3 exerts its immunosuppressive effect via internalization or modulation of the CD3 receptor with comodulation of the antigen receptor. After an initial dose of OKT3 (usually 5 mg in adults), CD3-reactive T cells virtually disappear from the circulation, while other T-cell receptors (CD4, CD8, and CD2) disappear transiently and then return. Prospective, randomized comparisons have suggested equal efficacy for ALG/ATG preparations and OKT3 when used as prophylactic agents. Patient and graft survivals, incidence of rejection, and time to onset of rejection are similar. Toxic side effects with OKT3 occur, however, with an overall higher incidence. The major difficulties encountered with OKT3 clinically are its toxic side effects and immunogenicity (Table 9.4). OKT3 activates T cells and generates the production of various cytokines including IL-2, interferon gamma, and tumor necrosis factor alpha, which mediate these adverse reactions. Fever, headache, hypertension or hypotension, dyspnea, nausea/vomiting, aseptic meningitis, seizure, rash, pruritus, and angina have been noted with the first two doses. This symptom complex does not appear to be altered significantly by pretreatment with antipyretics, steroids, or histamine receptor blockade. The use of specific anticytokine monoclonal therapy may prevent some of these side effects.

Another significant problem with OKT3 is its immunogenic potential. Approximately 50% of patients develop anti-OKT3 antibodies following initial treatment. Factors identified as predictors of success with OKT3 retreatment for rejection include the time elapsed after the first treatment, the absence of antibody production after a first OKT3 treatment, effective T-cell CD3 modulation, and anti-OKT3 antibody titer of less than 1:1000.

Another new MCA is directed at activated mononuclear cells. The IL-2 receptor is transiently expressed on all activated but not resting

CD4+ and CD8+ T cells. IL-2 receptors may also be expressed on monocytes and activated B lymphocytes. Activated T cells express a high, and significantly greater, number of low-affinity IL-2 binding sites. The effectiveness of IL-2 receptor-directed therapy as a prophylactic adjunct has been demonstrated in rodents, primates, and humans. Like CsA, anti-IL-2 receptor monoclonal antibody therapy may be effective only in preventing rejection.

Other promising MCAs include T10B9.1A-31 (directed at the alpha/beta chains of CD3 with less toxicity) and OKT4A directed at CD4. The rapid development of monoclonal antibody technology will lead to the introduction of new specific antibodies, immunoconjugates (agents constructed using genetic engineering to develop antibodies conjugated to various cellular toxins), and chimeric agents combining the specificity of murine antibodies with the safety of human protein. The mechanisms of action and side effects of the commonly used immunosuppressive agents are summarized in Table 9.4.

NEW IMMUNOSUPPRESSIVE AGENTS

A number of new drugs hold promise as immunosuppressive agents in clinical, solid-organ transplantation (Table 9.7).

FK506

FK506 is a potent immunosuppressive agent isolated from mycelia and fermentation broth of a soil fungus. in vitro, it inhibits lymphocyte IL-2, IL-3, transferrin, and interferon gamma production. FK506 inhibits IL-2 receptor expression, MLR, and cytotoxic T-cell generation, and prolongs skin, heart, bowel, and kidney allografts in rodents. FK506 is effective in vitro and in vivo at significantly lower doses than cyclosporine. CsA and FK506 share similar biomolecular mechanisms, although FK506 appears to bind to a cytoplasmic protein other than cyclophilin.

The immunosuppressive and toxic effects of FK506 have some degree of species specificity. Toxic effects in animal transplant models have been variable. Initial reports utilizing FK506 in large-animal models were discouraging. However, subsequent reports have been encouraging, and toxicity in humans appears to be minimal. Controlled, randomized trials comparing FK506 to cyclosporine in kidney transplantation are currently being performed.

15-Deoxyspergualin

15-deoxyspergualin (DSG) is an antitumor antibiotic extracted from the culture filtrate of a bacillus and subsequently found to be immunosup-

Table 9.7: New Immunosuppressive Agents

Drug	*Mechanism of Action*	*Toxicity*
FK506	Macrolide derived from streptomyces species Binds to FK506 binding protein Inhibits lympokine (IL-2, etc.) production	Nephrotoxic, neurotoxic
Rapamycin	Macrolide antibiotic Uncouples IL-2 binding, aborts activation pathways	?
RS-61443	Inhibits inosine monophosphate dehydrogenase Ester of mycophenolic acid Selective antiproliferative effect on lymphocytes	Gastrointestinal
Deoxyspergualin	Antitumor antibiotic Suppresses macrophage activation, Class II antigen expression, and cytotoxic T-cell induction and proliferation *Increases* IL-1 and IL-2 production	Bone marrow suppression Gastrointestinal
Mizoribine	Imidazole antibiotic Purine metabolism inhibition Similar action to azathioprine	Bone marrow suppression

pressive in a variety of animal allograft models. Like FK506, it appears to be species-specific with regard to toxicity. However, studies in animals and humans have revealed minimal toxicity and a potent immunosuppressive effect. As antirejection therapy, DSG reverses steroid, ALG, and anti-CD3-resistant rejection episodes.

DSG appears to have a unique mechanism of immunosuppressive action, which may explain its effectiveness in both humoral and cellular-mediated immune events. It suppresses monocyte/macrophage activation, class II antigen expression, cytotoxic T-cell induction and proliferation, and the differentiation of hematopoietic stem cells. Paradoxically, DSG increases, rather than inhibits, the production of IL-1 and IL-2 by macrophages and lymphocytes, and increases the response to IL-3 and macrophage colony stimulating factor. The effects of DSG are reversible by exogenous interferon gamma, but not by IL-2. Currently, its mechanism appears to be via the inhibition of macrophage-assisted clonal T-cell amplification and the amplification and differentiation of B cells to plasma cells.

The toxicity and complications of DSG in clinical transplantation appear mild and consist of perioral and facial numbness, variable gastrointestinal complaints, mild to moderate reversible leukopenia, anemia, and thrombocytopenia. None of these side effects has required the discontinuation of therapy. The most promising characteristic of DSG is its ability to reverse or prevent humorally mediated rejection not amenable to commonly employed agents such as Csts, CsA, ALG, or OKT3.

Mizoribine

Mizoribine (Bredinin-MZ) is an antibiotic isolated from a fungal culture medium. Its immunosuppressive mode of action is similar to that of AZA. MZ inhibits RNA and DNA synthesis by interfering with purine biosynthesis. MZ has been used in Japan for nearly a decade for adult living-related and cadaveric renal transplantation. MZ has equal or greater effectiveness than AZA. Large trials have yet to be done in Europe and North America, although the Japanese results demonstrate effectiveness equal to that of AZA with reduced toxicity.

RS61443 (Mycophenolic Acid Morpholinoethylester)

RS61443 is a derivative of the fungal antibiotic, mycophenolic acid. It is a noncompetitive, reversible inhibitor of guanosine monophosphate biosynthesis, and, like MZ, it interferes with the purine synthesis in T and B cells. RS61443 inhibits B-cell and T-cell lymphoproliferative responses to mitogens and alloantigens in vitro. Animal studies have shown it to be an effective immunosuppressant for the prevention and treatment of allograft rejection. RS61443 holds significant promise as an adjunctive agent and is ideally suited for combination therapy with the currently used immunosuppressives. Phase I trials have been encouraging, and clinical trials comparing it to AZA in cadaveric renal allograft recipients are currently underway.

Rapamycin

Rapamycin is a macrolide antibiotic produced by a mycelium and related to FK506. Its mechanism of action is not completely known, but it inhibits growth of human T-cell and B-cell lines via a reduced sensitivity to IL-2 and it has a significant inhibitory effect on major metabolic pathways. Effectiveness in preventing organ allograft rejection in animals has been demonstrated. It has also been noted to produce indefinite survival in rat heart and kidney allografts after discontinuation. Toxicity, consisting of vasculitis affecting the gastrointestinal tract, was an early concern with this drug but is species-specific. Rapamycin awaits future application in clinical organ transplantation.

ISSUES IN TRANSPLANTATION

The most distressing issue in clinical, solid-organ transplantation is the growing shortage of cadaver donor organs. Approximately one-third of patients on hemodialysis could be rehabilitated by transplantation. The number of cadaver donor kidney transplants in 1989 actually decreased from the previous year by nearly 200. The average waiting time nationwide for a cadaver kidney has almost doubled in the last 5 years, with over 3000 patients waiting for more than 3 years to receive a cadaver kidney. The average retrieval rate in the United States is approximately 15 donors per million inhabitants, an embarrassingly low number compared to that in Europe, which is nearly twice as high. Some smaller organ procurement agencies within the United States have retrieval rates exceeding 30 donors per million. This may reflect the success achievable with a local community-level approach to organ donation.

The relative lack of availability of cadaver organs has led to new approaches. The successful use of previously considered marginal organ donors has prompted the use of kidneys previously considered inadequate for transplantation. The use of kidneys from donors over 55 years of age is now common, and some centers even use donors over 65 years of age. The reported success rates are equivalent to those for donors in the optimal age group (15 to 45 years). Another controversial group of marginal donors is younger donors, especially those under 2 years of age. Although some centers have demonstrated adequate graft survival using these kidneys, others have shown a detrimental effect on graft survival. A further method of increasing the donor pool, used successfully in Europe, is the use of non-heartbeating donors. Another issue in renal transplantation involves sharing of kidneys over long distances based on HLA matching. Paradoxical results and interpretation of multi-center and single-center studies regarding the benefits of HLA matching have been reported. Thus the controversy remains as to whether sharing of kidneys to provide a good HLA match is in the best interest of the patient and the transplant community.

CANCER IN TRANSPLANT RECIPIENTS

Significant immunosuppression induced by drugs, radiation, or disease inevitably leads to the development of certain cancers. Interestingly, transplant patients do not frequently develop the common neoplasms such as lung, colon, prostate, and breast. Conventional immunosuppression (CIT), that is, AZA/prednisone, is associated with a marked increase in skin cancer (Table 9.8). The overall incidence is 10 to 20 times that in the

Table 9.8: Cancer in Transplant Recipients

	CsA	*CIT*
Time after Transplant	*26 months (1–223 months) (% of patients)*	*64 months (1–253 months) (% of patients)*
Skin/lip[a]	22	40
Lymphomas[b]	29	12
Kaposi's sarcoma	11	3
Lower anogenita (vulva, perineum, external genitalia)	1	3
In-situ cervical	2	6
Renal cell	6	3

[a]Skin cancer tends to be more malignant (squamous) with CIT
[b]Extranodal and CNS involvement more common with CIT

general population, and many of the tumors are aggressive (squamous cell carcinomas) with increased metastases and mortality. Non-Hodgkin's lymphoma (NHL) with frequent CNS involvement, Kaposi's sarcoma (KS), cancer of the lower anogenital area (vulva, perineum, external genitalia), in-situ cervical cancer, and renal cell carcinoma are also increased in patients treated with conventional immunosuppression.

CsA therapy changed the type and incidence of post-transplant malignancy (Table 9.8). In CIT patients, the mean time to develop a neoplasm is 64 months, with CsA therapy this is significantly shortened to 26 months. The occurrence of NHL, KS, and renal cell carcinoma is increased two to fourfold in CsA-treated transplant recipients. In contrast, the incidence of skin, cervical, and lower anogenital cancers is two to fourfold less in CsA-treated patients.

Several types of malignancy merit discussion. Lymphomas occur at 2.5 times the frequency with CsA therapy versus CIT and are 30 to 50 times more frequent than in the general population. The time to appearance is four times shorter in CsA patients, with a mean of 12 months. However, the malignant potential appears to be less with CsA therapy, with less than half the extranodal and CNS involvement seen in CIT patients. Reticulum cell sarcoma and B-cell lymphomas predominate with both types of therapy. The occurrence of NHL has also been associated with additional immunosuppressive therapy, particularly ALG and OKT3. Phenytoin use has been associated with the appearance of lymphomas and pseudolymphomas. B-cell lymphoma has been associated with the Epstein-Barr virus. Lymphomas in CsA-treated patients seem to respond more readily to therapy such as reducing or discontinuation of immunosuppression, acyclovir, radiation, surgery, and chemotherapy.

Kaposi's sarcoma (KS) is nearly four times more common with CsA therapy and 400 to 500 times that seen in the general population. Presenting as a reddish-blue macule or plaque on the skin or the oropharyngeal mucosa, it may also involve the internal viscera. KS may be related to CMV infection.

Acquired cystic disease develops in 50% of patients on hemodialysis, with a reported 7 to 20% incidence of renal cell cancer (RCC). Acquired cystic disease does, however, regress after transplantation. RCC in either the native kidneys or the allograft occurs in 3% and 5%, respectively, of CIT- and CsA-treated patients, a significantly higher incidence than in the general population. Aggressive screening and therapy is advocated, as these tumors have significant malignant potential.

Why do transplant patients develop these neoplasms? Carcinogenic metabolites have been proposed to account for the high incidence of skin cancers. The development of impaired immunoregulatory feedback mechanisms resulting in unrestrained proliferation and the activation of endogenous oncoviruses has been investigated. Lymphomas may result from chronic antigenic stimulation with resultant hyperplasia and neoplasia, as well as depressed NK cell activity. It is likely that a combination of all of these mechanisms plays a role in the development of post-transplant malignancy.

In summary, while the incidence of malignancy does not appear to differ in CsA versus CIT patients, the types and clinical behavior of cancers in CsA-treated patients suggest a more life-threatening potential in these patients. Future immunosuppression, although likely to be more specific, will need to address this clinical problem.

CONCLUSION

Clinical organ transplantation has made considerable progress over the past two decades. In the 1990s the desirability for clinical transplantion without the need for chronic immunosuppression will continue. However, it is more likely that within this decade more specific immunosuppressive agents will be introduced that will enable transplant physicians and surgeons to prevent organ allograft loss with considerably less morbidity. The introduction and application of the techniques of molecular biology will undoubtedly contribute in many ways, ranging from advances in tissue typing to the genetic engineering of new and more effective agents for transplant immunosuppression.

SUGGESTED READINGS

Strom TB, Carpenter CB. Immunobiology of kidney transplantation. In: Brenner BM, Rector FC Jr, eds. The kidney, ed. 4. Philadelphia: WB Saunders, 1991: 2336.

Comprehensive review of most aspects of transplantation immunobiology. An in-depth review written in an easily understood manner, providing an excellent reference for those with or without a background in this discipline.

Tilney NL. Renal transplantation. Curr Prob Surg 1989; 26(9):601.

Overview highlighting most aspects of immunobiology, immunosuppression, and clinical renal transplantation. Some degree of emphasis placed on the peritransplant period with regard to donor and recipient management.

Halloran PF, Cockfield SM, Madrenas J. The molecular immunology of transplantation and graft rejection. Immunol Allergy Clin North Am 1989; 9:1.

Excellent in-depth discussion of the role of various immune cells and their products in the allograft response.

Darby JM, Stein K, Grenurk A, Stuart SA. Approach to the management of the heartbeating "brain dead" organ donor. JAMA 1989; 261(15):2222.

Concise, detailed, systematic discussion of organ donor management. Approach to assessment and mangement of the multiorgan donor is covered. The physiologic rationale behind the management and a discussion of experimental therapy also presented.

Belzer FO, Southard JH. Principles of solid organ preservation by cold storage. Transplantation 1988; 44:673.

Classic and still current discussion of the chemistry and physiology of organ preservation written by international authorities.

Novick AC. Surgery of renal transplantation and complications. In: Novick AC, Straffon R eds. Vascular problems in urologic surgery, ed. 1. Philadelphia: WB Saunders 1982:233.

Discussion of the technical aspects of renal donor procurement, recipient transplantation, and surgical complications.

Johnson CP, Simmons RL, Sutherland DER, et al. A randomized trial comparing cyclosporine with anti-lymphoblast globulin-azathioprine for renal allograft recipients. Transplantation 1988; 45:380.

Report comparing the use of Minnesota ALG/AZA/prednisone with CsA/prednisone in a randomized prospective fashion. The results highlight the efficacy of both protocols, their toxicities, advantages, and disadvantages.

Steinmuller DR. Cyclosporine nephrotoxicity. Clev Clin J Med 1989; 56(1):89.

Concise, focused discussion of the mechanism of CsA nephrotoxicity and its clinical implications.

Lake KD. Management of drug interactions with cyclosporine. Pharmacotherapy 1991; 11(5):110S.

Detailed coverage of the various pharmacologic interactions of CsA. Complete list of references included.

Stratta RJ, D'Alessandro AM, Armbrust MJ, et al. Sequential antilymphocyte globulin cyclosporine immunosuppression in cadaveric renal transplantation. Transplantation 1989; 47:96.

Report focusing on results of use of a popular immunosuppressive protocol with important implications noted regarding CsA nephrotoxicity, infection associated with combined ALG/OKT3 or prolonged ALG therapy, and rejection therapy.

Lewis RM, Janney RP, Golden DL, et al. Stability of renal allograft function associated with long-term cyclosporine immunosuppressive therapy: five year follow-up. Transplantation 1989; 47:266.

Report of the results using another commonly employed immunosuppressive protocol with analysis of long-term results and factors correlating with graft loss.

Norman DJ. The clinical role of OKT3. Immunol Allergy Clin North Am 1989; 9:95.

Discussion of the immunology, clinical use, and toxicity of OKT3 written in a clear, comprehensive fashion by a leading authority.

Soulilou JP, Jacques Y. Monoclonal anti-IL-2 receptor in organ transplantation. Transplant Int 1989; 2:46.

Report summarizing the research, clinical uses, and mechanism of action of the anti-IL-2 receptor antibodies.

Penn I. Risk of cancer in the transplant patient. In: Flye MW ed. Principles of organ transplantation, ed 1. Philadelphia: WB Saunders, 1989; 634.

Excellent summary covering most aspects on this subject written by the world's leading authority.

CHAPTER 10

Urinary-Tract Infections

Grannum R. Sant
Edwin M. Meares Jr.

Infections of the urinary tract are common and present a number of diagnostic and treatment challenges to the urologist. Twenty percent of adult women experience a urinary-tract infection (UTI) during their lifetime, and women with acute, uncomplicated UTIs account for more than 5 million office visits annually in the United States. Most women with simple cystitis undergo laboratory testing and drug treatment estimated at costing more than $1 billion annually. As many as 250,000 UTIs are bouts of acute pyelonephritis, often leading to hospitalization and the use of parenteral antimicrobial therapy. After an initial infection, about 20% of women develop recurrent cystitis, which causes significant disability and discomfort. UTIs in pregnancy can lead to both maternal and fetal morbidity. Other major risk groups for UTIs include the elderly, men with prostatic obstruction, catheterized patients, and young school-aged girls.

A clear understanding of the pathogenesis of UTIs is critically important to the clinician. This chapter reviews current information concerning the epidemiology, microbiology, and pathogenesis of UTIs. A synthesis of the pathophysiologic aspects of UTIs provides the clinician a clear conceptual framework to recognize, understand, and treat these infections.

EPIDEMIOLOGIC CONCEPTS

Except in neonates and the elderly, the prevalence of UTIs is much greater in females than in males (Table 10.1). In the neonatal period, boys have a higher rate of infection than girls. Subsequently, the ratio of females to males increases to about 25:1. This ratio continues into puberty, adolescence, and adulthood.

Table 10:1: Prevalence of UTIs

Age Group	*%*	*Male to Female Ratio*
Neonatal	1	1.5:1
Preschool	2–3	1:10
School-age	1–2	1:30
Reproductive age	2.5	1:50
Elderly	20–30	1:5–10

Congenital genitourinary (GU) tract disorders (e.g., vesicoureteral reflux, urethral valves) are found in about 40% of male bacteriuric infants—an incidence double that found in bacteriuric girls. Other factors contributing to male neonatal infections include incomplete bladder emptying and fecal contamination of the prepuce and urethral meatus in uncircumcised infants. Indeed, uncircumcised boys are 10 to 40 times more likely than circumcised boys to develop UTIs during the first year of life, as a result of bacterial colonization of the prepuce and ascending infection. The normal physiologic separation of the foreskin from the underlying glans penis that occurs after infancy permits better hygiene and reduces the risk of bacterial colonization. This and early surgical correction of congenital GU-tract abnormalities explains the low prevalence of bacteriuria in boys over 1 year old. Bacteriuria in adult males is uncommon until the fourth or fifth decade, when prostatic disease and lower urinary-tract instrumentation increase the risk of bacteriuria. Recurrent infections in men are usually associated with anatomic or functional abnormalities of the lower urinary tract (e.g., prostatism, bacterial prostatitis).

Neonatal UTIs can involve the kidney but go unrecognized because symptoms, such as high fever and failure to thrive, are non-specific. Unrecognized and untreated bouts of pyelonephritis in infancy often lead to renal scarring, hypertension, and eventual renal failure, requiring dialysis or transplantation. Urographic imaging helps to detect abnormalities of the GU tract and prevent recurrent pyelonephritis and renal failure.

The prevalence of bacteriuria is significantly higher in preschool girls (4.5%) than in boys (0.5%), and this bacteriuria often is associated with vesicoureteral reflux. During childhood kidney development, reflux and infection more readily cause renal damage than in adult kidneys. In school-aged children, bacteriuria occurs in about 1.2% of girls but in only 0.03% of boys. Many of these infections are asymptomatic, and most are not associated with severe GU-tract abnormalities.

In women of childbearing age, the prevalence of bacteriuria is about 5%, which significantly exceeds that of adolescent boys and men. This is a result of bacterial colonization of the vaginal introitus and distal urethra with subsequent ascending infection of the lower urinary tract. Antimicrobial treatment of uncomplicated UTIs usually cures the symptoms and eradicates the causative organisms from the urine. However, recurrences develop in about 20% of women, and many experience multiple recurrent episodes of UTIs. Three percent of women experience more than 1 UTI per year, and most have a fairly constant rate of infection (average = 3 UTIs annually). These infections almost always are reinfections caused by uropathogenic bacteria migrating from the rectum to the vagina, the urethral meatus, and into the urinary bladder.

A variety of terms are used to categorize recurrent UTIs. Relapse is defined as the isolation of the original infecting pathogen following antimicrobial therapy. Relapses usually occur within weeks of completion of therapy due to poor patient compliance, inadequate courses of treatment, upper-tract involvement, or the presence of underlying urologic or renal disease. Urologically, relapses are caused by either bacterial persistence or unresolved bacteriuria. With the latter, the infection fails to respond to treatment because of bacterial resistance from prior antibiotic therapy or R-factor mediated resistance, poor antibiotic delivery, azotemia, or medullary concentrating defects, (e.g., papillary necrosis) or a large bacterial "inoculum" (e.g., "infected" struvite renal calculi). Bacterial persistence results in relapse of infection with the original infecting pathogen. The usual causes are "infected" renal calculi (both sexes) and chronic bacterial prostatitis (men). Both of these conditions are relatively uncommon but are the only correctable causes of recurrent UTIs. Patients (men and women) with suspected bacterial persistence should undergo complete radiologic and urologic evaluation.

The most frequent cause of recurrent UTIs is reinfection—the isolation of a new bacterial strain following eradication of the original infecting strain. These infections do not recur as quickly as cases of bacterial persistence because the bacteria arise from outside of the GU tract (i.e., perineum, vagina). This scenario commonly occurs in adult women who have bacterial colonization of the introitus and vagina and in uncircumcised boys who have preputial bacterial colonization. Bacterial reinfections usually do not require radiologic or cystoscopic evaluation except in men and in children (Table 10.2).

The rates of bacteriuria and UTIs increase markedly in the elderly. The ratio of females to males of between 25 and 30:1 in young adults changes significantly in those over 65 years of age to about 2:1. The reasons for this high prevalence of infection in the geriatric age group is discussed in the section dealing with infections in the elderly. Aging men develop alterations in prostatic size due to benign prostatic hyperplasia or

Table 10.2: Bacterial Persistence versus Bacterial Reinfection

	Bacterial Persistence	*Bacterial Reinfection*
Time interval	Weeks	Months to years
Bacterial species	Same	Different
Source bacteria	GU tract	Outside GU tract
Frequency	Uncommon	Common
Evaluation	All patients	Men, children
Causes	Chronic bacterial prostatitis, infected calculi—renal, prostatic	Bacterial adherence (introitus, prepuce)
Surgically correctable	Often	No

prostate carcinoma as well as alterations in the composition of their prostatic fluid. Furthermore, many elderly men undergo urethral catheterization or lower-tract instrumentation. These factors contribute to the high prevalence of bacteriuria in men.

MICROBIOLOGICAL CONSIDERATIONS

Escherichia coli is responsible for most commonly acquired UTIs and 80% of recurrent UTIs in women. *Staphylococcus saprophyticus*, a gram-positive, coagulase-negative, novobiocin-resistant, nonhemolytic coccus accounts for 10 to 20% of UTIs in sexually active women. Other aerobic, gram-negative bacteria causing cystitis include *Klebsiella* species, Enterococcus, *Proteus mirabilis* and Pseudomonas. In hospital-acquired infections, *Pseudomonas aeruginosa*, *Proteus mirabilis*, *Staphylococcus epidermidis*, and *Enterococcus* are the most common pathogens. These bacteria frequently exhibit drug resistance, and the infection often is polymicrobial.

The common urinary pathogens are capable of causing UTIs despite an anatomically normal GU tract. However, some less virulent bacteria cause infection only when natural host defenses are impaired (e.g., following instrumentation, catheterization, immunosuppression). These less "aggressive" organisms include *S. epidermidis*, fungi, *Gardnerella vaginalis*, lactobacillus, and *Ureaplasma urealyticum*. Uropathogenicity is therefore a function of specific virulence factors present in certain bacteria.

Diagnosis of a UTI relies on symptoms and confirmation of infection. Dysuria is the main symptom of cystitis, but many patients experience frequency, urgency, nocturia, pain, and voiding in small amounts. The symptoms of acute pyelonephritis include flank and back pain, abdominal pain, and symptoms of systemic infection, such as fever, malaise, nausea, vomiting, and sweats. Clinical evaluation is insufficient to clearly delineate lower- from upper tract infections. Indeed, many patients (10 to 50%) with cystitis have subclinical pyelonephritis, as shown by sophisticated localization culture techniques. Upper UTIs are more difficult to treat, have higher complication rates, and require prolonged treatment, including frequent hospitalization. The definitive techniques to localize infections are ureteral catheterization (Stamey test) and the bladder washout (Fairley) test, but both are invasive, complex procedures that are not commonly used. Noninvasive localization techniques include the antibody-coated bacteria (ACB) test, which is positive in tissue infections (e.g., pyelonephritis, prostatitis), and urinary beta$_2$-microglobulin, which is increased in upper UTIs as a result of renal tubular damage. These techniques are largely research tools and are not available to the practicing physician.

Pyuria, defined as over 10 WBC/mm^3 of urine, is a sensitive indicator of infection; it correlates with a urinary leukocyte excretion rate of 400,000 leukocytes per hour and quantitative bacterial counts of over 10^5 colonies per milliliter of urine. Pyuria can also be detected by "dipstick" chemical detection of leukocyte esterases and by use of a hemocytometer cell-counting chamber. Although bladder urine is normally sterile, voided urine can be contaminated by distal urethral and perineal organisms. Quantitation of bacteria in voided urine often distinguishes contamination from true infection. Following its initial description by Kass, significant bacteriuria has been defined as over 10^5 bacteria per milliliter of urine. However, recent studies in acutely dysuric women with symptoms of cystitis show that one-third have colony counts of 10^2 to 10^4 cfu (colony forming units) per milliliter of urine (Table 10.3). This has redefined "significant" bacteriuria as more than 10^2 colonies of uropathogenic bacteria per milliliter of urine in a symptomatic patient. Reasons for these low bacterial counts include urinary frequency or states of diuresis, which prevent bladder stasis, and multiplication of the bacteria. Likewise, fastidious organisms and slow-growing gram-negative bacteria may not reach counts of over 10^5 CfU/ml in urine. In catheter-associated bacteriuria, bacterial counts of less than 10^5 CfU/ml usually indicate a UTI.

Direct microscopic examination of a gram-stained uncentrifuged urine showing one bacterial organism per oil-immersion field, or an unstained centrifuged urine showing any bacteria, correlates with a colony count of over 10^5 CfU/ml of urine. The bacterial enzyme, nitrate reductase, produces nitrite from urinary nitrates and is the basis of a quick dipstick test for bacteriuria. A new bioluminescence assay detects bacterial ATP in urine and confirms the presence of bacteria. These rapid methods for the detection of bacteriuria are specific but not very sensitive, especially when bacterial counts are less than 10^5 CfU/ml.

Table 10.3: Causes of Acute Dysuria in Women

Classic Bacteriuria

>10^5 CfU/ml
30–40% patients
E. coli, *Staph. saprophyticus*

Low Count Bacteriuria

10^2–10^4 CfU/ml
30% patients
E. coli, *Staph. saprophyticus*

Vaginitis

0–10^2 CfU/ml bacteria
10–20% patients
Gardnerella, trichomonads, yeast

Urethritis

0–10^2 CfU/ml bacteria
5–10% patients
Herpes simplex, gonococcus, chlamydia

Other Causes

Interstitial cystitis
Irritation
Trauma

In sexually active young women, especially those with multiple sexual partners, the symptoms of cystitis can be mimicked by sexually transmitted diseases (STDs) or vaginitis. Vaginitis can be caused by candidal fungal species, trichomonas, or *Gardnerella vaginalis*. The common STD pathogens are *Neisseria gonorrhoeae*, *Chlamydia trachomatis*, and Herpes simplex viruses (Table 10.3). In the past, symptomatic women with low-count bacteriuria and urethritis were diagnosed as having the urethral syndrome.

Some bacteria produce urease, an enzyme that hydrolyzes urea to ammonia, with resultant alkalinization of the urine. This causes decreased solubility of magnesium and calcium phosphate and leads to the formation of struvite triple-phosphate and apatite renal calculi. Urease-producing bacteria, frequently embedded and incorporated within these stones, are a common cause of bacterial persistence. Complete removal of these "infection" stones is necessary to cure these infections. Common uropathogens producing urease include *Proteus species*, Klebsiella, Pseudomonas, *S. epidermidis*, *S. saprophyticus*, and *Ureaplasma urealyticum* (Table 10.4). The urinary pH in patients with "infection" stones is usually alkaline (>7.5).

Table 10.4: Common Urease-Producing Bacteria

Proteus species
Klebsiella species
Pseudomonas
Staph. Saprophyticus
Staph. aureus
Ureaplasma urealyticum
Corynebacteria

PATHOGENESIS OF URINARY-TRACT INFECTIONS

Considerable progress has been made in understanding the pathogenesis of UTIs. The critical balance that exists between bacterial virulence factors and host defense mechanisms determines whether UTIs develop. Virulence factors are especially important in the pathogenesis of UTIs in patients who have no anatomic or functional abnormalities of the GU tract (Table 10.5). In complicated UTIs, virulence factors play a lesser role than altered host defenses (e.g., chronic bacterial prostatitis).

Most UTIs are a result of ascending infection in which urethral organisms spread to infect the bladder. Only infrequently do these infections arise via hematogenous or lymphatic pathways. The work of Stamey clearly demonstrates that bacteria (e.g., *E. coli*) from the fecal flora initially colonize the perineum and vaginal introitus and then ascend through the urethra into the bladder. The density of a uropathogen in the fecal flora contributes to the frequency with which it causes UTIs. The common urinary pathogens (Enterobacteriaceae, enterococci) are found in large numbers in the colon (10^6 to 10^8 per gram of colonic contents). The short length of the female urethra and its frequent bacter-

Table 10.5: Uropathogenicity: Virulence Factors

Bacterial adherence
Bacterial adhesins
Uroepithelial cell receptors
Bacterial biofilm
Hemolysin production
Aerobactin production
Capsular K antigen
Bacterial lipopolysaccharide (O antigen)

ial colonization contribute to the high incidence of UTIs in women. In men, the long urethra and antibacterial properties of prostatic antibacterial factor (PAF) appear to effectively blunt bacterial ascent and lower the incidence of male UTIs. In contrast to other mucosal sites in the body, the urinary tract is sterile above the urethral level. Following urethral catheterization, ascending UTIs develop in 1% of outpatients. In contrast, all patients with indwelling catheters develop bacteriuria within 5 to 7 days of catheterization. Once bacteria gain access to the bladder, the determinants of whether an infection develops are specific bacterial virulence characteristics, bacterial density ("inoculum size"), and the integrity and adequacy of the host defenses.

Bacterial Adherence

Although more than 170 O-serotypes of *E. coli* are known, most UTIs are caused by only a few serotypes (O1, 2, 4, 6, 7, 11, 18, and 75). Serotyping and biotyping of *E. coli* urinary isolates have identified clones of bacteria harboring specific virulence factors. Perhaps the most critical virulence factor is bacterial adherence to uroepithelial cells. This is a prerequisite for colonization, persistence, and infection, especially in the urinary tract with its continuous flow and emptying mechanisms. There is considerable evidence that uropathogenic strains of *E. coli* have unique virulence factors that enable them to infect the lower or upper urinary tracts. Bacterial fimbriae or pili are the most common surface adhesins (or ligands) responsible for attachment to uroepithelial cells. These adherence pili are proteinaceous appendages, arising from the bacterial cell surface (Figure 10.1). Typically, 150 to 200 are present on each cell. The pili have been characterized by electron microscopy and their ability to agglutinate erythrocytes. Agglutination of *E. coli* type-1 fimbriae is inhibited by mannose (mannose sensitive, MS). Type 1 MS fimbriae are thought to play an important role in acute uncomplicated cystitis and catheter-associated UTIs. A second fimbrial type, the P fimbriae, binds to P blood group antigens on red blood cells and urothelial cells. These are mannose resistant (MR) and are variably expressed on certain *E. coli* serotypes. Other recently described mannose-resistant adhesins include X, S, G, M, and IC adhesins. Type-1 fimbriae are commonly expressed by bacteria colonizing the vaginal introitus and lower urinary tract, whereas bacteria associated with pyelonephritis, bacteremia, and urosepsis more frequently express P and X fimbriae. Similar virulence factors have been observed in non-*E. coli* uropathogens such as *Staph. saprophyticus*, *Klebsiella* species, and *Proteus* species. *Staph. epidermidis*, a frequent cause of catheter-associated UTIs, attaches to and forms a biofilm on foreign bodies. Some infecting strains of bacteria lack pili, and these strains occur in patients with abnor-

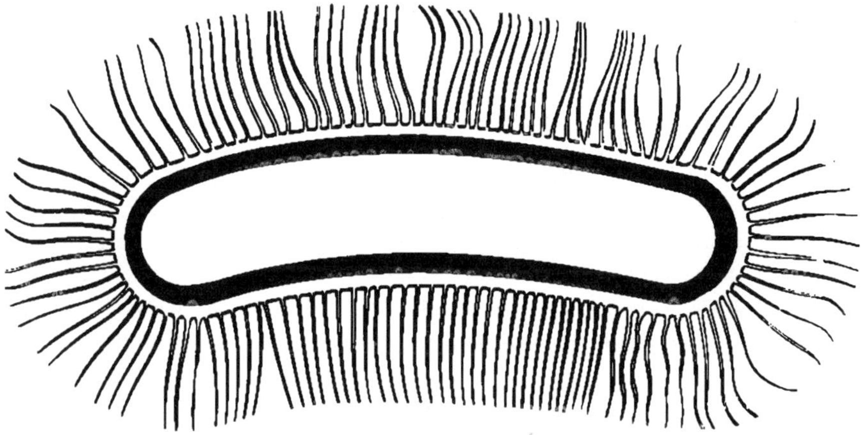

Figure 10.1: Enterobacillus showing the pili. *Reproduced with permission from Blandy J. Lecture Notes on Urology 4th ed. Oxford: Blackwell Scientific Publications, 1991:173.*

malities of the GU tract, indwelling catheters, or reflux, and in women who use the diaphragm for contraception.

Adherence is the end result of the interaction between adhesins present on bacterial cell surfaces and the epithelial receptivity of vaginal and urothelial cells. Increased receptivity has been demonstrated in females with recurrent UTIs during and between episodes of infection, and this receptivity is more pronounced in the first half of the menstrual cycle. *E. coli* adherence to vaginal cells is paralleled in buccal mucosal cells, suggesting that epithelial cell receptivity is a systemic, possibly genetically determined, risk factor for UTIs. Genetic factors associated with an increased risk of UTIs include the P1 blood group with an increased risk of pyelonephritis, especially in children, and blood group (e.g., Lewis) nonsecretors with an increased risk of recurrent cystitis in women. The nonexpression of blood group antigens in nonsecretors may allow the unmasking of receptors for *E. coli* and increase the likelihood of adherence and colonization by uropathogens. In animal models, bacterial adherence can be altered by oligosaccharides and monoclonal fimbrial antibodies. Immunization of animals with fimbrial antigens can alter the pyelonephritic responses to infection. These data further corroborate the pathogenetic roles of bacterial surface fimbriae/antigens and epithelial cell receptivity in the genesis of UTIs.

Bacterial adhesins attach to disaccharide moieties on glycoproteins present on epithelial surfaces. The P fimbriae of uropathogenic *E. coli* attach to specific Gal 1-4 Gal disaccharide receptors present in the globoseries glycolipids of epithelial cells lining the urinary tract and vagina. Tamm-Horsfall protein (uromucoid), which is excreted from the ascending limb of the loop of Henle, is a normal urinary constituent rich in mannose residues. Type 1 fimbriated *E. coli* avidly bind to uromucoid, and the elimination of this uromucoid during micturition serves as an antibacterial defense mechanism in the lower urinary tract. Beyond specific receptor binding, there is nonspecific cell attachment based on cell surface changes, such as hydrophobicity and surface charge characteristics. Certain bacterial species, (e.g., Pseudomonas) can produce a bacterial biofilm on mucosal or foreign body (e.g., catheter) surfaces. This biofilm is formed from bacterial exopolysaccharide and host extracellular matrix proteins. Bacteria growing in the biofilm (sessile bacteria) are protected from the effects of antibodies whereas bacteria in the urine (planktonic bacteria) are not. The bacterial biofilm prevents or retards the diffusion of antimicrobials, and this explains the difficulty in eradicating infections associated with genitourinary prostheses and indwelling catheters. Bacterial biofilms have been well documented in catheter-associated UTIs.

In addition to adherence, other virulence factors play a role in the pathogenesis of UTIs (Table 10.5). These include the lipopolysaccharide of gram-negative bacteria containing O antigens, which are highly toxic and inflammatory; the K antigens of the capsular polysaccharides, which encapsulate bacteria and help resist phagocytosis; hemolysin production, which releases iron from lysed erythrocytes and destroys phagocytic and inflammatory cells; and aerobactin, which is an iron acquisition and transport system that facilitates growth of *E. coli* in iron depleted media, such as urine. Strains of bacteria causing acute pyelonephritis are more likely to produce hemolysin and aerobactin, to express O and K antigens and to show increased adherence to uroepithelial cells, compared with strains causing cystitis.

Host Defense Mechanisms

Bacterial virulence factors are not the sole determinants of UTIs. Numerous host defense mechanisms operate at various sites of the urinary tract to counteract bacterial virulence (Table 10.6). The adequacy of these host defenses and the size of the bacterial "inoculum" determine the type and anatomic level of an infection.

Regular, efficient bladder emptying is an important defense against the development of UTIs. The periodic washing effect of micturition eliminates infecting organisms from the bladder (Figure 10.2). Emptying of the bladder removes the bulk of contaminated urine, which is then subsequently diluted by the addition of fresh urine from the upper tract. If postvoid residual volumes are high, bacteria tend to persist and proliferate.

Table 10.6: Host Defenses Against UTIs

Mechanical effects of voiding
Bacterial inhibitory properties of urine
Immune mechanisms
Ureteral peristalsis
Antiadherence mechanisms
Bacterial interference
Uromucoid (Tamm-Horsfall protein)
Mucosal glycosaminoglycans (GAGs)
Secretory IgA (SIgA)

This is seen in patients with bladder outlet obstruction and neuropathic bladder dysfunction. Because of the shearing forces associated with voiding, bladder emptying may mechanically interfere with bacterial adherence.

Although urine normally promotes bacterial growth, at times it inhibits bacterial growth and is bactericidal against small numbers ("inocula") of uropathogens. The factors contributing to inhibition are high osmolality, high urea concentration, low urinary pH, and high organic acid content. "Osmoprotectant" substances (e.g., betaine, choline, proline, and

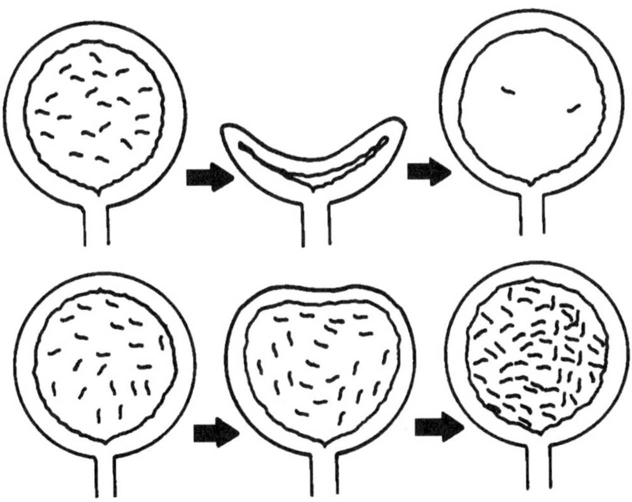

Figure 10.2: The chief natural defense of the bladder against infection is to keep itself regularly emptied. *Reproduced with permission from Blandy J. Lecture Notes on Urology, 4th ed. Oxford: Blackwell Scientific Publications, 1991:173.*

glutamine), synthesized in the renal papillae, protect the distal tubular epithelium from the hyperosmolar effects of urine in the renal medulla. These substances may also protect bacteria and contribute to the increased susceptibility of the renal medulla to bacterial infections, compared with the renal cortex. Glucose in the urine provides an enhanced medium for growth and multiplication of *E. coli* and may account for the increased frequency and severity of UTIs in diabetic patients.

Antiadherence mechanisms exist throughout the urinary tract (i.e., urinary oligosaccharides, Tamm-Horsfall protein, urinary immunoglobulins) or at specific sites (e.g., bacterial interference in the vagina, mucopolysaccharides, and mechanical flushing in the bladder). Commensal vaginal lactobacilli can adhere to epithelial cells and competitively prevent adherence of pathogenic bacteria. The glycosaminoglycan (GAG) moiety of the mucopolysaccharide lining of the bladder wall also apparently plays an important role in discouraging bacterial adherence. This hydrophilic layer attracts an aqueous film of water or urine onto its surface and prevents adherence. Experimentally, acid treatment destroys this layer, but it regenerates within 24 hours. Tamm-Horsfall (T-H) protein ("urinary slime") occurs in the urine as a coating on exfoliated cells and in a free-floating form. This T-H protein contains mannose residues that agglutinate *E. coli* harboring type 1 fimbriae. Probably, this agglutination/binding of organisms in conjunction with the flushing effect of micturition is an important defense against the development of UTIs. It is known that reduced levels of uromucoid occur in elderly patients, a group particularly prone to infection.

Renal infections generate systemic and local antibody responses. These antibodies are directed against a variety of antigens (including the O, K, type 1, and P fimbrial antigens) and are of the IgM, IgG, and IgA varieties). These antibodies are thought to reduce local tissue damage, resist bacterial spread, and prevent reinfection by the same bacterial strain. Secretory IgA (SIgA) in the urine reportedly helps prevent pyelonephritis, whereas reduced levels of urinary SIgA are associated with an increased risk of cystitis. Ureteral peristalsis ensures the flow of urine from the kidney to the bladder. If it is inhibited or diminished (e.g., during pregnancy, by a ureteroplegic factor produced by certain uropathogens, vesicoureteral reflux) infection of the upper tract is enhanced. Obstruction alone, however, probably does not increase the risk of upper tract infection. The changes in intrarenal blood flow associated with hydronephrosis, especially medullary blood flow, probably are important in development of infection. The medulla is much more prone than the renal cortex to develop infection because of relatively slow blood flow, hyperosmolality, low pH, and high concentrations of ammonia.

URINARY-TRACT INFECTIONS IN SPECIAL GROUPS

Recurrent UTIs in Females

Recurrent UTIs are relatively common in young women who have anatomically and functional normal GU tracts. These UTIs are a result of reinfection, not persistent infection. The infecting organisms reach the bladder via perineal/introital colonization from the rectum (Figure 10.3). Longitudinal studies have shown more frequent and prolonged colonization in women with recurrent UTIs than in normal women. Thus, increased bacterial adherence, not GU tract abnormalities, is the fundamental factor in the genesis of these UTIs. This is a result of a genetic predisposition that enhances bacterial adherence to vaginal and urethral mucosal cells. Moreover, this genetic tendency is associated with certain HLA phenotypes (HLA-A3) and blood group nonsecretors (Lewis and ABO groups) (Table 10.7).

Acquired risk factors for UTIs in women include sexual activity and the use of the diaphragm and spermicidals. Diaphragms and spermicidals may contribute to as many as one-third of all acute UTIs. Sexual intercourse leads to bacteriuria because pathogenic bacteria colonize the vagina. This vaginal colonization generally is mild in women using oral contraceptives but more marked in those using spermicidal foams and diaphragms. Nonoxynol-9, the active ingredient in most spermicides, has significant antimicrobial activity against sexually transmitted bacteria,

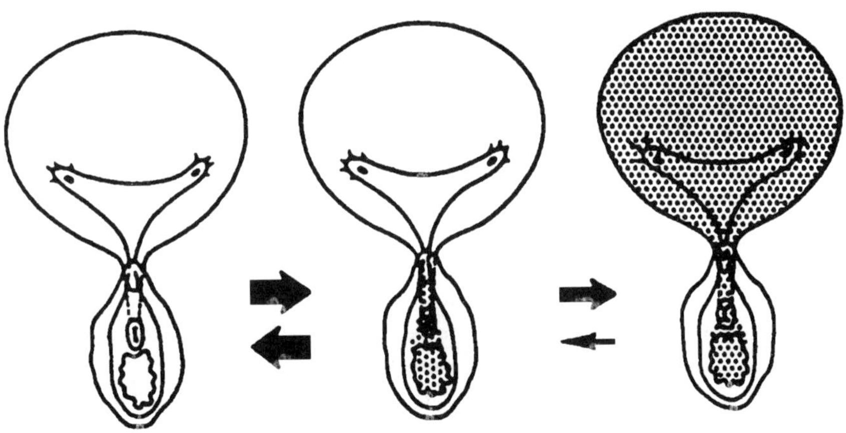

Figure 10.3: Pathogenesis of urinary reinfection in females. Colonization of the vaginal mucosa by gram-negative bacilli from the fecal reservoir is a dynamic process. If bacteriuria does develop the infection may resolve spontaneously.

Table 10.7: Risk Factors for UTIs in Women

Inherited	*Acquired*
Blood Group nonsecretors	Sexual activity
HLA-A3 phenotype	Diaphragm use
	Spermicidal use

Gardnerella vaginalis, viruses, and lactobacilli, but little activity against *Enterococcus*, *Klebsiella*, and *E. coli*. It has been shown that spermicide use significantly alters the normal vaginal flora and encourages vaginal colonization with uropathogenic bacteria. Diaphragms may also partially obstruct the urethra, interfere with normal voiding, and increase the risk of infection in women using spermicidals.

Based on known pathogenetic mechanisms, the following approaches have been used to control recurrent UTIs in women: competitive colonization of the vagina with lactobacilli; immunization with antigens produced from uropathogenic bacteria or fimbriae; postintercourse micturition and long-term, low-dose, prophylactic antimicrobials; and postcoital antimicrobial prophylaxis. Continuous, low-dose antibiotic prophylaxis for 3 to 12 months has successfully reduced UTI infection rates from 2 or 3 to less than 0.15 infections per patient year. It is important that antibiotics used for prophylaxis are safe, cheap, and unlikely to select resistant bacteria from the bowel flora. Trimethoprim-sulfamethoxazole (TMP-SMX) and the new fluoroquinolones eradicate most uropathogens from the bladder as well as the fecal stream. Other agents, which are completely absorbed in the upper gastrointestinal tract, do not reach the colon, and, therefore, are less likely to cause resistance in bowel bacteria, include cephradine, cefaclor, and nitrofurantoin macrocrystals. The frequency of infection and the interval between infections are reduced with these regimens. Adverse side effects from TMP-SMX are low, but the emergence of resistant organisms and the development of enterococcal infections can be problematic. One-quarter of the usual therapeutic dose of the drug is usually given in a single night-time dose (e.g., 100 mg nitrofurantoin or 1/2 DS tablet TMP-SMX). This allows for better compliance and reduces the likelihood of troublesome side effects. Continuous prophylaxis is used in patients with more than 3 UTIs per year. If the infections are temporally related to sexual intercourse, postcoital prophylaxis may be considered.

Urinary-Tract Infection in Pregnancy

The prevalence of asymptomatic bacteriuria during pregnancy is about

5% (range 4 to 7%), a rate similar to that in nonpregnant women. Asymptomatic bacteriuria in women rises at a prevalence rate of 1% for each decade of life beyond age 5 years. Prevalence rates in pregnant women increase with age, sexual activity, parity, and low socioeconomic status. The fact that 98% of pregnant women who are bacteriuric are at their first prenatal visit must be emphasized. Gestation itself is not responsible for bacteriuria because less than 1% of pregnant women with negative urine cultures at initial screening acquire bacteriuria later in pregnancy.

Asymptomatic bacteriuria in a pregnant woman, left untreated, can progress to pyelonephritis. The hormonal and mechanical changes that occur during pregnancy significantly increase the risk of pyelonephritis. The most impressive change is dilatation of the collecting system (hydroureter of pregnancy), which develops as early as the eighth week of gestation. Hyperestrogenism is thought to contribute to the dilatation, which is usually worse on the right side because of mechanical factors (e.g., right-sided placenta, etc.). Ureteral peristalsis is also reduced, and bladder capacity increases as the bladder moves out of the pelvis into the abdomen. Other physiologic changes, such as urinary stasis, reduced renal concentrating ability, aminoaciduria, and gestational glycosuria, all increase the risk of pyelonephritis, especially during the third trimester.

Asymptomatic bacteriuria, common during pregnancy, usually is a reflection of prior colonization, not the development of the bacteriuria during pregnancy. Approximately 30% of untreated women with asymptomatic bacteriuria detected in early pregnancy later develop acute pyelonephritis (Table 10.8). Pyelonephritis, the most common medical complication of pregnancy occurs in 1 to 2% of all pregnancies. The risk of pyelonephritis is facilitated by profound physiologic and anatomic changes that occur in the urinary tract during pregnancy. Moreover, pyelonephritis of pregnancy, is associated with significant maternal and fetal risks. Premature labor often results, possibly due to bacterial liberation of arachidonic acid metabolites from phospholipids in the amniotic and chorionic membranes and due to the production of prostaglandins E_2 and

Table 10.8: UTIs in Pregnancy

Asymptomatic bacteriuria 5%
>98% bacteriuria discovered at first antenatal visit
Pyelonephritis in 30% of untreated patients
Maternal, fetal risk
GU anomalies in 20% when UTIs are recurrent

F_2. Treatment of asymptomatic bacteriuria prevents the acute pyelonephritis in about 90% of pregnant women. The association of prematurity and low birth weight with asymptomatic bacteriuria is less well defined than with symptomatic pyelonephritis. Since most symptomatic UTIs develop in women who have asymptomatic bacteriuria detected in early pregnancy, all bacteriuric pregnant women should be treated to reduce the risks of prematurity, premature labor, low birth weight, and other fetal complications. Women should be screened at their first prenatal visit, and those with positive cultures should receive an appropriate antimicrobial agent, (e.g., ampicillin or nitrofurantoin macrocrystals). *E. coli* and *Klebsiella-Enterobacter* species account for 80 to 90% of the UTIs in pregnancy. Recurrence or persistence of UTI following treatment suggest an anatomic abnormality, bacterial persistence, stones, or renal parenchymal infection. These patients should undergo a full urologic evaluation following parturition. About 20% have structural abnormalities of the kidney, ureter, or bladder.

UTIs in the Elderly

The incidence and prevalence of bacteriuria is highest in the elderly. In women of reproductive age, the prevalence of bacteriuria is about 5%, compared with only 0.1% in age-matched men. This marked female prevalence fades with increasing age. Indeed, in adults over 65 years of age, bacteriuria is found in 20% of women and 10% of men. These prevalence figures are even higher for elderly patients residing in nursing homes, extended-care facilities, or hospitals. Studies show that this bacteriuria is usually intermittent and seldom is persistent.

Although *E. coli* is still the most common uropathogen in the elderly, there is an increased rate of infection with *Proteus*, *Klebsiella*, *Enterobacter*, *Serratia*, *Pseudomonas*, and *Enterococcus*. Interestingly, elderly men may have a high incidence of urethral catheterization, cystoscopy, hospitalization, and antimicrobial agents. Many of these infections are polymicrobial, especially in hospitalized or institutionalized elderly patients.

Various factors contribute to this high rate of bacteriuria in the elderly (Table 10.9). Micturition may be impaired as a result of prostatic enlargement in men or bladder prolapse in women. The levels of prostatic antibacterial factor (PAF)—a zinc substance—decline with increasing age. Perineal soiling from fecal incontinence, the use of urethral catheterization, and reduced host defense mechanisms, (e.g. T-H protein) also predispose to bacteriuria. Both indwelling and condom catheters contribute to bacteriuria in the elderly; this is discussed in the section dealing with catheter-associated infections.

Table 10.9: UTIs in the Elderly

Prevalence: 20–50%
Female to Male ratio: 2–3:1

Risk factors
- Immobilization, instrumentation
- Hospitalization, age, systemic disease
- Fecal incontinence, neurogenic bladder dysfunction
- Catheters (Foley, condom)
  - Men: Benign prostatic hyperplasia
    - Prostate cancer
    - Loss of prostatic antibacterial factor
  - Women: Bacterial colonization introitus, perineum
    - pH changes

Bacteriology
- Polymicrobial; intermittent bacteriuria
- More noncoliform infections
- Gram-positive infections in men

Asymptomatic bacteriuria is common in the elderly, but whether this leads to excessive mortality or morbidity remains controversial. The risks of adverse drug reactions and the emergence of resistant bacterial strains may outweigh the benefits of the routine treatment of asymptomatic bacteriuria. Urine cultures in the elderly with symptomatic UTIs do not always show more than 10^5 bacteria per milliliter of urine—a situation similar to that found in sexually active women. Pyuria is a less significant marker for bacteriuria in the elderly than in the young. However, the absence of pyuria suggest insignificant bacteriuria. Studies using the antibody coated bacteria test and the Fairley washout technique have show upper urinary-tract infection in about 50% who have asymptomatic bacteriuria. Moreover, the typical clinical signs and symptoms (e.g., fever, flank pain) are often absent in patients with documented pyelonephritis.

Relapse of infection after appropriate treatment of either lower- or upper-tract infection may indicate renal involvement, anatomic abnormality of the GU tract, or chronic bacterial prostatitis.

Catheter-Associated Urinary-Tract Infections

Catheter-associated bacteriuria, the most common hospital-acquired infection, accounts for 40% of annual nosocomial infections. Moreover, catheterization (indwelling or "in and out") and instrumentation account for about 80% of all nosocomial UTIs. It is estimated that 15 to 20% of all hospitalized patients undergo urinary-tract catheterization, and 1 to 3% of these patients develop bacteremia with a mortality rate of about 10%. Most catheters are left in-situ for short periods of time—mean duration of 2 days and median of 4 days. The incidence of bacteriuria associated with indwelling urethral catheterization increases about 5% per day. Thus, bacteriuria universally develops within 3 to 4 weeks, even when closed urinary drainage is strictly used.

Bacteria can enter the bladder at the time of catheter insertion, through the lumen of the catheter or along the periurethral space between the catheter and the urethral mucosa (Table 10.10). The distal urethra is normally colonized by bacteria, and catheter insertion leads to bacteriuria in 1% of ambulatory patients and as many as 20% of hospitalized patients. Intraluminal contamination is a result of ascending infection from the drainage bag or breaks in the system of closed drainage. The main route of infection, however, is the periurethral space. Meatal colonization precedes bladder bacteriuria in about two-thirds of patients who have indwelling catheters. Once bacteria reach the bladder, their persistence and proliferation depend on factors such as bacterial adherence, the antibacterial effect of surface glycosaminoglycans, and the development of bacterial biofilm on the catheter surface. Organisms trapped within biofilms theoretically are protected from the mechanical flow of urine, antibiotics, and other host defense mechanisms. Condom catheter drainage in incontinent men is also associated with an increased risk of bacteriuria. Poorly fitted catheters can cause urethral obstruction and impair bladder emptying. In addition, bacteria from the perineum can colonize the condom portion of the catheter and act as a reservoir for ascending infection.

Risk factors for the development of bacteriuria in catheterized patients include prolonged catheterization, inadequate care of the drainage

Table 10.10: Catheter-Associated UTIs

Catheter-Associated UTIs
40% of all nosocomial infections
Significant causes:
Periurethral migration
Bacterial biofilm
Altered bladder defenses (GAGs, etc.)
Less significant causes:
Retrograde spread from distal urethra
Drainage bag contamination
Break in closed drainage system

bag and closed drainage system, the female gender, systemic diseases (e.g., diabetes mellitus), renal failure, and systemic immunosuppression. Many patients in nursing homes have indwelling urethral catheters to treat urinary incontinence or prostatic obstruction. Some bacteria (e.g., *Providencia stuartii* and *Staph. epidermidis*) adhere readily to catheter surfaces and frequently cause catheter associated bacteriuria. Moreover, urease-producing bacteria hydrolyze urea to ammonia, increase urinary pH, and predispose to the formation of struvite and apatite stones. In addition, bladders catheterized for more than 10 years frequently show metaplasia and have an increased incidence of bladder cancer compared with noncatheterized bladders.

Catheter-associated UTIs can be reduced by limiting the duration of catheterization and using alternative methods of drainage (e.g., intermittent catheterization, suprapubic tubes). The use of closed drainage systems is mandatory (Figure 10.4). Methods that postpone bacteriuria in catheterized patients include the use of drainage bag antibacterial addi-

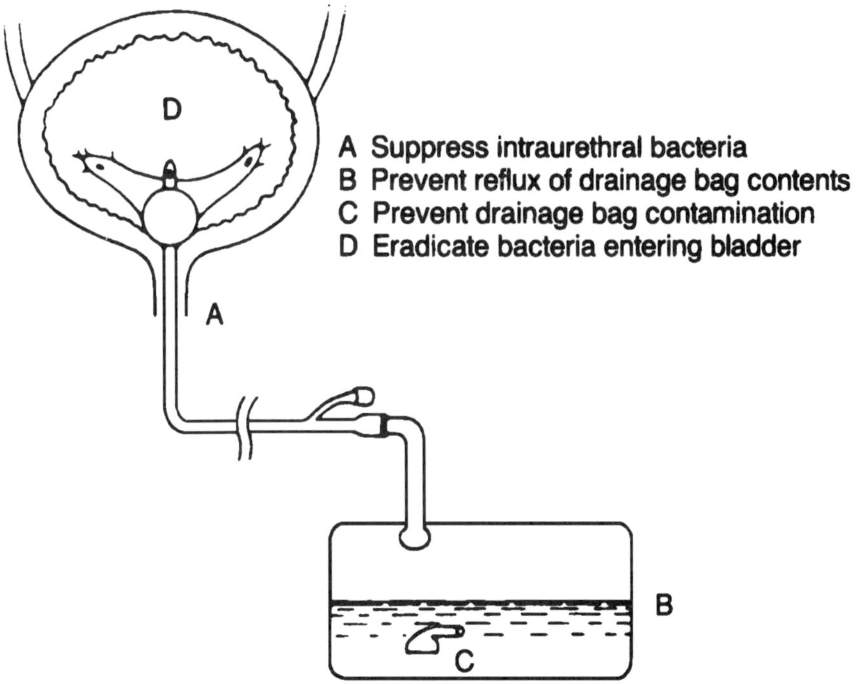

Figure 10.4: Measures to prevent urinay tract infection during closed-catheter drainage

tives (e.g., hydrogen peroxide, povidone), meatal care with soaps and antibiotic ointments, silver-coated catheters, hydrophilic catheters and antibiotics, either systemically or by bladder irrigation. Unfortunately, studies show that these methods fail to affect, or delay significantly, the development of bacteriuria. Asymptomatic bacteriuria in patients with indwelling catheters, except bacteriuria due to urease-producing bacteria, should not be routinely treated with antimicrobial agents.

Urinary-tract Infections in Men

The prevalence of UTIs in men is low but increases with age. In women, rectal bacteria initially colonize the perineum and vaginal introitus, enter the urethra and bladder, and then cause ascending infection. In men, the situation is different. The male urinary meatus is far removed from the perineum and is surrounded by dry epithelium of the glans penis. This results in a microbial environment that differs significantly from the moist vaginal introitus. Both the long male urethra and normal levels of prostatic antibacterial factor in prostatic fluid are thought to confer added protection to men.

In general, UTIs in men are considered complicated infections, usually associated with structural or functional abnormalities of the GU tract. The prostate gland is the most important structure involved in the pathogenesis of UTIs in men. Prostatic enlargement interferes with efficient voiding and increases the likelihood of infection. In addition, the evaluation of prostatism frequently involves bladder catheterization and cystoscopy, which increase the risk of infection. As men grow older, the level of PAF in their prostatic secretions decreases, which probably increases their susceptibility to GU infection. Relapsing recurrent UTI in men usually is a result of chronic bacterial prostatitis (CBP). CBP probably develops from spread of bacteria from the urethra or bladder via the prostatic ducts into the prostate as a result of intraprostatic urinary reflux. Prostatic calculi, common in middle-aged men and almost universal in elderly men, can become secondarily infected (comparable to infection stones of the kidney), and this makes eradication of infection difficult. Other GU-tract abnormalities associated with bacteriuria include neurogenic bladder dysfunction, indwelling catheters, tumors, and foreign bodies. It has also been shown that homosexual men are at increased risk for the development of UTIs as a consequence of anal insertive intercourse.

The growth in urine culture of more than 10^3 colony forming units per milliliter of uropathogens indicates bacteriuria and probably GU infection. A major problem associated with UTIs in men is the localization of the site and source of the bacteria (Table 10.11). The only reliable means other than complicated antigen-specific antibody studies, of

Table 10.11: Prostatic Localization Cultures

Techniques

Meares-Stamey test
  Four specimens
  VB_1, VB_2, VB_3, EPS
Microscopic examination of expressed prostatic secretions (EPS)
  Leukocytes
  Oval fat bodies

Findings

Chronic bacterial prostatitis (CBP)
  VB_3, EPS bacterial counts highest
  Leukocytes, oval fat bodies
Nonbacterial prostatitis
  Negative localization cultures
  Leukocytes, oval fat bodies
Prostatodynia
  Normal EPS/localization cultures
  Abnormal videourodynamic findings

diagnosing CBP is the prostatic localization test (the 4-glass or Meares-Stamey test). Four specimens are collected for quantitative culture, including three from the voided urine (VB_1, VB_2, and VB_3) and one from the expressed prostatic secretions (EPS) obtained by prostatic massage (Figure 10.5). The test confirms bacterial prostatitis if the EPS or VB_3 (the prostatic specimens) cultures show greater colony counts than

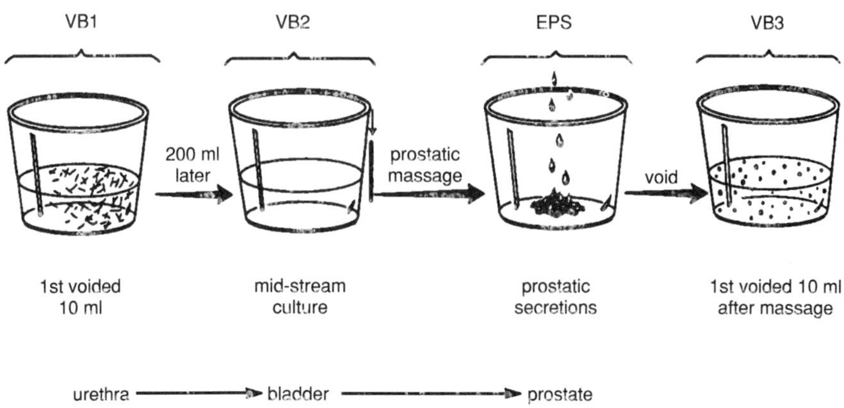

Figure 10.5: Bacteriologic localization cultures in the diagnosis of chronic bacterial prostatitis

the VB_1 (urethra) or VB_2 (bladder) specimens. A 10-fold increase in counts is regarded as significant. In patients in whom all cultures show more than 10^5 CFU/ml, definite localization is impossible until the bladder urine is sterilized with an antibiotic (e.g., ampicillin or nitrofurantoin) that does not penetrate into the prostate fluid. Changes in numbers of leukocytes, enzymes, or immunoglobulins in prostatic fluid also help to localize infections to the prostate. Other than demonstration of elevated antigen-specific antibodies in the EPS, however, these methods are not as accurate as the Meares-Stamey test.

Both gram-negative enteric bacteria and gram-positive bacteria cause UTIs in men. Men with relapsing bacteriuria usually have CBP, infected urinary stones, or anatomic or functional abnormalities of the GU tract. These are regarded as complicated UTIs, require prolonged treatment with antimicrobials (at least 1 month), and deserve full urologic evaluation. Single-dose antibiotic treatment, successful in many women with simple cystitis, has not been adequately studied in men. However, treatment of men with CBP is difficult because most antibiotics penetrate poorly into prostate fluid (Figure 10.6). Antibiotics that do achieve adequate prostatic fluid levels include trimethoprim and the new fluoroquinolones. Patients may respond favorably to these antibiotics unless infected prostatic calculi are present. The surgical removal of all infected stones and tissue via radical transurethral prostatectomy may be required for cure of the infection.

In contradistinction to women, a single episode of bacteriuria in a

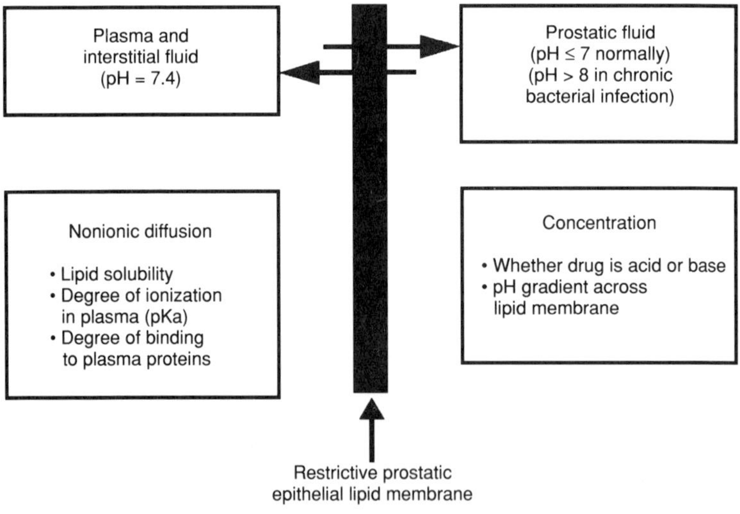

Figure 10.6: Drug transfer from plasma to prostatic fluid

man warrants full urologic evaluation. Genitourinary tract abnormalities are frequent in bacteriuric male patients, occurring in 25% of young men and as many as 70 to 80% of elderly men. Many of these abnormalities affect the upper tract. Uroradiologic studies, (e.g. urography, ultrasonography) are always indicated in men who experience recurrent or complicated UTIs.

Only about 10% of men with symptoms of "prostatitis" have positive prostatic bacterial localization cultures. The remaining 90% or so have either nonbacterial prostatitis (NBP) or prostatodynia. Leukocytes and oval-fat bodies (lipid-laden macrophages) may be present in the EPS in nonbacterial prostatitis. However, it is usually difficult to separate patients with prostatodynia from those with nonbacterial prostatitis. An infectious etiology for NBP (e.g., Chlamydia, mycoplasma) has been postulated but not proven. It may well be that NBP and prostatodynia are both caused by a cascade of prostatic reflux of sterile urine, sterile prostatic inflammation, and prostatic/pelvic floor spasm. The last changes are manifested on videourodynamic testing as abnormal urethral pressure profiles (UPP) and reduced urinary flow rates.

INTERSTITIAL CYSTITIS

Evaluation of the symptom complex of urinary frequency, urgency, suprapubic discomfort, suprapubic, pelvic or perineal pain, and dyspareunia in women is difficult and frequently unrewarding. Interstitial cystitis (IC), a cause of this symptom complex, was thought to be rare because of the infrequent occurrence of ulceration (Hunner's ulcers) in patients with irritative symptoms and pain. However, in 1978, the nonulcer variety of IC was described and its prevalence emphasized. This led to the more frequent diagnosis of IC and the recognition of two subtypes of the disease—the uncommon Hunner's ulcer disease, and the vastly more common (10:1) early or nonulcer variety. Diagnosis is usually made on the basis of patient symptomatology, urologic evaluation including cystoscopy, and exclusion of other recognizable bladder diseases. Mucosal glomerulations are the endoscopic hallmark of the condition. The lack of specific diagnostic criteria for IC means that diagnosis frequently depends on the awareness, interest, and personal bias of the physician.

The natural history of IC is variable. Symptoms usually develop subacutely, progress to the classic symptom complex in a relatively short time, and then plateau. Clinical experience suggests that progression from the nonulcer to the classic Hunner's ulcer variant is rare. The two forms of the disease may well have separate causes that result in end-organ bladder inflammation.

The absence of clear-cut histologic markers has led to various theories of IC causation, including infection, vascular obstruction, autoimmunity, lymphatic obstruction, neurogenic and hormonal factors, genetics, defects in bladder cytoprotection, the presence of toxic substances in the urine, and even psychiatric causes (Table 10.12). Currently, the etiology is thought to be multifactorial, with IC a clinical syndrome rather than a specific disease. Studies have failed to isolate bacteria, mycobacteria, fungi, or viruses in IC. A recent study that used specialized culture techniques for urine and bladder biopsy tissue identified fastidious bacteria (*Gardnerella vaginalis*, *Lactobacillus sp.*) in patients with sterile urine and symptoms suggestive of IC and suggested that the urethral syndrome and IC represent the early and late stages of the same disease process. However, the lack of symptomatic improvement with antibiotic treatment argues against a bacterial etiology of IC.

The bladder surface glycosaminoglycans (GAGs) are an important defense against bacterial adherence and a protective layer against injury from toxic substances (chemicals, carcinogens, allergens) in the urine. The beneficial effects of sodium pentosanpolysulfate (Elmiron), a highly sulfated, exogenous, orally administered GAG, suggest that impaired cytoprotection plays a role in the pathogenesis of IC. Bladder wall permeability is increased in IC, probably due to defective intercellular junctions. Increased urea absorption from the bladder is further evidence of a “leaky” urothelium in IC. A leaky urothelium results in bladder wall inflammation, which can be toxic, allergic, or immunologically induced. Tamm-Horsfall protein, produced in the renal tubules, is not normally present in the bladder wall. Its identification beneath the bladder epithelium in IC is indicative of an abnormality of the bladder lining.

Table 10.12: Current Etiologies Regarding Pathogenesis of IC

Infection
Fastidious bacteria
Latent viruses
Dysfunctional bladder epithelium
Defective GAG cytoprotection
Abnormal intercellular junctions
Toxic substances in urine
Allergic/immune/autoimmune causes
Neurogenic disturbances
Bladder mastocytosis
Psychosomatic
Others
Food intolerance
Endocrine causes

Antibiotics (nitrofurantoin and tetracycline) have been proposed to alter the bladder glycocalyx and cause a leak of urine into the bladder wall. Animal studies have failed to implicate antibiotics as a cause of IC. Substances in the urine (e.g., food, metabolites, food additives, drugs, environmental pollutants) may play a role in the pathogenesis of IC. They may gain access to the bladder wall through a defective GAG layer, or via direct destruction of the normal GAG layer.

An association between IC and autoimmune diseases such as polyarteritis nodosa, rheumatoid arthritis, ulcerative colitis, lupus erythematosus, and thyroiditis has been proposed. The weak association with other autoimmune disorders, the lack of a strong or consistent association between IC and HLA phenotypes, and the inability to reproduce the disease by syngeneic transfer of circulating autoantibodies suggest that autoimmunity plays a less than compelling role in the pathogenesis of IC.

Increased submucosal nerve density, perineural fibrosis, and inflammation have been described in IC. Vasoactive intestinal peptide (VIP) and substance P have been demonstrated in the sensory nerve plexus of the bladder, within the lamina propria and submucosa. Neurogenic inflammation is inhibited by dimethyl sulfoxide, which destroys C fibers or substances (e.g., capsaicin) that cause axonal degeneration of C fibers.

Histamine release from mast cells was suggested in the 1950s as a cause of IC. Two mast cell subsets are present in IC. Cells with the phenotypic appearance of connective tissue mast cells predominate in the detrusor muscle layers, and those with features of mucosal mast cells are increased in the mucosa and submucosa. Patients with IC have been shown to have more activated detrusor mast cells. Light microscopy reveals mastocytosis in only 30 to 50% of IC patients. However, electron microscopy has demonstrated increased activation rather than increased numbers of mast cells in a significant proportion of patients. The factors responsible for the migration and proliferation of mast cells in IC are unknown, and there is no evidence of a parasitic cause. However, an allergic reaction to an allergen located in the urine (toxic urine) or bladder tissue is a possibility.

THE URETHRAL SYNDROME

Prior to the description of the nonulcer variety of interstitial cystitis, the urethral syndrome was frequently diagnosed in women with frequency and urgency. Up to one-third of women presenting with symptoms of cystitis have negative urine cultures—that is, less than 100,000 bacteria per milliliter of urine—and are diagnosed as having urethral syndrome. Many of these patients have pyuria and low levels of bacteriuria—counts between 10^2 and 10^5 bacteria per milliliter (Table 10.3). The sexually transmitted organisms—chlamydia, mycoplasmas, herpes viruses, etc.—also cause pyuria and irritative voiding symptoms. It is possible that infection or inflammation of the urethral glands contributes to the pathogenesis of the urethral syndrome, and this may be the reason that urethral dilatations sometime help patients with frequency or urgency.

The distinction between the urethral syndrome and interstitial cystitis can be clinically blurred, as symptoms are similar in both conditions. However, the presence of pain (suprapubic, pelvic) and dyspareunia is a useful clue as to the likelihood of IC. Pyuria and/or low count bacteriuria suggests the diagnosis of the urethral syndrome. Treatment consists of antibiotics with broad activity against gram-negative (e.g., coliforms) and gram-positive (e.g., *Staph. epidermidis*, enterococcus) uropathogens that frequently cause urinary-tract infections. If the urine culture is negative for bacteria but pyuria is present, an empiric treatment with doxycycline, minocycline, or erythromycin is indicated for presumed chlamydial/mycoplasmal infection. Specific cultures for these sexually transmitted pathogens are not routinely performed but reserved for research studies.

Noninfectious etiologies have also been proposed for the urethral syndrome. These include spasm of the external striated sphincter, bladder neck spasm (internal sphincter dyssynergia), and pelvic floor tension myalgia. The precise contributions of these pathogenetic mechanisms in the causation of the urethral syndrome have not been clearly elucidated. Treatment approaches based on these putative theories include urethral dilatation, pharmacologic therapy with smooth muscle relaxants, alpha-adrenergic blockers (e.g., minipress, terazosin), pelvic floor relaxation, and biofeedback. In spite of the use of repeated urethral dilatations in patients with symptoms of IC or the urethral syndrome, the urethral lumen is of normal caliber in the majority of women so treated.

SUGGESTED READINGS

Lipsky BA. Urinary-tract infections in men: epidemiology, pathophysiology, diagnosis and treatment. Ann Intern Med 1989; 110:138.

Comprehensive review of male urinary-tract infections, with emphasis on pathophysiology. Strong discussion of prostatitis and infections in uncircumcised boys.

Parsons CL. Pathogenesis of urinary-tract infections: bacterial adherence, bladder defense mechanisms. Urol Clin North Am 1986; 13:563.

Complete summary of the relative contributions of antibacterial host factors and bacterial virulence characteristics to the development of urinary-tract infections.

Sant GR. Interstitial cystitis. Monog Urol 1991; 12:37.

Overview of interstitial cystitis with emphasis on pathogenesis and potential etiologies of this enigmatic bladder disease.

Meares EM Jr. Acute and chronic prostatitis: diagnosis and treatment. Infect Dis Clin North Am 1987; 1:855.

Critical review of the prostatitis syndromes. Diagnosis and treatment are emphasized, with particular emphasis on drug pharmacokinetics in prostatic disease.

Stamm WE, Wagner KF, Ansel R, et al. Causes of the acute urethral syndrome in women. N Engl J Med 1980; 303:409.

Careful, microbiological study of the urethral syndrome. The concept of low-count bacteriuria emphasized.

Stamey TA, Timothy M, Millar M, Mihara G. Recurrent urinary infections in adult women. The role of introital enterobacteria. Calif Med 1971; 115:1.

Seminal paper describing the role of bacterial adherence in the pathogenesis of recurrent urinary-tract infections in women.

Ramsey JW, Garnham AJ, Mulhall AB, et al. Biofilms, bacteria and bladder catheters. A clinical study. Br J Urol 1989; 64:395.

Concise overview of the role of the bacterial biofilm in the pathogenesis of catheter-associated urinary-tract infections. Implications for antibiotic therapy also discussed.

Schaeffer AJ, Chmiel JS. Urethral meatal colonization in the pathogenesis of catheter-associated bacteriuria. J Urol 1983; 130:1096–1099.

Excellent discussion of role of bacterial meatal colonization in the causation of catheter-associated infection.

Parsons CL, Stauffer C, Schmidt J. Bladder-surface glycosaminoglycans: an efficient mechanism of environmental adaptation. Science 1980; 208:605.

A concise review of the anti-infective and protective properties of the bladder glycosaminoglycans. Their putative roles in the geneses of bladder disease are cogently discussed.

Sheinfeld J, Schaeffer AJ, Cordon-Cardo C, Pagatko A, Fair WR. Associa-tion of the Lewis blood-group phenotype with recurrent urinary-tract infections in women. N Engl J Med 1989; 320:773.

Elegant study suggesting that blood group antigens on the surface of urothelial cells influence bacterial adherence and susceptibility to urinary-tract infection. Absence of these antigens is a marker of increased bacterial colonization.

Hooton TM, Hillier S, Johnson C, Roberts PL, Stamm WE. *Escherichia coli* bacteriuria and contraceptive method. JAMA 1991; 265:64.

Emphasizes the concept that intercourse is associated with bacteriuria. The roles of spermicides and the diaphragm in the causation of urinary-tract infections in women are also discussed.

CHAPTER 11

Antimicrobials in Urology

Mary Lee
Roohollah Sharifi

Knowledge of the pharmacologic actions and pharmocokinetic properties of antimicrobial agents is fundamental to their optimal use. This chapter reviews a select group of antibiotics and antiseptics that are effective for the treatment of urinary-tract infections. The mechanism of action, antimicrobial spectrum, pharmocokinetics, and adverse reactions of individual drugs are summarized and the relative benefits and potential risks discussed. This chapter is not an exhaustive review, but rather a concise overview of the antibiotics commonly used in urologic practice.

PENICILLINS

Penicillins are bactericidal and bind to transpeptidase and carboxypeptidase receptors located between the cytoplasmic membrane and the outer bacterial cell wall. Once attached to penicillin binding protein sites 1 and 3, they inhibit synthesis of peptidoglycans, an integral component of bacterial cell walls. Penicillins also activate the autolytic system of bacteria. Both mechanisms result in loss of cell wall integrity, osmotic rupture, and death of actively replicating bacterial cells. There are four main types of penicillins: natural, penicillinase-resistant, aminopenicillins, and antipseudomonas (Table 11.1).

Natural Penicillins

The natural penicillin group includes penicillins G (benzylpenicillin) and V (phenoxymethyl penicillin)—the drugs of choice for infections caused by group A streptococci and *Strep. pneumoniae.* Because of its high level of renal excretion, penicillin G has been recommended as an effective broad-spectrum antibiotic for treatment of community acquired bacterial cystitis.

Table 11.1: The Penicillins

Types
Natural
Penicillinase-resistant
Aminopenicillins
Antipseudomonas
Adverse Reactions
Hypersensitivity
Anaphylaxis, skin rash
Gastrointestinal
Diarrhea (ampicillin)
Hematologic
Hemolytic anemia (penicillin G)
Platelet dysfunction (carbenicillin)
Electrolyte
Sodium overload (carbenicillin)
Hypokalemia (penicillin G, carbenicillin)
Neurologic
Seizures (penicillin G)
Renal
Interstitial nephritis (methicillin)

At doses of 500 mg orally every 6 hours, penicillin G achieves urine concentrations of 100 μg/ml, which are effective against 80% of *Escherichia coli* strains, and 100% of *Proteus mirabilis* and *Streptococcus fecalis.*

Penicillin V has better oral bioavailability than penicillin G. It is not destroyed by gastric acid and is well absorbed even in the presence of food. Penicillin G is acid labile and should be prescribed 1 hour before or 2 hours after meals. Both agents have short plasma half-lives (30 minutes) and are rapidly excreted by the kidneys as unchanged drug. Penicillins undergo glomerular filtration and tubular secretion. The latter is delayed by probenecid (Benemid), which may be added to oral or intramuscular penicillin therapy to increase serum drug levels. In general, penicillins achieve effective urinary concentrations even in the face of severe renal dysfunction, that is, creatinine clearances less than 10 ml/min.

Penicillinase-Resistant Penicillins

Methicillin, nafcillin, oxacillin, dicloxacillin, and cloxacillin are the drugs of choice for infections due to penicillinase-producing *Staphylococcus aureus.* These drugs are therapeutically equivalent and interchangeable.

If *Staph. aureus* is resistant to one of these agents, it is usually resistant to others in this group, and vancomycin therapy is indicated.

Differences in product formulation, kinetics, and adverse reaction profile dictate prescribing preferences. Oral bioavailability is best for cloxacillin and dicloxacillin, because of better absorption and resistance to gastric acid. With the exception of methicillin, these agents undergo extensive hepatic metabolism and subsequent renal elimination; therefore, dose modification is not necessary in renal failure. Methicillin is the drug in this group most often associated with the development of interstitial nephritis.

Aminopenicillins

Ampicillin and amoxicillin are as active as penicillin G against group A streptococcus and *Strep. pneumoniae* but more active against *Strep. fecalis.* They are the drugs of choice for urinary-tract infections due to *Strep. fecalis* (enterococcus) used singly (mild to moderate infections) or in combination with aminoglycoside (severe infections).

Only 30 to 60% of an oral dose of ampicillin is absorbed. The large amounts left unabsorbed in the colon can alter the normal bacterial gut flora. Diarrhea and development of ampicillin-resistant organisms are therefore common complications of therapy. Amoxicillin has better oral bioavailability with plasma concentrations twice that of ampicillin. Thus, the dosing interval for amoxicillin is longer than that for ampicillin: every 8 hours rather than every 6 hours. Diarrhea occurs less frequently with amoxicillin than with ampicillin. Both drugs are primarily excreted by the kidney, and the dosing interval should be increased when the creatinine clearance falls below 30 ml/min.

Antipseudomonas Penicillins

The drugs in this group are the extended spectrum penicillins—for example, carbenicillin and ticarcillin—and the ureidopenicillins—for example, piperacillin, azlocillin, and mezlocillin. They are effective against most uropathogens. However, nosocomial infections require high plasma concentrations of these antibiotics, and bacterial resistance and infection relapse are not uncommon. Based on their spectrum of activity, high percentage of renal excretion of unchanged drug, and minimal nephrotoxicity, these agents are useful alternatives to aminoglycosides for the treatment of multidrug resistant pathogens. When high plasma concentrations are needed for bactericidal effect, mezlocillin or piperacillin may be preferred because they are the most potent and can be administered in smaller daily doses. This decreases the risk of platelet dysfunction, sodium overload, and hypokalemia.

With the exception of the indanyl sodium salt of carbenicillin, extended-spectrum penicillins are not absorbed orally. Once absorbed, the salt is hydrolyzed to free carbenicillin, which is renally excreted. It does not provide effective plasma or tissue concentrations for extragenitourinary-tract infections. Although FDA-approved for the treatment of prostatitis, carbenicillin indanyl sodium does not achieve optimal concentrations in chronically inflamed prostates, and this explains its lack of clinical efficacy in the treatment of chronic bacterial prostatitis. Compared to carbenicillin and ticarcillin, the newer ureidopenicillins generally exhibit lower protein binding and a larger volume of distribution. All of these agents undergo hepatobiliary and renal excretion. Dosage adjustments are therefore required in patients with renal dysfunction and in patients with hepatic and renal failure. Penicillins share similar adverse reaction profiles, which are summarized in Table 11.1.

CEPHALOSPORINS

These bactericidal antibiotics are similar to penicillins, in that they inhibit synthesis of the peptidoglycan strands of bacterial cell walls. The first-generation cephalosporins are therapeutically equivalent to each other. When compared to ampicillin, first-generation cephalosporins have similar gram-positive and gram-negative antibacterial activity. They are ineffective against *Strep. fecalis* (enterococcus). They are particularly useful for surgical prophylaxis during the insertion of genitourinary prostheses.

Compared to first-generation cephalosporins, the second-generation agents are less active against gram-positive cocci, and selected agents are more active against gram-negative bacilli and *Bacteroides fragilis.* Second-generation cephalosporins are used in the treatment of urinary-tract infections due to multidrug-resistant pathogens that are shown to be sensitive to these agents, especially when other less expensive or more toxic agents cannot or should not be used. Cefoxitin and the longer-acting cefotetan are convenient and cost-saving agents, compared to traditional antibiotic combinations, for example, metronidazole and gentamicin used for prophylaxis of intra-abdominal or transrectal procedures.

The third-generation drugs have inferior gram-positive cocci and superior gram-negative bacilli coverage when compared to the other cephalosporins. Ceftazidime and cefoperazone are the most potent against *Pseudomonas aeruginosa*, with comparable activity to piperacillin. Moxalactam and ceftizoxime are the most active against *Bacteroides fragilis* and are comparable in potency to cefoxitin or cefotetan.

In elderly patients with nosocomial urinary-tract infections or those with pre-existing renal impairment, cephalosporins are a good alternative to aminoglycosides. Cephalosporins do not require plasma-concentration monitoring or dosage modification unless the creatinine clearance is less than 30 ml/min, and they do not exacerbate renal dysfunction. Cefoxitin, ceftizoxime, or cefotetan monotherapy is as efficacious as and less expensive than such drug combinations as an aminoglycoside plus metronidazole or clindamycin for the prophylaxis or treatment of mixed intra-abdominal or pelvic infections.

Pharmocokinetic differences influence cephalosporin choice. Cefazolin's half-life is twice as long as cephalothin's (1.5 hours versus 0.6 hours), and it can be administered parenterally at 8-hour intervals for serious infection, compared to 4-hour intervals for cephalothin. Newer second- and third-generation cephalosporins, for example, cefonicid and ceftriaxone, can be administered once or twice daily in most patients. All cephalosporins, except for cefoperazone and ceftriaxone, require some dosage adjustments when the creatinine clearance falls below 30 ml/min, because they are excreted unchanged by the kidneys. Cefoperazone and ceftriaxone may require dosage modification in patients with combined hepatic and renal failure.

Adverse reactions to cephalosporins are similar to those of the penicillins. However, a unique set of side effects is linked to agents possessing a methylthiotetrazole (MTT) side chain (Table 11.2). These agents exert a warfarin-like effect by noncompetitively inhibiting vitamin K dependent carboxylase. Carboxylation (activation) of coagulation factors 2, 7, 9, and 10 is halted, hence hypoprothrombinemia and bleeding may occur. Disulfiram reactions have also been described, probably because the MTT side chain may inhibit aldehyde dehydrogenase.

AZTREONAM: A MONOBACTAM ANTIBIOTIC

Aztreonam is a monobactam, or monocyclic beta lactam, that binds to penicillin binding protein 3 and inhibits bacterial cell wall synthesis. It is bactericidal. The aerobic gram-negative bacilli spectrum of activity of aztreonam rivals that of the third-generation cephalosporins, ureidopenicillins, and the aminoglycosides. Moreover, it is synergistic with aminoglycosides against *Pseudomonas* species. Aztreonam has no activity against

Table 11.2: Cephalosporins with Methylthiotetrazole (MMT) Side Chain

Cefamandole
Cefmetazole
Cefoperazone
Cefotetan
Moxalactam

aerobic gram-positive cocci or *Bacteroides fragilis.* Superinfections are most often due to *Strep. fecalis* or resistant gram-negative bacilli.

Aztreonam does not affect the anaerobic gut flora or undergo extensive hepatobiliary excretion. Therefore, pseudomembranous colitis and antibiotic-induced diarrhea are both uncommon. Aztreonam is a poor inducer of beta lactamase and is resistant to virtually all plasmid and chromosomally mediated beta lactamase enzymes. Emergence of resistance is rare. It has no cross allergy with the penicillins or cephalosporins.

Aztreonam is not absorbed after oral administration. Intramuscular and intravenous bioavailability are equivalent. Its half-life is 1.5 to 2.0 hours, with 88% of each dose excreted unchanged by the kidney. Dosage should be reduced in renal failure. Adverse reactions to aztreonam are similar to those of the penicillins.

IMIPENEM-CILASTATIN

Imipenem, a derivative of thienamycin, is a carbapenem that possesses a beta lactam ring that is chemically distinct from that of the penicillins. Imipenem is catabolized by the brush border renal tubular dipeptidase enzyme. Therefore, cilastatin, a reversible competitive inhibitor of dipeptidase, is added to the formulation. Cilastatin increases the amount of active imipenem in the urine to about 70% of the administered dose.

Imipenem binds to penicillin binding proteins 1 and 2, inhibits cell wall synthesis, and is bactericidal. It is active against most gram-negative aerobic bacilli, including *Pseudomonas aeruginosa*, and is comparable in activity to third-generation cephalosporins, aztreonam, and ureidopenicillin. It is as active against *Bacteroides fragilis* as metronidazole and clindamycin, and equivalent to penicillin G against *Strep. fecalis.* Imipenem is inactive against other *Strep.* species, methicillin-resistant *Staph. aureus* and *Staph. epidermidis.*

Imipenem induces beta lactamase enzyme production among gram-negative rods with the likelihood of drug resistance. A significant number of *Pseudomonas aeruginosa* strains become resistant during therapy. Currently, imipenem-cilastatin should be reserved for infections caused by susceptible pathogens, and for patients who would otherwise receive more toxic or expensive antibiotics. Imipenem-cilastatin should not be used for prophylaxis or as empiric treatment.

Imipenem is not absorbed orally. Its short half-life (1 hour) is attributed to rapid renal elimination, although approximately 25% of each dose undergoes nonrenal elimination. The usual dose of 0.25 to 1.0 g Q 6 to 8 hours requires reduction when the creatinine clearance falls below 70 ml/min.

A syndrome of nausea, vomiting, dizziness, and diaphoresis may follow rapid intravenous infusion of imipenem-cilastatin, and this can be ameliorated by slower infusion. Seizures may occur as a result of a lowering of the seizure threshold. Risk factors include previous head injury, a history of alcoholism, seizure disorder, brain tumor, and renal failure. The daily dose should be limited to 2 g in patients with renal impairment. The drug should not be used in patients with hypersensitivity reactions to penicillins, as it has induced skin rashes in such patients.

AMINOGLYCOSIDES

Aminoglycoside antibiotics include gentamicin, netilmicin, tobramycin, amikacin, kanamycin, neomycin, streptomycin, and spectinomycin. Streptomycin and spectinomycin are not discussed because their use is restricted to the treatment of tuberculosis and gonorrhea, respectively.

Aminoglycosides are bactericidal. They bind to the 30s and 50s bacterial ribosomes, interfere with messenger RNA codons, and block protein synthesis. Aminoglycosides are effective against all aerobic gram-negative bacilli, and *Staph. aureus*, including penicillinase-resistant strains. Aminoglycosides exert a bacteriostatic effect against *Strep. fecalis*, but are bactericidal when combined with ampicillin. *Bacteroides fragilis* is resistant to the aminoglycosides.

Resistance to aminoglycosides may be mediated chromosomally, or, more commonly, by plasmids. Plasmids produce aminoglycoside-modifying (inactivating) enzymes that block passage of the antibiotic across the bacterial cell membrane or inhibit antibiotic binding to ribosomes. Amikacin is least susceptible to this enzymatic inactivation, gentamicin most susceptible, and netilmicin and tobramycin exhibit intermediate susceptibility. In general, bacteria resistant to gentamicin are usually cross-resistant to netilmicin and tobramycin, but sensitive to amikacin. Amikacin should be reserved for treatment of infections that cannot be treated with other aminoglycosides.

Aminoglycosides share similar pharmacokinetic properties (Table 11.3). They are not absorbed orally, have a plasma half-life of about 2 hours, and are excreted unchanged by the kidney. In the absence of hypotension, intramuscular injections have excellent bioavailability, comparable to that achieved by intravenous administration. Peak plasma concentrations occur within 30 to 60 minutes of intramuscular injections.

The usual dosage of gentamicin, netilmicin, and tobramycin is 1.5 to 2.0 mg/kg as a loading dose, followed by maintenance doses that vary according to creatinine clearances. Dosing should result in therapeutic peak plasma concentrations of 4 to 10 μg/ml, and trough concentrations less than 2 μg/ml. For amikacin, the usual dose is 7.5 mg/kg as a loading dose, followed by maintenance doses adjusted for the patient's level of renal function. Therapeutic peak and safe trough plasma amikacin concentrations are 20 to 35 μg/ml and 5 to 10 μg/ml, respectively (Table 11.3).

Various normograms and kinetic formulas are used to estimate proper aminoglycoside dosage for patients with renal impairment. We prefer the Hull and Sarubbi nomogram because of its ease of use. These methods provide dosing estimates, and because of interpatient variation in drug handling, plasma drug concentration monitoring is essential. Peak plasma aminoglycoside concentrations should be estimated 30 minutes after complete intravenous infusion or 60 minutes after an intramuscular dose. Specimens for trough plasma concentrations should be obtained just prior to the next dose. Plasma monitoring is required in patients after 7 to 10 days of continuous aminoglycoside treatment and in patients at increased risk of nephrotoxicity. The latter includes patients with underlying renal impairment or changing renal function, patients who are on dialysis, the elderly, and those who are hypotensive or volume contracted. In these patients, plasma aminoglycoside levels should be obtained within the first 48 to 72 hours of the start of treatment, or within 4 to 5 plasma half-lives after the maintenance dose of aminoglycoside has been started.

Table 11.3: Pharmacokinetic Properties of Selected Aminoglycosides

	Amikacin	*Gentamicin*	*Netilmicin*	*Tobramycin*
% oral bioavailability	0	0	0	0
Half-life (hours)	2.0–3.0	2	2.0–3.0	2.0–3.0
% protein bound	0–3	0	0	0
Therapeutic peak plasma concentration (μg/ml)	20–35	4–10	4–10	4–10
Safe trough plasma concentration (μg/ml)	5–10	2	2–4	2
% urine recovery of unchanged drug after 24 hours	99%	99%	99%	99%
Removed by hemodialysis	Yes	Yes	Yes	Yes
Removed by peritoneal dialysis	Yes	Yes	Yes	Yes

Adverse Reactions

Nephrotoxicity and ototoxicity are the most important adverse reactions associated with aminoglycoside use. The incidence of aminoglycoside-induced nephrotoxicity, defined as an increase in serum creatinine concentrations of at least 0.5 mg/dl, ranges from 8 to 26%. Following glomerular filtration, aminoglycosides enter the renal proximal tubular cells, where they block ATP production and cause the failure of the sodium-potassium ATPase pump. Failure to maintain normal intracellular concentrations of sodium and potassium ions then causes proximal tubular cell death. Aminoglycosides may also sequester in lysosomes, release hydrolytic enzymes, and produce cell injury. Clinically, mild, nonoliguric acute renal failure may develop after 5 to 7 consecutive days of treatment. Signs include a loss of renal concentrating ability, proteinuria, presence of casts in urine, and renal enzymuria. Progressive increases in serum creatinine and trough plasma aminoglycoside concentrations are late markers of aminoglycoside injury and indicate significant tubular injury. Discontinuation of the aminoglycoside is usually followed by complete recovery of renal function, although this may take up to 2 months.

The following are recommended to prevent nephrotoxicity in patients who require aminoglycoside antibiotics for more than 5 to 7 days: every other day monitoring of serum creatinine concentrations and blood urea nitrogen (BUN); screening urine for the presence of casts and protein and serial trough plasma drug concentrations. There are many risk factors for aminoglycoside-induced nephrotoxicity (Table 11.4). Patients with these risk factors should be monitored closely. The degree of proximal tubule injury is directly related to the cumulative dosage. Thus, prolonged treat-

Table 11.4: Aminoglycoside Nephrotoxicity: Risk Factors

Prolonged therapy, greater than 5–7 days
Type of aminoglycoside: amikacin and gentamicin accumulate in renal cortex to a greater extent than tobramycin or netilmicin
Dehydration
Concomitant furosemide or other nephrotoxic drugs, e.g., cephalothin, vancomycin, etc.
Pre-existing renal impairment or hepatic disease
Hypotension
Elderly patients
Trough serum levels
>10 μg/ml for amikacin
>2 μg/ml for other aminoglycosides
Previous or recent aminoglycoside therapy

ment with large daily doses for more than a week is likely to result in significant intracellular accumulation of aminoglycosides.

Aminoglycosides can produce vestibular or cochlear ototoxicity. Vestibular toxicity typically manifests as vertigo, ataxia, or nystagmus; cochlear toxicity is associated with tinnitus, deafness, or unilateral or bilateral high-frequency hearing loss (detectable by audiogram). Ototoxicity is irreversible in one-third of patients, and it may progress or develop weeks after the offending drug is stopped. Aminoglycosides can damage the eighth cranial nerve by interference with the ionic transport systems necessary for maintenance of the normal chemical composition of labrinthine fluid, or by irreversible damage to hair cells within the organ of Corti or the crista ampullaris. Streptomycin and kanamycin are the most ototoxic aminoglycosides. Gentamicin, tobramycin, and amikacin have intermediate toxicity, and netilmicin has the least. The type of ototoxicity varies (Table 11.5). Factors associated with increased ototoxicity include the specific aminoglycoside, age greater than 40 years, duration of treatment more than 10 days, pre-existing renal impairment, concomitant or previous exposure to aminoglycosides or other ototoxins (e.g., furosemide, ethacrynic acid, or bumetamide), and peak plasma concentrations over 10 to 12 μg/ml for gentamicin, tobramycin, and netilmicin or over 35 to 40 μg/ml for amikacin.

TETRACYCLINES

Tetracyclines are classified on the basis of their durations of action. The short-acting agents, tetracycline and oxytetracycline, have low protein binding, are excreted unchanged by the kidneys, and are of low to intermediate lipophilicity. Their plasma half-lives are short, and they are not extensively deposited in soft tissues. The long-acting agents, doxycycline and minocycline, exhibit considerable protein binding, are slowly excreted

Table 11.5: Type of Ototoxicity Caused by Aminoglycosides

	Vestibular	*Cochlear*
Amikacin	+	++
Gentamicin	++	+
Kanamycin	+	++
Netilmicin	+	++
Neomycin	+	++
Streptomycin	++	+
Tobramycin	+	+

by active secretion into the bowel lumen, and are highly lipophilic. These agents have long plasma half-lives and achieve excellent tissue concentrations. The tetracyclines are bacteriostatic. They bind to the 30s ribosomal subunit, prevent effective interaction between the messenger-RNA-ribosome complex and transfer RNA, and inhibit protein synthesis. Tetracyclines cross human cell membranes and are effective against intracellular organisms such as chlamydia trachomatis.

The tetracyclines have similar antibacterial activity as penicillin G and are useful against staphylococci, streptococci, and community-acquired gram-negative uropathogens. Tetracyclines are also effective against chlamydia species, *Mycoplasma hominis* and pneumoniae, *Hemophilus ducreyi*, *Neisseria gonorrhoeae*, and ureaplasma. However, tetracyclines are ineffective against *Strep. fecalis* (enterococcus). Bacteria that are resistant to one tetracycline are generally cross-resistant to the others.

Tetracycline is a useful alternative for the management of community-acquired cystitis in the penicillin-allergic patient. Because of superior lipophilicity, doxycycline is preferred for tissue infections such as epididymitis or prostatitis. Tetracycline and doxycycline are the drugs of choice for chlamydia and ureaplasma genitourinary-tract infections. Minocycline has a similar pharmacodynamic profile to doxycycline, but its vestibular toxicity limits its usefulness.

The renal excretion of tetracyclines is variable, although doxycycline and minocycline are least excreted by this route. Doxycycline is secreted into the bowel lumen and excreted as inactive conjugates; minocycline undergoes extensive enterohepatic recirculation. Doxycycline and minocycline can be administered without dosage modification in patients with renal failure. Tetracyclines share many adverse reactions, although some side effects are more frequent with particular agents (Table 11.6).

SULFONAMIDES, INCLUDING SULFAMETHOXAZOLE-TRIMETHOPRIM

Although long-acting sulfonamides cause crystalluria and renal tubular obstruction in patients with renal insufficiency, the currently prescribed short-acting sulfonamides are more water soluble and more rapidly excreted by the kidneys. Sulfonamides are bacteriostatic, and they competitively inhibit the conversion of para-aminobenzoic acid (PABA) to dihydrofolic acid. Trimethoprim, which is not a sulfonamide, blocks conversion of dihydrofolic acid to tetrahydrofolic acid. It is bacteriostatic at low doses and bactericidal at high doses. When used together, sulfamethoxazole-trimethoprim causes a sequential inhibition of bacterial folic acid production, thereby blocking DNA synthesis (Figure 11.1).

Table 11.6: Common Adverse Reactions to Tetracyclines

Tetracycline
Diarrhea, esophageal ulcers
Azotemia (in patients with renal impairment)
Fatty liver (during pregnancy)
Teeth discoloration (children ≤ 8 years of age, fetus)
Pseudotumor cerebri (infants)
Minocycline
Nausea, vomiting
Blue-gray skin and mucous membrane pigmentation
Hemolytic anemia
Vestibular toxicity
Doxycycline
Photosensitivity

Sulfonamides are effective as single-agent therapy for community-acquired *Escherichia coli*, *Klebsiella species*, *Enterobacter species*, *Proteus mirabilis*, indole-positive *Proteus sp.*, and *Staphylococcus aureus* infections. However, variable minimum inhibitory concentrations (MICs) have been noted, probably due to increasing bacterial resistance in patients treated for recurrent or chronic urinary-tract infections. As a single agent, trimethoprim has similar antibacterial activity to the sulfonamides. An expanded spectrum results from the sulfamethoxazole-trimethoprim combination. The only organisms with variable sensitivity or resistance include *Serratia marcescens*, *Streptococcus fecalis*, *Bacteroides fragilis*, *Pseudomonas aeruginosa* and ureaplasma.

Sulfonamides or trimethoprim are first-line agents for the treatment

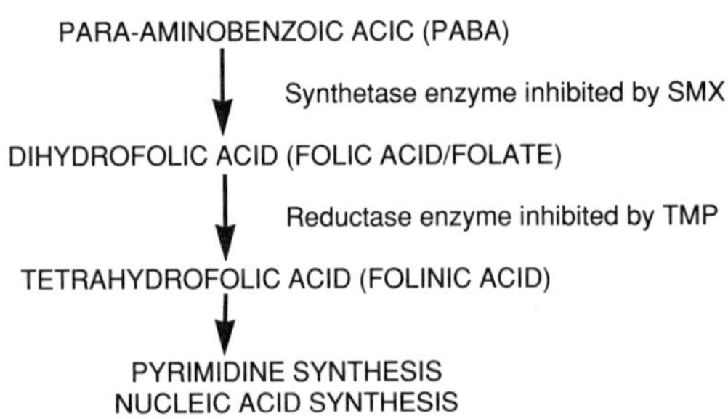

Figure 11.1: Sulfamethoxazole (SMX)/Trimethoprim (TMP) Actions

of community acquired urinary-tract infections. With the exception of *Strep. fecalis*, these agents have better antibacterial activity than ampicillin. Trimethoprim is a safe alternative in patients with sulfonamide allergy. Sulfamethoxazole-trimethoprim is a mainstay in the treatment of recurrent or chronic urinary-tract infections. The combination is widely employed for long-term, low-dose antimicrobial prophylaxis against recurrent infections. Bacterial resistance is less likely to develop than with a sulfonamide or trimethoprim alone.

The pharmacokinetic properties of the sulfonamides and trimethoprim are summarized in Table 11.7. Sulfamethoxazole and trimethoprim are rapidly absorbed after oral administration and undergo extensive tissue distribution. Trimethoprim's greater lipophilicity and lower protein binding facilitate its penetration into prostatic, vaginal, colonic, and other soft tissues. Protein displacement interactions with other highly protein-bound drugs, for example, methotrexate, warfarin and hypoglycemic agents, are a significant problem with sulfamethoxazole and can cause increased therapeutic/toxic activity of these agents. Sulfamethoxazole undergoes extensive hepatic conjugation and conversion to inactive metabolites. Trimethoprim undergoes little hepatic metabolism and is largely excreted unchanged by the kidneys. In patients with creatinine clearances less than 30 ml/min, the dosage of these agents should be modified to minimize the risk of sulfonamide crystallization in the renal tubules.

Adverse gastrointestinal effects and hypersensitivity reactions are the most common untoward reactions of sulfonamides and trimethoprim (Table 11.8).

Table 11.7: Pharmacokinetic Properties of Sulfamethoxazole and Trimethoprim

	Sulfamethoxazole	*Trimethoprim*
Oral bioavailability	Good	Good
Serum half-life (hours)		
Normal renal function	10–12	8–11
Renal failure (creatinine clearance <10 ml/min)	20–50	26
% protein bound	70	44
% excreted unchanged by kidneys	20–30	50–80
% hepatically metabolized	70	<20
Distribution into/across		
Prostatic tissue	Poor	Good
Placenta	Yes	Yes
Breast milk	Yes	Yes

Table 11.8: Adverse Sulfonamide, Trimethoprim Reactions

Gastrointestinal
Nausea
Vomiting
Diarrhea
Hypersensitivity
Skin Rash
Eosinophilia
Drug fever
Dermatologic
Skin rash
Stevens-Johnson syndrome
Toxic epidermal necrolysis
Photosensitivity reactions
Renal
Increased creatinine, BUN
Crystalluria
Interstitial nephritis
Tubular obstruction
Hematologic
Hemolytic anemia (G-6-PD deficiency)
Thrombocytopenia
Megaloblastic anemia
Agranulocytosis
Hepatic
Elevated liver enzymes
Chloestatic jaundice
Hepatic necrosis

METRONIDAZOLE

The nitro group of metronidazole is reduced to produce toxic, unstable, intermediate metabolites that bind to and inhibit DNA synthesis in susceptible bacteria. Metronidazole is bactericidal against all *Bacteroides* and *Clostridia species*, *Trichomonas vaginalis*, *Entamoeba histolytica*, and *Giardia lamblia*. It is ineffective against facultative anaerobes and aerobic gram-positive or gram-negative uropathogens. Metronidazole is the drug of choice for the treatment of serious infections due to *Bacteroides fragilis*, for example, strains resistant to clindamycin penicillin, or cefoxitin. It is also the drug of choice for trichomoniasis and amebiasis, and an alternative to vancomycin for the treatment of pseudomembranous colitis.

Metronidazole is almost completely absorbed following oral administration, and it has a serum half-life of 6 to 10 hours. Its low molecular weight and low degree of protein binding allow it to cross most semipermeable membranes. Tissue concentrations approach plasma levels in cerebrospinal fluid, bile, seminal fluid, vaginal secretions, and other body fluids. More than 80% of each dose undergoes hepatic metabolism to form five major products, two of which have antibacterial activity. Fifteen percent of each dose is excreted unchanged by the kidneys, and no dosage modification is required in renal failure. However, supplemental doses are recommended in patients undergoing hemodialysis or peritoneal dialysis. Doses should be empirically reduced in patients with hepatic failure. Metronidazole enhances the hypoprothrombinemic effect of warfarin by slowing catabolism of the S(-) isomer of the anticoagulant. Phenobarbital and phenytoin enhance hepatic catabolism and reduce the antibacterial effect of metronidazole. The adverse effects of metronidazole are summarized in Table 11.9.

VANCOMYCIN

Vancomycin interrupts synthesis of bacterial cell wall phospholipids and peptidoglycan strands, damages cytoplasmic membranes, and inhibits RNA synthesis. These multiple actions account for its bactericidal effect and for the low level of primary or acquired bacterial resistance.

Vancomycin's antibacterial spectrum is limited to *Staph.* species, including methicillin-resistant strains, and *Strep.* species, including *Strep.*

Table 11.9: Adverse Reactions to Metronidazole

Gastrointestinal
Furry tongue, metallic taste, nausea, anorexia, diarrhea
Neurologic
Sensory polyneuropathy (usually reversible)
Disulfiram reaction
Avoid alcohol for 24–48 hours after last metronidazole dose
Renal
Dysuria
Red-brown urine discoloration (harmless)
Hypersensitivity
Skin rash, urticaria

fecalis. Vancomycin is ineffective against *Bacteroides fragilis* and aerobic gram-negative bacilli that commonly cause urinary-tract infections. It is the drug of choice for serious staphylococcal or streptococcal infections in patients with penicillin or cephalosporin hypersensitivity and for patients with methicillin-resistant *Staph. epidermidis* or aureus infections. For these infections, vancomycin is often combined with aminoglycosides because of their synergistic activity. The combination is used for the preoperative prophylaxis of dental, upper respiratory tract, gastrointestinal, and genitourinary-tract procedures in penicillin-allergic patients.

Vancomycin is the oral drug of choice for *C. difficile*-associated pseudomembranous colitis. Oral vancomycin is poorly absorbed and is used for its local disinfecting effect on the bowel. Vancomycin pharmacokinetics exhibit wide interpatient variation, such that terminal serum half-lives range from 3 to 13 hours in patients with normal renal function, volume of distribution ranges from 0.5 to 1.0 L/kg, and protein-bound fraction ranges from 10 to 60%. Greater than 95% of each dose is renally excreted as unchanged drug. In patients with renal impairment, vancomycin half-life is significantly prolonged, for example, 7 to 8 days in patients who are functionally anephric. The drug is not significantly eliminated by hemodialysis or peritoneal dialysis.

The Matzke nomogram facilitates vancomycin dosing in patients with renal impairment and allows initial treatment until plasma drug level monitoring can be used to fine-tune therapy. This nomogram is valid for all levels of renal dysfunction, although it should not be used for patients undergoing hemodialysis or peritoneal dialysis. In such patients, serum concentrations should guide dose modifications. In serious infections, peak concentrations should be 20 to 40 μg/ml, with trough levels of 5 to 10 μg/ml. Peak plasma levels should be measured 1 to 2 hours following vancomycin infusion.

Adverse reactions are less frequent than previously reported because of the availability of more purified formulations of vancomycin. Nephrotoxicity and ototoxicity (cochlear and vestibular) can be avoided by plasma monitoring of trough and peak vancomycin levels, respectively. Phlebitis, the red man (neck) syndrome, and reversible neutropenia also occur.

QUINOLONES

The first-generation quinolones are nalidixic acid and cinoxacin. Norfloxacin, ciprofloxacin, ofloxacin, and lomefloxacin are second-generation agents. In 1992, temafloxacin, another second-generation quinolone, was withdrawn from the U.S. market because of adverse reactions, including severe hypoglycemia, hemolytic anemia, renal and hepatic impairment, and anaphylactic reactions. Therefore, it is not discussed. Unlike their predecessors, second-generation fluoroquinolones achieve bactericidal concentrations in urine and plasma and are effective for both urinary-tract and extragenitourinary-tract infections. The second-generation agents have an expanded antibacterial spectrum that includes *Pseudomonas aeruginosa*, *Neisseria gonorrhea* and *Strep. fecalis* (Table 11.10). DNA replication and protein synthesis are blocked by the quinolones via interference with the bacterial enzyme, DNA gyrase.

Major differences exist between first-generation quinolone agents and the fluoroquinolones. Nalidixic acid and cinoxacin are effective against community-acquired gram-negative uropathogens but are ineffective against gram-positive cocci (including *Strep.* and *Staph.* species), *Pseudomonas aeruginosa*, *Serratia Marcescens*, indole-positive *Proteus* species, and *Bacteroides fragilis*. The fluoroquinolones, particularly ciprofloxacin, exhibit an expanded spectrum against gram-negative bacilli, gram-positive cocci, and *Neisseria gonorrhea*. At usual doses, these agents are used to treat nosocomial urinary-tract infections due to multidrug-resistant, gram-negative organisms, *Strep. fecalis*, or *Staph. aureus*. Organisms that are resistant to norfloxacin or ofloxacin are usually cross-resistant to ciprofloxacin, and vice-versa. However, nalidixic acid resistant strains generally remain susceptible to the fluoroquinolones.

Table 11.10: Fluoroquinolone Bacterial Susceptibility

Highly susceptible
Enterobacteriaceae
Neisseria gonorrheae
Hemophilus ducreyi
Moderately susceptible
Pseudomonas aeruginosa
Acinebacter species
Staphylococci
Chlamydial species (Ofloxacin only)
Mycoplasmas
Enterococcus
Minimally susceptible
Anaerobes
Some pseudomonas species, e.g., maltophilia
Gardnerella vaginalis
Candida species
Ureaplasmas

Nalidixic acid and cinoxacin are second-line agents for treatment of community-acquired urinary-tract infections because of the high rate of bacterial resistance and the potential for adverse neurologic side effects. The fluoroquinolones are less expensive, oral alternatives to parenteral antibiotics for the treatment of urinary-tract infections due to susceptible organisms. *Pseudomonas aeruginosa* infections, which usually require hospitalization for intravenous aminoglycoside treatment, can now be treated orally with the fluoroquinolones. These agents are also indicated for the treatment of complicated or recurrent urinary-tract infections. Due to the aforementioned factors responsible for the low rate of resistance among aerobic gram-negative bacteria, fluoroquinolones will probably be useful for chronic prophylaxis against recurrent urinary-tract infections. The enhanced soft-tissue penetration of ciprofloxacin, lomefloxacin, and ofloxacin are particularly useful for the treatment of bacterial prostatitis and pyelonephritis.

The fluoroquinolones have significant advantages over nalidixic acid (Table 11.11). A higher percentage of each dose is excreted renally; the serum half-lives are longer, allowing once or twice a day dosing; and they exhibit lower protein binding and greater soft-tissue penetration than nalidixic acid and cinoxacin. In patients with renal impairment, second-generation fluoroquinolones will be delivered into urine in adequate concentrations; however, their daily dosage should be reduced to prevent drug accumulation. For nalidixic acid, the accumulation of potentially neurotoxic hepatic metabolites poses a significant risk. Hence, nalidixic acid is contraindicated in patients with creatinine clearances less than 30 ml/min.

Gastrointestinal upset, vomiting, and diarrhea are common side effects of the quinolones. Nausea may be ameliorated by advising the patient to take antibacterial doses with food, which delays but does not decrease drug absorption. Central nervous system reactions include headache, visual color disturbances, insomnia, restlessness, seizures, toxic psychosis, and increased intracranial pressure. The hepatic metabolite(s) of nalidixic acid may be responsible for the CNS effects since the drug undergoes extensive first-pass hepatic catabolism. However, the gamma-aminobutyric acid inhibitory effect of quinolones may be causative. Because of the severity of these neurologic reactions, nalidixic acid should not be used in patients with creatinine clearances less than 30 ml/min. Likewise, other quinolones should be used cautiously in patients with seizure disorders. Hemolytic anemia has been reported with nalidixic acid in patients with glucose-6-phosphate dehydrogenase (G-6-PD) deficiency. To decrease the risk of renal tubular obstruction from fluroquinolones, each dose should be taken with a full glass of water, and the daily dosage should be reduced when the creatinine falls below clearance 30 ml/min.

Table 11.11: Fluoroquinolone Pharmacokinetics

	Nalidixic Acid	*Cinoxacin*	*Norfloxacin*	*Ciprofloxacin*	*Ofloxacin*	*Lomefloxacin*
Half-life (hr)	1–2.5	1–1.5	4	4	5	7–8
Absorption (%)	96	100	40	75	100	95–100
Metabolism (%)	95	30–40	20–30	15–20	4	30–40
Urinary recovery (%)	2–3	60–65	30–40	40–50	70–80	60–70
Dose reduction in renal failure	Avoid	Yes	Yes	Yes	Yes	Yes

Arthropathy and cartilaginous lesions have been documented in beagle puppies, and the quinolones are therefore considered unsafe for use in pregnant women or in children with incomplete skeletal growth.

Antacids, iron salts, and sucralfate inhibit quinolone absorption; therefore, these antibiotics should be taken 2 hours before or after antacid doses. These antibacterial agents inhibit the P-450 hepatic microsomal enzyme system, thereby slowing catabolism of theophylline and caffeine. Sequential monitoring of serum theophylline levels is recommended when initiating fluoroquinolone therapy in patients taking theophylline. Likewise, quinolones may enhance the hypoprothrombinemic effect of warfarin. Probenecid decreases renal tubular secretion of fluoroquinolones. As a result, serum concentrations of these agents will increase while urinary concentrations decrease. The clinical importance of this interaction remains to be defined.

NITROFURANTOIN

Like nalidixic acid and cinoxacin, nitrofurantoin is a urinary-tract antiseptic, and it achieves bactericidal concentrations only in urine. Although its precise mechanism of action is unknown, nitrofurantoin may inhibit bacterial acetyl coenzyme A and interfere with carbohydrate metabolism. It may also disrupt cell wall synthesis.

Nitrofurantoin's antibacterial spectrum includes all *Staph.* and *Strep.* species, (including *Strep. fecalis*) and the community-acquired gram-negative uropathogens. *Pseudomonas aeruginosa*, *Klebsiella*, *Enterobacter*, *Serratia*, and indole positive *Proteus* species are usually resistant. Bacteria rarely develop resistance to nitrofurantoin, probably because the drug does not achieve significant concentrations in intestinal or vaginal fluids or tissues, does not alter normal gut flora, and does not select resistant flora. Nitrofurantoin is useful for community-acquired cystitis, particularly in pregnant patients during the first and second trimesters because it does not appear to be a teratogen. It is also used for long-term prophylaxis in patients with recurrent urinary-tract infections.

Nitrofurantoin is well absorbed orally and undergoes extensive first-pass hepatic catabolism. Its antibacterial effect is therefore due to the small percentage of unchanged drug that reaches the urine. Sixty percent of nitrofurantoin is protein bound. The serum half-life in patients with normal renal function is 20 minutes; this may be prolonged to 60 minutes in anephric patients. Since insufficient drug is delivered into urine once the creatinine clearance is less than 30 ml/min and toxic hepatic metabolites accumulate, nitrofurantoin is not recommended for use in patients with compromised renal function.

Oral nitrofurantoin is formulated in two forms: microcrystalline and macrocrystalline. The latter is less water soluble, more slowly absorbed, and produces less nausea than the microcrystalline form. The macrocrystalline form is preferred for patients who experience gastrointestinal intolerance to other oral formulations of nitrofurantoin. Although an intravenous formulation is available, nitrofurantoin's short plasma half-life produces only transient bactericidal plasma concentrations. The adverse reactions of nitrofurantoin are listed in Table 11.12.

METHENAMINE AND ITS SALTS

Methenamine, a urinary-tract antiseptic, is inactive until converted to formaldehyde. This conversion takes 2 to 3 hours at optimal urine pH levels, that is, less than 5.5. Several methods have been employed to promote this reaction, for example, use of acid salts of methenamine, such as methenamine mandelate or methenamine hippurate, and the concomitant administration of urinary acidifiers or cranberry juice. These adjuvants are of dubious value and have not been shown to be more effective than methenamine base alone.

Formaldehyde is bactericidal for the gram-positive cocci and gram-negative bacilli that cause urinary-tract infections. However, in the presence of urease-producing bacteria (e.g., *Proteus species*, *Klebsiella*, *Serratia*, *Pseudomonas*), the alkaline pH of urine may inhibit conversion of

Table 11.12: Adverse Reactions to Nitrofurantoin

Reaction	*Special Notes*
Gastrointestinal	Take drug with meals
Anorexia	Use macrocrystalline formulation
Nausea, vomiting	
Diarrhea	
Pulmonary	
Acute pneumonitis	? hypersensitivity reaction
Pulmonary fibrosis	? toxic reaction; occurs 1–6 months after start of therapy
Hepatotoxic	Association with treatment > 1 year duration
Chronic active hepatitis	
Hemotologic	Occurs in patients with G-6-PD deficiency
Hemolytic anemia	
Neurologic	
Peripheral neuropathy	In elderly patients receiving prolonged therapy; in patients with renal failure

methenamine to formaldehyde. Methenamine should not be used in patients with chronic indwelling catheters, as urine is not retained long enough in the bladder to allow conversion to formaldehyde.

Methenamine is indicated for treatment of mild chronic urinary-tract infections and prevention of recurrent infections. It should not be used for acute infections since steady-state formaldehyde concentrations are achieved slowly, that is, 2 to 3 days after the start of treatment. Methenamine is rapidly absorbed after oral administration and is enteric-coated to prevent conversion to formaldehyde in the stomach. The plasma half-life is 3 to 6 hours. Because of its low molecular weight, methenamine distributes readily throughout body fluids. In the genitourinary tract, conversion to formaldehyde only occurs in the bladder, since urine transit time through the renal tubules and collecting system is rapid. Bactericidal effects in the bladder are maintained for up to 6 hours or until the bladder is emptied.

Methenamine is probably delivered into urine in adequate concentrations in patients with renal impairment; however, it is not recommended in patients with creatinine clearances less than 30 ml/min because it may present an additional metabolic acid load.

Methenamine produces few adverse reactions. Large doses cause nausea, vomiting, and bladder irritation. Dysuria, frequency, and hematuria have been reported after prolonged high-dose treatment (up to 8 grams per day). Methenamine mandelate oral suspension, which is formulated in a vegetable oil base, has caused lipoid pneumonia when aspirated. To avoid this, methenamine water-soluble granules have been used when tablets cannot be swallowed. Methenamine and its salts should be avoided in patients with gout or uric acid stones since it may precipitate uric acid lithiasis. Methenamine is contraindicated in patients with hepatic failure because it may worsen hyperammonemia.

TISSUE VERSUS URINE LEVELS OF ANTIBIOTICS

Antimicrobial agents used for the treatment of urinary-tract infections are divided into two groups: antiseptics and systemic antibiotics. This classification has perpetuated several beliefs. Antiseptics are indicated for treatment of lower urinary-tract infections since they produce therapeutic urine drug levels. They are ineffective for upper urinary-tract infections because of subtherapeutic serum concentrations. In contrast, systemic antibiotics produce effective serum concentrations, are excreted predominantly by the kidney, and achieve urine concentrations many times greater than that in serum. Thus, systemic antibiotics are indicated for both upper and lower urinary-tract infections.

Systemic antibiotics produce better soft-tissue levels than antiseptics because the serum antibiotic diffuses readily across semipermeable membranes and into tissues. Theoretically, it follows that soft-tissue infections (e.g., pyelonephritis) should respond better to systemic antibiotics than antiseptics.

These generalizations have, however, produced some controversy. Some investigators have successfully used antiseptics (nitrofurantoin in particular) to treat upper urinary-tract infections and believe that therapeutic urine concentrations alone are adequate. Also, data collected from human cadavers and canine models suggest that some systemic antibiotics, including aminoglycosides, fail to achieve therapeutic tissue levels in the face of diseased kidneys. This suggests that therapeutic antibiotic tissue levels may not be necessary to eradicate upper-tract infection.

Nonetheless, it is generally agreed that antibiotics that produce high urine concentrations that exceed the minimum inhibitory concentrations of the infecting organisms are effective for lower, and possibly upper, urinary-tract infections. Systemic antibiotics that produce therapeutic serum levels are preferred for upper urinary-tract or soft-tissue (e.g., prostate, kidney) infections.

ANTIBIOTIC EFFECT ON HOST BACTERIAL FLORA

Bacterial flora in the vaginal vault and rectum are believed to cause recurrent urinary-tract infections. When exposed to antibiotics, susceptible resident flora are replaced by drug-resistant bacteria, which cause recurrent, drug-resistant infections. This phenomenon has been commonly reported after treatment with tetracycline, ampicillin, amoxicillin, cephalexin, and sulfonamides.

To avoid repeated episodes of cystitis, several strategies have been employed: the use of antibiotics that eradicate all (or nearly all) *Enterobacteriaceae* in the rectum and vagina (e.g., trimethoprim-sulfamethoxazole); the use of antibiotics that are not delivered into the vaginal vault or rectum (e.g., antiseptics), and the use of antibiotics that maintain constant therapeutic urine levels to eradicate bacteria introduced into the urinary tract (e.g., chronic, low-dose prophylactic antibiotic therapy).

Thus, it is generally believed that trimethoprim-sulfamethoxazole is an excellent agent for treatment and prophylaxis of recurrent urinary-tract infections. It is ion-trapped in vaginal secretions and delivered to the bowel, thereby eradicating potential pathogens from the reservoirs for urinary-tract infections. Urinary-tract antiseptics are excellent agents for prophylaxis of recurrent urinary-tract infections since they do not induce antibiotic resistance among introital and rectal flora. The quinolones are intermediate in their effect in that they are know to affect rectal flora but not vaginal flora. Their safety regarding development of bacterial resistance after long-term use remains to be evaluated.

SUGGESTED READINGS

Stamey TA, Govan DE, Palmer JM. The localization and treatment of urinary-tract infections: the role of bactericidal urine levels as opposed to serum levels. Medicine 1965; 44:1.

Key article that explains the clinical efficacy of antibiotics for genitourinary-tract infections based on serum and urine concentrations of antibiotics.

Bennett WM. Guide to drug dosage in renal failure. Clin. Pharmacokinet. 1988; 15:326.

Excellent, practical guide for making dose and interval dosing adjustments of antibiotics and other drugs in patients with renal impairment.

Meares EM Jr. Acute and chronic prostatitis: diagnosis and treatment. Infect Dis Clin North Am 1987; 1:855.

Excellent overview of pharmacokinetic and pharmacodynamic properties of antibiotics that affect drug penetration into prostate tissue.

Sarubbi FA, Hull JH. Amikacin serum concentrations: predictions of levels and dosage guidelines. Ann Intern Med 1978; 89 (part1): 612.

Useful dosing nomogram for gentamicin, tobramycin, and amikacin. Applicable for estimating initial dosage regimens for patients with renal impairment.

Matzke GR, McGrory RW, Halstenson CE, Keane WF. Pharmacokinetics of vancomycin in patients with various degrees of renal function. Antimicrob Agents Chemother 1984; 25:433.

Useful dosing nomogram for initial maintenance dose estimates in patients with renal impairment.

Farber BF, Moellering RC. Retrospective study of toxicity of preparations of vancomycin from 1974–1981. Antimicrob Agents Chemother 1983; 23: 138.

Review of vancomycin nephrotoxicity with a discussion of the synergistic nephrotoxicity of vancomycin and aminoglycosides.

Hooper DC, Wolfson JS. Fluoroquinolone antimicrobial agents. N Engl J Med 1991; 324: 384.

Excellent overview of the fluoroquinolones with insightful recommendations for their clinical use.

Stamey TA. Recurrent urinary-tract infections in female patients: an overview of management and treatment. Rev Infect Dis 1987; 9:195S.

Excellent analysis of pharmacologic and pharmacodynamic aspects of antibiotics used for prophylaxis of recurrent cystitis in women.

Wright AJ, Wilkowske CJ. The penicillins. Mayo Clin Pro 1991; 66: 1047.

Up-to-date overview of all the penicillins with emphasis on clinical indications, pharmacology, kinetics, adverse effects, and drug interactions.

Gurtaferro CA, Steckelberg JM. Cephalosporin antimicrobial agents and related compounds. Mayo Clin Proc 1991; 66:1064.

Review of the cephalosporins with excellent critical section on indications and cost comparisons with other antimicrobials.

CHAPTER 12

Calculi

Howard M. Price
Mani Menon

Despite advances in therapy, urolithiasis remains a common and significant cause of morbidity. In the United States, the constant annual incidence is 70 to 200 per 100,000, with regional variations. Epidemiological studies suggest that a white American male has a 1 in 8 chance of developing a renal stone by age 70. The morbidity of ureteral colic is considerable, and up to 20% of patients require surgical intervention. The total burden to society includes not only the costs of medical care but also the cost of days lost from work—particularly important as this condition commonly afflicts patients of working age. These costs are estimated at one billion dollars per year.

The morbidity from renal stones has been reduced by improved surgical therapy over the last 15 years. Recent emphasis has turned to understanding the pathophysiologic mechanisms underlying stone formation rather than just improving therapy. The ultimate justification for this emphasis is that medical intervention successfully reduces stone recurrences and decreases expense and morbidity. The cause of stone disease can now be determined in greater than 95% of patients with recurrent stones.

In this chapter, the normal metabolism of the compounds of interest in stone formation is reviewed, followed by a discussion of the pathophysiology of stone formation and metabolic aspects of therapy.

PHYSIOCHEMISTRY

The central event in stone formation is supersaturation. The solubility produce, K_{sp}, is a constant, equal to the product of the concentrations of the pure chemical components at which the solid and dissolved states are in equilibrium in *water* at standard conditions and temperature. For calcium oxalate monohydrate, the K_{sp} in distilled water at 37° C is 2.34×10^{-9}. If the product of the calcium and oxalate concentrations exceeds this, calcium oxalate crystals precipitate. Urine contains inhibitors and other molecules that raise the concentrations at which stone constituents precipitate. A second higher constant, the formation product, or K_f, describes precipitation in urine. The concentrations of most urinary stone components are in the "metastable" range between K_{sp} and K_f; thus, the question really is not why some people form stones, but why most do not (Figure 12.1).

Once calcium oxalate concentration exceeds its K_{sp}, crystallization occurs by the process of homogeneous nucleation. Crystallization may develop before the K_{sp} is reached, if particulate matter (e.g., cells, tubular fragments, other crystals) acts as a nucleus for precipitation. This heterogeneous nucleation occurs in vivo more commonly than does homogeneous nucleation. Crystal enlargement then follows by crystal growth and/or crystal aggregation.

Whether a precipitated crystal becomes a stone depends on its

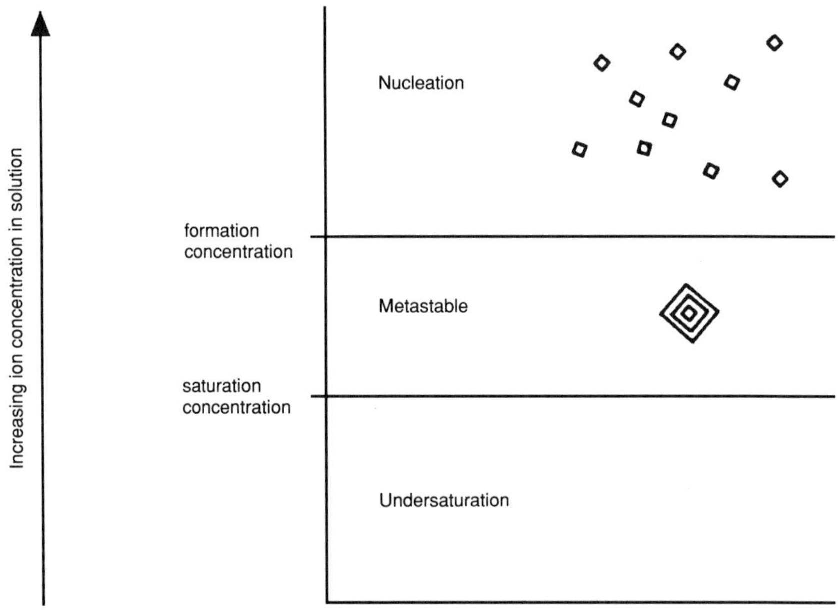

Figure 12.1: Effects of increasing ion concentration in urine. *Reproduced with permission from Blandy J. Lecture Notes on Urology, 4th ed. Oxford: Blackwell Scientific Publications, 1991:80.*

retention time within the kidney. Free crystals are washed out into the bladder, whereas crystals adherent to cellular or papillary surfaces grow to become stones. Reduced urinary flow may contribute to stone formation (e.g., the dilated renal pelvis of ureteropelvic junction obstruction or the dilated tubules of medullary sponge kidney).

Inhibitors counteract the tendency to crystallization. The most important urine inhibitors are citrate, pyrophosphate, magnesium, and glycosaminoglycans. Mechanisms of inhibitor action include reduction of ionic activity by formation of complexes (i.e., citrate for calcium or magnesium for oxalate) and "poisoning" of the crystal lattice (i.e., pyrophosphate or citrate). A number of kidney proteins (e.g., nephrocalcin, Tamm-Horsfall mucoprotein, and uropontin) are known to inhibit the different phases of stone crystallization.

Stones are identified by their appearance under polarized-light microscopy, infrared spectroscopy, or x-ray diffraction, and receive mineralogic names based on their state of hydration. Little is known about the differences in hydration of crystal components, although this does carry clinical significance; that is, the many-faceted crystals of calcium oxalate dihydrate tend to fragment more easily following lithotripsy than the more compact monohydrate (Fig. 12.2). The comparative incidences of stone types in the United States are shown in Table 12.1.

NORMAL MINERAL HOMEOSTASIS

Calcium Homeostasis

Serum calcium levels are maintained at a remarkably constant level. Extracellular fluid calcium levels range between 8.5 and 10.5 mg/dl, represent-

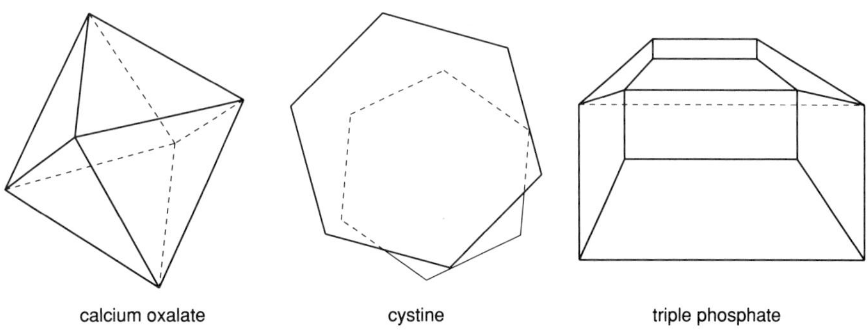

Figure 12.2: Crystals with characteristic shapes of which oxalate, cystine, and triple phosphate are the common types. *Reproduced with permission from Blandy J. Lecture Notes on Urology, 4th ed. Oxford: Blackwell Scientific Publications, 1991:12.*

Table 12.1: Stone Composition

Stone Type	*As Predominant Constituent (%)*	*As Contributing Constituent (%)*
Calcium oxalate monohydrate	31.7	43.0
Calcium oxalate dihydrate	41.4	61.0
Calcium phosphate (apatite)	2.3	38.4
Calcium phosphate (brushite)	1.4	2.6
Urate	7.6	9.4
Cystine	0.9	0.9
Struvite	9.2	15.7
Carbonate	4.5	23.1
Matrix	<1	100
Other	<1	<1
Nonbiologic	<1	<1

ing 1000 to 2000 mg of calcium in 11 L of extracellular fluid. However, 99% of the body's calcium is in the bones, a store of 1000 to 2000 g. Dietary calcium intake is variable and averages 500 to 1200 mg/day. Because of vitamin D's feedback, intestinal absorption of calcium is generally inversely proportional to dietary calcium intake. Less than half of the dietary intake is absorbed, the remainder passing directly into the feces. There is an obligatory and apparently unregulated secretion of calcium into the gut of 100 to 200 mg/day, and a balanced turnover of calcium from the bone stores of approximately 500 mg/day. Renal glomerular filtration of calcium is 5000 to 10,000 mg/day, yet the normal adult loses only 100 to 300 mg/day with the remainder being reabsorbed. This remarkable preservation of calcium is under tight hormonal control, and failure of this control is central to the pathogenesis of some calcium stones. Calcium reabsorption in the proximal tubule and medullary ascending limb of the loop of Henle is passively linked to sodium reabsorption, while in the distal tubule calcium is actively reabsorbed under hormonal control, independent of sodium.

The hormonal control of calcium metabolism is primarily by parathyroid hormone (PTH) and D 1,25-dihydroxy-vitamin. DPTH increases serum calcium by multiple mechanisms: bone resorption by direct activation of osteoclasts and inactivation of osteoblasts, decreased tubular reabsorption of phosphate and increased tubular reabsorption of calcium via ATPase stimulation, and stimulation of the renal conversion of vitamin D to its active form. Vitamin D (cholecalciferol) is a steroid hormone formed from precursors by the action of ultraviolet light on the skin, or obtained directly from dietary sources. The liver hydroxylates cholecalciferol to 25-OHD, the major circulating metabolite. Renal, and to a much lesser extent, cartilage, mitochondrial hydroxylases then convert it to either inactive 24,25-$(OH)_2D$ or active 1,25-$(OH)_2D$ (called calcitriol). 1,25-$(OH)_2D$ stimulates calcium and phosphate absorption across the jejunal mucosa, and acts synergistically with PTH to increase bone reabsorption. Calcitonin, despite its effect on the kidney to reduce calcium and phosphate reabsorption has not been implicated in stone formation.

Oxalate Homeostasis

Ninety percent of the body's oxalate is synthesized as the useless metabolic end-product of endogenous and dietary compounds; the remaining 10% is obtained directly from dietary sources. Half of the synthesized fraction is created from ascorbic acid and the remainder from the oxidation of glyoxylate, an intermediary in the metabolism of the amino acids alanine, glycine, and hydroxyproline.

Intestinal oxalate absorption occurs by passive diffusion without hormonal control. The colon is the primary site, but there is some absorption throughout the gastrointestinal tract. Oxalate normally complexes with calcium in the bowel lumen to precipitate as insoluble compounds, making the oxalate unavailable for absorption. Foods with high oxalate content include spinach and other dark green vegetables, nuts and seeds, tea and chocolate. However, only 2 to 5% of the oxalate content of food is actually absorbed. Average dietary oxalate content is 80 to 100 mg/day; 10 mg/day are lost in the feces, 70 to 100 mg/day are destroyed by bowel bacteria, and 4 to 6 mg/day are absorbed. Endogenous production contributes 15 to 45 mg/day.

The normal serum oxalate is only about 0.02 mg/dl. Normal renal excretion is less than 44 mg/day. In the absence of bowel disease, dietary oxalate excesses rarely contribute significantly to urine oxalate levels. Oxalate is freely filtered at the glomerulus, and reabsorbed and secreted by the proximal tubule. Tubular secretion may be abnormally increased in some patients with nephrolithiasis.

Phosphate Homeostasis

The skeleton is a reservoir of phosphorous, containing 85% of the body's total, a store of 1000 grams. The extracellular fluid level is maintained at 3.0 to 4.5 mg/dl, or 800 mg absolute. Daily oral intake is variable (600 to 2000 mg). However, intestinal absorption is highly efficient, increasing to up to 90% at low levels of intake. There is a small and insignificant level of phosphate secretion into the gut. The bone stores undergo a balanced turnover of approximately 300 mg/day. Glomerular filtration of phosphate if 4000 to 6000 mg/day, but 85 to 90% is reabsorbed, predominantly in the proximal tubule by a sodium-linked process, resulting in the daily loss of only 500 to 1100 mg. Markedly elevated serum calcium and phosphate levels may result in metabolic calcification.

Hormonal control of phosphate metabolism is exerted by parathyroid hormone and vitamin D. PTH acts by increasing bone resorption, thereby releasing phosphate, and by decreasing renal tubular phosphate reabsorption. Vitamin D increases phosphate and calcium uptake across the intestinal mucosa.

Hydrogen Ion (Acid) Homeostasis

Acid is normally added to the blood by (a) oxidative metabolism producing CO_2, which is hydrated to the weak acid H_2CO_3 (carbonic acid), and (b) "fixed" acids released from the catabolism of proteins (sulfuric acid) or phospholipids (phosphoric acid), from anaerobic metabolism (lactic acid), and in certain pathologic states. This acid load is handled sequentially by initial bicarbonate buffering and (to a limited extent) serum proteins, respiratory compensation by CO_2 excretion, and finally by renal acid excretion. In addition to excreting these acids, the kidney retrieves the large quantities of bicarbonate that are continuously filtered through the glomerulus. This is achieved predominantly in the proximal tubule by active H^+ secretion, the H^+ being generated by carbonic anhydrase-catalyzed combination of CO_2 and H_2O to H_2CO_3, which then rapidly dissociates to the required H^+ and the retrieved HCO_3^- (actually a different molecule of bicarbonate than that which was filtered). Na^+ then follows passively to maintain electroneutrality.

The excretion of fixed acids requires the creation of a new bicarbonate ion for replenishment of the blood. Phosphoric acid is filtered into the urine as the neutral salt Na_2HPO_4. H^+, obtained from the carbonic anhydrase-catalyzed formation of H_2CO_3, is actively secreted throughout the tubule, combining with phosphoric acid to create the weak acid NaH_2PO_4, which is excreted. The bicarbonate ion formed from the dissociation of H_2CO_3 then diffuses back into the blood. Filtered sulfate is combined with secreted H^+ (again releasing a bicarbonate to the blood) and with ammonia derived from the degradation of glutamine and other amino acids. In a process known as "ion trapping," the ammonia, once combined with H^+ in the lumen, forms a charged molecule and can no longer freely diffuse back into the cell. It is then excreted with the sulfate as $(NH_4)_2SO_4$. There is a limit to the kidney's ability to maintain a pH gradient, as acid loading lowers the pH only to 5.5.

Citrate Homeostasis

Citrate is the best characterized stone inhibitor. It lowers calcium oxalate supersaturation by complexing calcium in the urine, reducing calcium's ionic activity, and it "poisons" the forming crystals of calcium salts, thereby inhibiting crystal growth.

Citric acid, $HOOC\text{-}CH_2\text{-}COH(COOH)\text{-}CH_2\text{-}COOH$, is ubiquitous in the body because of its role in the energy-producing citric acid cycle. Its normal serum concentration is about 2.7 mg/dl. It is freely filtered at the glomerulus, and 75% is reabsorbed in the proximal tubule, where it is metabolized for energy. The remaining 25% appears in the urine, at a normal level of about 320 mg/day.

Magnesium Homeostasis

Urinary magnesium complexes oxalate, reducing oxalate's ionic activity and hence the saturation of calcium oxalate. Long-term magnesium therapy decreases tubular reabsorption of citrate and increases its excretion. Serum magnesium is normally 2.0 to 3.0 mg/dl and urinary excretion over 60 mg/day.

Urate Homeostasis

Uric acid is the end product of purine metabolism. The normal diet contains purines that are converted to approximately 400 mg of urate per day, while catabolism contributes an equal amount. Uric acid, which is quite insoluble, is derived from the more soluble xanthine by xanthine oxidase. Humans (and dalmatian dogs) lack the enzyme uricase, which converts uric acid in other nonprimate mammals into the more soluble allantoin. In humans, enteric bacteria process urate to allantoin and allantoin acid, accounting for approximately 200 mg/day, or 25% of the daily production of urate. The normal serum uric acid level is 2.5 to 8.0 mg/dl. It is freely filtered at the glomerulus. Ninety-three percent is reabsorbed, but 92% is again secreted, only to be reabsorbed, leaving a daily excretion of 600 mg, or 75% of the daily production of urate.

Cysteine Homeostasis

Cysteine is formed by the spontaneous disulfide bridge linkage of two cysteine amino acids. Cysteine is obtained from the diet or from methionine, an essential amino acid. Cysteine is filtered at the glomerulus and almost completely reabsorbed, resulting in urinary loss of less than 20 mg/day.

PATHOPHYSIOLOGY OF STONE FORMATION

The conceptual analysis of the pathophysiology of stone formation that follows attempts to explain clinical observations. Controversy exists as to whether the various etiologies described below are distinct or represent a continuum. The mechanisms are complex and highly interrelated, and it is not surprising that they overlap and that combined clinical syndromes are common (Table 12.2). The pathophysiology is described for each stone type.

Calcium Oxalate Stones

Calcium oxalate is the most common component of urinary stones (Table 12.3). Pathologic conditions leading to hypercalciuria and hyperoxaluria increase concentrations of the constituents and lead to precipitation. Heterogeneous nucleation may be the determining factor in the initiation of stone growth. The concentration product of calcium and oxalate typically lies in the metastable range in the urine of normal and stone-forming patients. In normal urine the concentration of calcium oxalate salt is four times higher than its solubility. Thus, other factors such as inhibitors are important in preventing precipitation. Oxalic acid's pK_a (4.0) is too low for the solubility of calcium oxalate to be affected by urinary pH manipulation; thus no medications are available for dissolution of calcium oxalate stones.

Calcium oxalate crystals form as the monohydrate (whewellite) and

Table 12.2: Diagnostic Categories of Stone Disease

Category	*As Sole Etiology (%)*	*As Contributing Etiology (%)*
Absorptive hypercalciuria	20	40
Resorptive hypercalciuria	3	5
Renal leak hypercalciuria	5	8
Other hypercalciuria	15	25
Hyperoxaluria	2	15
HUCN	10	40
Hypocitraturia	10	50
Gouty hyperuricosuria	15	30
Cysteinuria	<1	<1
Infection stones	1	5
Hypomagnesiuria	5	10
Low volume	10	50
Unidentified and miscellaneous	<3	<3

Table 12.3: Etiologies of Calcium Stones

Predominant Stone Composition	*Etiology*
Calcium oxalate	Hypercalciuria
	Absorptive
	Resorptive
	Renal calcium leak
	Renal phosphate leak
	Vitamin D excess
	Other hypercalcemias
	Hyperoxaluria
	Primary
	Increased substrate
	Enteric
	Hyperuricosuria
	Hypocitraturia
	Chronic diarrhea
	Thiazide usage
	Idiopathic
	Incomplete distal RTA
	Complete distal RTA
Mixed	Low volume
	Hypomagnesiuria
Calcium phosphate	Distal RTA

the dihydrate (weddellite). There is little metabolic significance to this difference in hydration state. However, dihydrate stones are more easily fragmented by extracorporeal shockwave lithotripsy (ESWL), laser, and ultrasound.

The Hypercalciurias Hypercalciuria results from increased uptake of calcium from the gut, increased release from bone stores, or increased renal excretion of calcium (Table 12.4).

Absorptive hypercalciuria The primary defect, inherited as an autosomal dominant trait, is excessive passive mucosal absorption of calcium in the jejunum (Table 12.4). This defect is selective for calcium, as phosphate absorption is normal. The increased calcium uptake results in a slight, transient elevation of serum calcium, which then suppresses PTH secretion. This reduces vitamin D activation, and a new steady state is achieved with a high-normal serum calcium level and low-normal PTH and vitamin D levels. Renal tubular reabsorption of calcium (under PTH

Table 12.4: The Hypercalciurias

Type	*Primary Abnormality*
Absorptive (I,II)	Increased intestinal calcium absorption
Resorptive	Increased parathormone (PTH) activity
Renal calcium leak	Reduced renal tubular calcium reabsorption
Renal phosphate leak	Reduced renal tubular phosphate reabsorption
Vitamin D excess	Increased 1,25-vitamin D
Hypercalcemia	Increased serum calcium
Malignancy	
Sarcoidosis	
Milk alkali syndrome	
Hyperthyroidism	
Immobilization	
Paget's disease	

control) is inhibited; this, together with the increased filtered load, causes hypercalciuria. Fasting normalizes urinary calcium levels, whereas oral calcium loading produces an exaggerated increase in urine calcium levels. On a prolonged calcium-restricted diet, urine calcium remains abnormally high in the severe form of the disease (absorptive hypercalciuria type I); in the less severe variant (type II), urine calcium normalizes.

A slight increase in intestinal oxalate absorption may also be present in patients with absorptive hypercalciuria. The increased calcium absorption reduces the intraluminal pool available to complex oxalate; this effect is more pronounced in patients treated with either dietary calcium restriction or luminal calcium binders such as sodium cellulose phosphate.

Resorptive hypercalciuria This is due to stimulation of bone resorption, most commonly from primary hyperparathyroidism, but occasionally from PTH-like substances produced by malignancies (Table 12.4). The number of patients with hyperparathyroidism who present with stone disease is decreasing because of earlier detection of hypercalcemia by routine blood testing. The majority of patients with hypercalcemia who form stones have primary hyperparathyroidism. Parathyroid adenoma and hyperplasia both may cause resorptive hypercalciuria.

The elevated PTH augments bone resorption, thereby increasing serum calcium and the filtered load of calcium. This overwhelms the stimulatory action of PTH on the renal tubules to reabsorb calcium, resulting in an overflow of calcium into the urine and hypercalciuria. This is further augmented by the PTH-induced renal production of 1,25-$(OH)_2D$, which results in increased intestinal absorption of calcium. Hypercalciuria occurs in the fasting state, and is exaggerated after calcium loading.

Renal hypercalciuria In renal hypercalciuria ("calcium leak," or reabsorptive hypercalciuria) there is impaired renal tubular reabsorption of calcium (Table 12.4). The increased renal loss of calcium reduces the serum calcium level and causes a secondary elevation in PTH. This in turn increases bone resorption, promotes urinary phosphate loss, and activates vitamin D-mediated intestinal calcium absorption, all of which successfully return the serum calcium level to normal. After calcium starvation, the urine shows inappropriately high levels of calcium excretion, in the face of elevated serum PTH and vitamin D. In long-standing renal hypercalciuria, the persistently elevated PTH can result in measurable bone resorption, approaching the osteopenia of primary hyperparathyroidism. The PTH elevation can sometimes be missed if calcium starvation is inadequate, because enough dietary calcium is absorbed to block PTH secretion.

Renal phosphate leak The cause of this condition (previously called absorptive hypercalciuria type III) is thought to be an abnormally low tubular threshold of phosphate excretion that results in increased urinary loss of phosphate and hypophosphatemia (Table 12.4). The latter then directly stimulates the renal activation of vitamin D, which in turn causes increased calcium and phosphate absorption in the gut. Additional calcium may be contributed from the possible direct effect of vitamin D to increase bone resorption. Thus, the major laboratory difference between this and renal "calcium leak" hypercalciuria is a normal rather than elevated serum PTH.

Excess vitamin D Exogenous vitamin D or enhanced intrinsic synthesis of 1,25-$(OH)_2D$ results in a state resembling absorptive hypercalciuria, distinguishable mainly by an increased serum 1,25-$(OH)_2D$ level. Such a condition may occur in sarcoidosis. Active vitamin D stimulates intestinal absorption of calcium (and phosphate) and may augment bone reabsorption, resulting in increased calcium delivery to the glomerulus and suppression of PTH secretion. While it may be expected that calcium fasting would prevent the hypercalciuria, in fact the suppression of PTH and the loss of PTH-stimulated renal tubular reabsorption of calcium can result in fasting hypercalciuria.

Other causes of hypercalcemia Any pathologic state that induces hypercalcemia can result in nephrolithiasis because of the increased filtered load of calcium (Table 12.4). There are several common causes. With malignancy, osteolytic metastases release significant quantities of calcium. This is particularly true in multiple myeloma, which may also involve the action of an osteoclast activating factor. Certain cancers cause a pseudohyperparathyroidism by producing PTH or PTH-like substances, which result in resorptive hypercalciuria. 1 to 2% of patients with Sarcoid granulomatous disease of unknown etiology, have increased levels of 1,25-$(OH)_2D$, produced by mononuclear phagocytes in the granulomas. Increased intestinal absorption of calcium may lead to hypercalcemia in patients with advanced, disseminated disease. In milk-alkali syndrome, long-term calcium and absorbable antacid intake causes hypercalcemia with metabolic alkalosis, which results in renal calcium phosphate deposition. In hyperthyroidism, patients may have increased bone resorption of a type resembling osteoporosis, releasing excessive amounts of calcium and phosphate to the serum. Bone resorption increases with prolonged immobilization but is reversible with resumption of normal activity. Finally, the increased bone turnover in Paget's disease favors resorption, which leads to increased filtered calcium and even hypercalcemia.

The Hyperoxalurias Increased urinary oxalate arises from increased synthesis, increased provision of substrate, or increased absorption of oxalate. In these conditions, the elevated urinary concentration of oxalate exceeds the formation product for calcium oxalate precipitation and leads to crystallization (Table 12.5)

Primary hyperoxaluria The primary hyperoxalurias are rare inborn errors of metabolism that result in the excretion of abnormally increased amounts of oxalate in the urine, often exceeding 100 mg/day. The abnormality, seen in autosomal recessive homozygotes, is secondary to a decrease in the activity of the hepatic enzymes alanine:glyoxylate aminotransferase (primary hyperoxaluria-type I; not alpha-ketoglutarate:gly-

Table 12.5: The Hyperoxalurias

Type	*Primary Abnormality*
Primary hyperoxaluria	Oxalate overproduction
Increased substrate	Oxalate overproduction
Vitamin B_6 deficiency	
Ethylene glycol	
Methoxyflurane	
Enteric hyperoxaluria	Increased colonic absorption of oxalate

oxylate carboligase as previously thought) or D-glyceric acid dehydrogenase (type II). These enzymes degrade oxalate precursors to other compounds, and decreased activity results in greater amounts of oxalate in the blood (Table 12.5) and elevated urine levels of glycolic acid (type I) and L-glyceric acid (type II). Stone formation often begins in childhood, and death from renal failure secondary to tubulointerstitial nephropathy ensues by age 20. There is no successful medical therapy for primary hyperoxaluria.

Increased substrate A nonhereditary cause of increased oxalate synthesis occurs with pyridoxine (vitamin B_6) deficiency. Pyridoxine is a cofactor for the enzyme that converts glyoxylate to glycine, and a deficiency of pyridoxine causes increased conversion of glyoxylate to oxalate.

Exogenous oxalate can originate from the hepatic detoxification of inhalational anesthetics (such as methoxyflurane), or of ethylene glycol (wood alcohol) ingestion (Table 12.5). Ascorbic acid (vitamin C) ingestion is a potentially common cause of hyperoxaluria, although this remains controversial. In patients who do not form stones, urinary oxalate excretion can increase by 12 mg/day on a dose of 4 grams of vitamin C per day. Stoneformers may show an even more exaggerated response.

Enteric hyperoxaluria The most common cause of hyperoxaluria is colonic hyperabsorption of oxalate (enteric hyperoxaluria) (Table 12.5). Increased transit of bile salts and fatty acids from the small bowel to the colon occurs in conditions that reduce either the absorptive function of the small bowel (regional enteritis, small bowel bypass or resection) or the absorption of fats or bile salts in the small bowel (chronic pancreatitis, pancreatectomy, celiac sprue). The increased amounts of bile salts and fatty acids in the colon result in (a) increased permeability of the colon to oxalate, and (b) complexing of fatty acids with luminal calcium to form soaps, which reduce the availability of calcium to bind oxalate in the intestinal lumen. Increased amounts of oxalate are then absorbed, leading to increased urinary excretion. An intact colon is essential to this mechanism of stone formation, since oxalate absorption occurs primarily in the colon. Thus, enteric hyperoxaluria can resolve in patients with inflammatory bowel disease following colectomy. Urinary stones form in 7 to 10% of patients with malabsorption syndromes (e.g., intrinsic disease, resection, jejunoileal bypass).

While the intestinal absorption of oxalate is increased, that of calcium may be decreased by the intraluminal complexing of calcium by fatty acids, by the decreased calcium absorptive ability of bowel wall exposed to fatty acids, and possibly by vitamin D deficiency resulting from fat malabsorption. The decreased calcium absorption may lead to an elevated serum PTH.

Other factors also contribute to stone formation in patients with enteric hyperoxaluria. Fecal fluid loss in short bowel syndromes results in reduced urine volumes, which predispose to stone precipitation. Increased intestinal loss of bicarbonate in diarrhea may lead to metabolic acidosis, which leads to urinary acidosis and urate precipitation. Metabolic acidosis also contributes to hypocitraturia, and magnesium absorption is reduced by intraluminal soap complexes. Thus, the urinary levels of two major inhibitors of stone formation are reduced.

Hyperuricosuric Calcium Oxalate Stones The mechanisms leading to hyperuricosuria are considered in more detail in the section on urate stones. The only demonstrable metabolic abnormality in some patients with calcium oxalate stones is hyperuricosuria, with a normal urine pH. Monosodium urate may supersaturate and precipitate, leading to calcium oxalate deposition by heterogeneous nucleation. Alternatively, uric acid may reduce the inhibitory potential of crystal growth inhibitors, particularly the glycosaminoglycans. In contrast to the hyperuricosuria in patients with urate stones, the underlying abnormality is commonly dietary purine overindulgence.

Hypocitraturia Hypocitraturia, found in 19 to 63% of patients with stones, may contribute to both calcium oxalate and calcium phosphate stone formation by virtue of decreased inhibitor activity. The etiologies of hypocitraturia are discussed below.

Calcium Phosphate Stones

Calcium phosphate appears in two crystal forms: hydroxyapatite ($Ca_5(PO_4)_3OH$), and the rare brushite ($CaHPO_4 \cdot 2H_20$). Although the urinary concentration of all species of phosphate ion is high, the concentration of the trivalent phosphate ion that forms hydroxyapatite is markedly affected by the pH. Poorly defined inhibitors also play a role in preventing phosphate precipitation.

Pure apatite stones account for 6.8% of stones and pure brushite for only 1.7%, although calcium phosphate is present as a minor constituent in a much larger percentage (28.9%). Because of the pronounced decrease of calcium phosphate solubility at high pH, distal (type I) renal tubular acidosis should be suspected if pure brushite stones occur.

Renal Tubular Acidosis In proximal, or type II, RTA, there is a defect of bicarbonate retrieval caused by poorly characterized mechanisms in the renal tubules (Table 12.6). Proximal RTA is not usually associated with nephrolithiasis. Bicarbonate (HCO_3^-), loss in the urine leads to metabolic acidosis, until the serum HCO_3^- level drops low enough to decrease the filtered load of bicarbonate. A new steady state is reached at a serum HCO_3^- concentration of 15 to 20 mEq/dl. The effects on urine pH are variable; in the absence of bicarbonate loading, the urine is appropriately acid. Supplementation with bicarbonate does not correct the acidosis because the excess serum bicarbonate is filtered and unsuccessfully reabsorbed.

In distal, or type I, RTA, proximal tubular bicarbonate reabsorption is normal, but the distal tubule is not able to generate a steep H^+ gradient (Table 12.6). The etiologies and mechanisms of this dysfunction are varied and poorly understood at the molecular level, but the common denominator is renal tubular cellular dysfunction. In the most complete and severe forms, the inability to excrete the daily acid load results in a progressive nonanion gap metabolic acidosis and elevated urine pH. Partial but insufficient compensation occurs by increasing NH_3 production to ion-trap H^+ in the lumen. In contrast to proximal RTA, alkalinizing buffers such as sodium bicarbonate can correct the acidosis by providing more buffering in the urine. Laboratory findings include high serum Cl^- (chloride), low serum K^+ and CO_2, and urine pH > 6.8. The elevated urine pH favors calcium phosphate crystallization and the formation of calcium phosphate stones—the typical stones in patients with distal RTA (Table 12.6).

Table 12.6: Renal Tubular Acidosis (RTA)

Proximal (Type II) RTA

Not associated with urolithiasis
Proximal tubule unable to retrieve bicarbonate

Distal (Type I) RTA

May cause calcium oxalate or calcium phosphate stones
Specifically associated with brushite stones
Distal tubule unable to generate steep acid (H^+ ion) gradient
Urine pH > 6.8 (complete) or > 5.5 (incomplete)

Ammonium chloride test

Administer 100 mg/kg ammonium chloride orally
After 3 hours, measure urine pH and serum bicarbonate or pH:

Normal result	urine pH < 5.3
Incomplete distal RTA	urine pH > 5.4 and blood pH < 7.32 or serum bicarbonate < 16 meq/dl

Complete distal RTA also causes hypercalciuria because of the buffering of the metabolic acidosis by bone, with release of calcium and phosphate. Osteomalacia or rickets may ensue in serious cases. In the less severe "incomplete" form, the increased ammonia production successfully allows excretion of the entire acid load and prevents metabolic acidosis. However, the urine pH is inappropriately high for the level of the serum bicarbonate. Diagnosis is made by the ammonium chloride loading test: 100 mg/kg ammonium chloride is given orally; 3 hours later, urine pH over 5.4, blood pH less than 7.32, or serum bicarbonate less than 16 mEq/dl are indicative of incomplete distal RTA.

Hypocitraturia Hypocitraturia reflects several processes rather than a single entity, although idiopathic hypocitraturia does occur. The most common contributing factor is metabolic acidosis, which causes increased citrate uptake by tubular cell mitochondria and reduced urine levels of citrate. The opposite occurs in metabolic alkalosis. Hypocitraturia is the sole abnormality in 5% of stone patients, and it coexists with other abnormalities in an additional 50%.

Hypocitraturia has several causes. In distal RTA, the alkaline urine favors calcium phosphate precipitation, and the metabolic acidosis causes hypocitraturia and deprives the urine of a major stone inhibitor. RTA is unlikely in the absence of hypocitraturia. In chronic diarrheal syndrome, fecal loss of bicarbonate and potassium results in metabolic acidosis and hypocitraturia. In contrast to distal RTA, the kidneys continue to excrete the acid load and produce low pH urine. The low-volume state produced by diarrheal fluid loss also contributes to stone formation. Stone formation may be exacerbated by enteric hyperoxaluria. The hypokalemia induced by thiazide diuretics causes tubular intracellular acidosis and decreased urine citrate excretion. Other, idiopathic, causes of acidosis may contribute to decreased citrate excretion, for example, a diet rich in acids (such as animal proteins), or extreme exercise, which produces high levels of lactic acid. Isolated defects in citrate metabolism also occur. Some reports suggest that hypocitraturia is more common in women stone formers than men.

Uric Acid Stones

Uric acid stone formation results from supersaturation of urine with undissociated uric acid and occurs even in the absence of hyperuricosuria. The first dissociable proton in this weak acid has a pK_a of 5.5; thus precipitation is very pH dependent. This pH dependence offers a mechanism for the medical dissolution of urate stones. There is no known inhibitor of uric acid crystallization. On the contrary, crystals of uric acid and monosodium urate can act as heterogeneous nuclei for the deposition of calcium oxalate, and uric acid's crystal lattice is similar enough to calcium oxalate's to aid in epitaxy. Whether uric acid or calcium stones form on a urate nucleus depends on the urine pH; if it is persistently below pH 5.5. uric acid stones are favored. Interestingly, calcium oxalate stones are more common in hyperuricemia than are uric acid stones.

The most common cause of uric acid stones is gout, which occurs in 2 to 18% of the U.S. population (Table 12.7). Hyperuricemia is the hallmark of this condition, which is inherited as an autosomal dominant trait with variable penetrance. Approximately 20% of patients with gout develop uric acid nephrolithiasis, compared to only 0.01% of the population as a whole. Three metabolic defects, all of unknown mechanism, contribute to the clinical syndrome of gout: (1) urate overproduction by the shunting of precursors from nucleic acid synthesis toward urate synthesis; (2) production of urine with a pH consistently below 5.5., which contributes to uric acid precipitation even in the absence of hyperuricosuria; and (3) relative diminution of urate clearance. The incidence of urate nephrolithiasis correlates with the severity of the hyperuricosuria, approaching 50% in patients with urine urate levels greater than 1000 mg/day.

Other causes of hyperuricemia associated with hyperuricosuria include the inborn errors of metabolism such as hypoxanthine-guanine phosphoribosyl transferase deficiency (Lesch-Nyhan syndrome) and increased tissue catabolism, seen in myeloproliferative disorders and chemotherapy-induced cell necrosis. Hyperuricosuria without hyperuricemia can be due

Table 12.7: Etiologies of Uric Acid Stones

Hyperuricosuria
With hyperuricemia
Urine pH < 5
gout
Urine pH normal
Lesch-Nyhan syndrome
Cell necrosis
Myeloproliferative diseases
Chemotherapy
With normouricemia
Purine gluttony
Drugs, e.g., probenecid
Normouricosuria
Gastrointestinal fluid and bicarbonate loss

to uricosuric drugs which reduce the tubular reabsorption of urate, for example, probenecid, high-dose salicylates, or radiographic contrast agents. Hyperuricosuria also occurs in "purine gluttony" from meat overindulgence, and in some additional patients with excessive endogenous purine metabolism. However, these conditions rarely produce the low urine pH necessary to cause uric acid precipitation, and therefore usually cause hyperuricosuric calcium nephrolithiasis.

Uric acid stone formation, despite normouricosuria, is seen in several gastrointestinal disorders (ulcerative colitis, regional enteritis, ileostomy) associated with dehydration and acidic urine from diarrheal loss of bicarbonate.

Cystine Stones

Cystinuria is an autosomal recessive condition associated with a defect in the luminal transmembrane transport of cystine, ornithine, lysine, and arginine by renal tubular and intestinal cells. Decreased tubular reabsorption results in increased urinary levels of these amino acids (up to 250 mg/day for cystine). Cystine is the only one of these four amino acids whose solubility is low enough to precipitate and form calculi. The situation is complicated somewhat by evidence of separate transport mechanisms for the other amino acids in the kidney and the intestine.

The middle pK_a of cystine is 8.2; thus alkalinization increases its solubility by approximately 50% at pH 7.5. The cyanide-nitroprusside or similar screening test is used for screening and demonstrates urinary excretion levels greater than 75 mg/day. In up to 30% of patients with homozygous cystinuria, stones contain little or no cystine. Since cystine does not appear to contribute to heterogeneous nucleation, this suggests the coexistence of other metabolic abnormalities in cystinuric patients.

Infection Stones

The hallmark of an infection stone is the presence of struvite, $MgNH_4PO_4 \cdot 6H_2O$, and to a lesser extent carbonate apatite, $Ca_{10}(PO_4)_6 \cdot CO_3$. These stones have also been termed triple-phosphate stones because of the presence of three cations (Ca^{+2}, Mg^{+2}, and NH_4^+) with a single phosphate anion. Struvite crystallization requires a urine pH above 7.2 and the presence of free ammonia. These conditions are rarely met except by the action of bacteria containing urease, an enzyme that hydrolyzes urea into two molecules of ammonia and one of CO_2; the ammonia is hydrolyzed to ammonium with release of a hydroxyl ion ($pK = 9.03$), which raises the pH. The CO_2 is hydrolyzed to HCO_3^- ($pK = 6.33$) then to CO_3^{-2} ($pK = 10.1$) with release of two protons. These reactions result in a decidedly alkaline urine. The determinants of the balance between carbonate and struvite in stone composition remain unknown.

Proteus mirabilis, the classic urease-producing bacteria associated with struvite stones, accounts for up to 87% of infection stones. Urease has also been identified in all urinary pathogens (including Corynebacterium and Mycoplasma), with the exception of *E. coli*. However, some 13% of struvite stones show only *E. coli* infections, and another small percentage have negative urine cultures. Local influences in the kidney, such as the glycosaminoglycan layer or the mucoprotein matrix, may contribute to infection stone formation. Conditions that predispose to upper-tract infection with urea-splitting organisms (including neurogenic bladder, enteral diversion, indwelling catheters, and vesicoureteral reflux) are associated with an increased incidence of infection stones.

Enlargement of stones and difficulty with eradication are common, as the stone material entraps and shelters the bacteria, allowing the stone to fill the collecting system. However, the term *staghorn* is a radiologic description and is not synonymous with infection. Only 75% of staghorn stones consist of the struvite/carbonate apatite/matrix spectrum; the remainder can be of any composition.

Miscellaneous Stone Constituents

Several other inborn errors of metabolism result in urolithiasis, including adenine phosphoribosyl transferase deficiency (2,8-dihydroxyadenine stones) and xanthine oxidase deficiency (xanthine stones). Hypomagnesiuria, of dietary origin, may contribute to calcium oxalate stone formation in 4% of patients with stones. Iatrogenic causes of stones include triamterene, a potassium-sparing diuretic, and silica, found in silicate antacids.

Matrix is a mucoprotein constituent of all renal calculi. It is composed of cellular debris, bacterial degradation products, and excreted proteins. Occasionally, the only material found on surgical exploration is the gummy matrix, which is sufficient to predispose to stone recurrence if incompletely removed.

Structural abnormalities

Anatomic abnormalities predispose to clinical stone formation because of the effect of urine flow rate on crystal enlargement (see earlier discussion). Thus the relationship between obstructive lesions such as congenital ureteropelvic junction obstructions and stones. Of greater significance is the congenital condition of medullary sponge kidney, which consists of dilated collecting tubules in the renal medulla, and is found in 20% of patients with calculous disease. Recent research suggests that the increased incidence of stone disease in patients with radiologic findings of medullary sponge kidney is not due to associated metabolic abnormalities. Rather, the structure–flow relationship is the probable cause of stones in these patients.

Low Urine Volumes

A low urine volume contributes to stone formation by causing a relative increase in the formation product of the stone constituents, which makes precipitation more likely. Low urine volume is occasionally the only abnormality found, but more commonly is found combined with other metabolic abnormalities. Daily insensible losses, in the absence of excessive gastrointestinal loss or sweating, average 800 ml, while water obtained from solid food contributes 500 to 1000 ml/day. The goal in preventing stone recurrence is a urine output of at least 2000 ml/day; thus a patient on routine activity must drink at least 3 L per day.

METABOLIC EVALUATION

The evaluation of patients with urolithiasis is directed to the identification of medically treatable causes. Stone composition analysis is most informative and is pathognomonic for cystine, struvite, and iatrogenic stones. Metabolic evaluation is recommended, however, to exclude coincidental conditions that may predispose to stone formation after successful control of the primary condition. Improvements in laboratory methods, particularly assays for serum PTH and urine oxalate, have simplified the metabolic evaluation. Because the excretion of stone constituents varies over time, 24-hour urine collections have become standard. This, however, may obscure transient lithogenic conditions, such as a postprandial hypercalciuria. Many patients exhibit more than one metabolic abnormality, as outlined in Tables 12.8 through 12.10 and Figure 12.3.

Metabolic evaluation of the first-time stone former is controversial. However, the high lifetime recurrence rates and the cost of surgical therapy are cogent arguments for evaluation and medical intervention. This determination should be tempered by estimates of the patient's stone-forming activity and risk. High-risk groups include children, patients with multiple stones at the time of presentation, those with a positive family history, and patients with intestinal disease, gout, or noncalcium stones.

Evaluation starts with a careful medical history, with emphasis on medications (including nonprescription) such as vitamin C (hyperoxaluria), acetazolamide (hypocitraturia secondary to acidosis), calcium supplements, vitamin D (hypercalciuria), or triamterene. It is unusual for a moderate diet, without excesses or "gluttony," to play a significant causative role in lithiasis. Classic excesses are calcium-rich milk, cheese, and ice cream, and the oxalate-rich nuts and seeds. Dietary protein excess can lead to stone formation by virtue of the acidity of the high sulfate content of its amino acids, which lowers urine pH and decreases citrate excretion, and by providing substrate for conversion to uric acid. Serum levels of

Table 12.8: Metabolic Evaluation—Serum and Spot Urine

Finding	*Possible Diagnosis*	*Further Test*
Serum		
Calcium elevation	Resorptive	24 hr urine
Phosphate decrease	Renal phosphate leak	24 hr urine
Hyperchloremic acidosis	Distal RTA	24 hr urine
Uric acid elevation	Gout	24 hr urine
Spot Urine		
pH > 7.5 and/or positive culture	Urea-splitting infection	Urine culture
pH > 6.8, no infection, hyperchloremic acidosis	Complete distal RTA	
pH > 5.5, no infection, normal electrolytes	Incomplete distal RA	Ammonium chloride test
pH < 5.5	Gout	24 hr urine
Hexagonal crystals	Cystinuria	Cyanide-nitroprusside test 24 hr quantitative cystine

sodium, potassium, chloride, carbon dioxide, creatinine, calcium, phosphorous, and uric acid are checked and a urinalysis performed. Important findings are outlined in Table 12.8.

Full metabolic evaluation protocols vary. Patients can be tested on controlled or random diets. A 24-hour urine collection on the patient's

Table 12.9: Metabolic Evaluation—24 hr Urine

Finding	*Possible Diagnosis*	*Further Test*
Volume < 2000 ml	Inadequate fluid intake	
Sodium > 150 mg	Excessive sodium intake	
Oxalate > 80 mg, or > 60 mg with systemic signs	Primary hyperoxaluria	Evaluate for enzyme deficiency
Oxalate > 44 mg with intestinal disease	Enteric hyperoxaluria	
Citrate < 320 mg, no RTA	Chronic diarrhea Thiazide usage Idiopathic hypocitraturia	
Urate > 700 mg	Hyperuricosuria	See Table 12.7
Urate normal, with uric acid stones	Intestinal bicarbonate loss	
Calcium > 250 mg	Hypercalciuria	See Table 12.11

Table 12.10: Results of Metabolic Testing

			Hypercalciuria							*Hyperoxaluria*			*HUCN*
		Normal Values	*AH-1*	*AH-2*	*Resorptive*	*Renal Ca Leak*	*Renal P Leak*	*1,25-Vit. D excess*	*Other Hyper-calcemia*	*Primary*	*Increased Substrate*	*Enteric*	
Serum	*Ca*	8.5–10.5 mg/dl	N	N	↑	N	N	N	↑	N	N	N	N
	P	3.0–4.5 mg/dl	N	N	↓	N	↓	N		N	N	N	N
	PTH	0.29–0.85 pg/dl	N	N	↑	↑	N	N/↓	N/↓			↑	N
	CO_2	21–30 mEq/l								N	N	↓	
	Urate	2.5–8.0 mg/dl											N
	1,25-D	25–40 pg/dl	N	N	↑	↑	↑	↑					
	K	3.5–5.0 mEq/l								N	N	↓	
	Cl	98–106 mEq/l											
24-hr urine	*Ca (random diet)*	< 250 mg	↑	↑	↑	↑	↑	↑	↑	N	N	↓	N
	Oxalate	< 44 mg								↑	↑	↑	N
	Urate	< 700 mg											↑
	Citrate	> 320 mg								N	N	↓	N
	Ca (restricted diet)	< 200 mg	↑	N	↑	↑	↑	↑				↓	N

Table 12.10: continued

			Hypocitraturia				
		Normal Values	Chronic Diarrhea	Thiazide	Idiopathic	Incomplete Distal RTA	Complete Distal RTA
Serum	*Ca*	8.5–10.5 mg/dl			N	N	N
	P	3.0–4.5 mg/dl			N	N	N
	PTH	0.29–0.85 pg/dl			N	N	N
	CO_2	21–30 mEq/l	N/↓	↑		N	↓
	Urate	2.5–8.0 mg/dl					
	1,25-D	25–40 pg/dl			N		
	K	3.5–5.0 mEq/l	N/↓	↓		N	↓
	Cl	98–106 mEq/l	N/↑	↓		N	↑
24-hr urine	*Ca (random diet)*	< 250 mg	↓	↓	N		↑
	Oxalate	< 44 mg			N		N
	Urate	< 700 mg			N		N
	Citrate	> 320 mg	↓	↓	↓	↓	↓
	Ca (restricted diet)	< 200 mg			N		

usual diet and fluid intake is a good initial test (Table 12.9). This is checked for total volume, creatinine (allowing calculation of creatinine clearance), calcium, sodium, oxalate, citrate, magnesium and qualitative cystine if indicated (the cyanide-nitroprusside test). The 24-hour urine creatinine (normally 20 mg/kg) is a check on the completeness of the collection. Medication that may influence the values (i.e., thiazides or calcium antacids) should be continued if there is suspicion that they influenced stone formation. Litmus paper or test strips can be used to record urine pH at various times of the day. A repeat collection is often beneficial, as the levels of several stone components vary widely. The significant results of metabolic testing are summarized in Table 12.10. If a

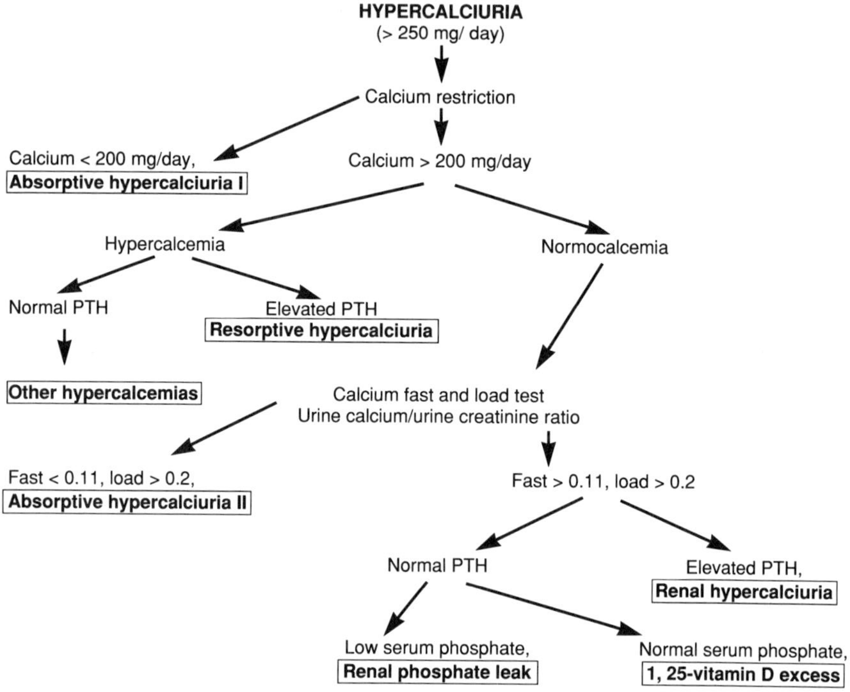

Figure 12.3: Hypercalciuria—Differential Diagnosis

patient has cystine stones or a positive cyanide-nitroprusside test, a 24-hour quantitative urine cystine assessment is obtained.

If a patient is hypercalciuric on a random diet (urine calcium > 250 mg/day), the patient is given a restricted diet containing 400 mg/day calcium 100 mEq/day sodium, and low oxalate, in preparation for the calcium, fast and load test. Calcium restriction can be augmented by adding sodium cellulose phosphate (5 gm t.i.d. with meals) for several days before the test. After 7 days of calcium restriction, a repeat 24-hour urine collection and fasting PTH and repeat blood tests are obtained, and a calcium load test is performed. The Dallas protocol for the calcium load test is as follows: the patient fasts beginning at 9 P.M. the night before, except for 300 ml distilled water at 9 P.M. and midnight. At 7 A.M., the patient voids, drinks 600 ml distilled water, and begins the 2-hour fasting urine collection. At 9 A.M., the patient receives 1 g of elemental calcium in a 250-ml liquid synthetic meal orally and begins the 4-hour post-load urine collection. The urine is tested for creatinine and calcium levels. Results are expressed as mg calcium/mg creatinine, reflecting renal function and controlling for muscle mass. The normal fasting ratio is less than 0.11, and a post-load value greater than 0.2 is significant (Table 12.11).

Table 12.11: Medical Therapy of Stones

	Condition	*Therapy*	*Problems*
Hypercalciuria	AH-1	SCP and magnesium citrate	Hypomagnesiuria Hyperoxaluria
		Thiazide	Escape Hypocitraturia
	AH-2	Ca restrict	
	Resorptive	Surgery	
	Renal	Thiazide	Hypocitraturia Impotence
	Renal phosphate leak	Orthophosphate	GI
	1,25-vitamin D excess	Thiazide	
	Other hypercal-cemia	Treat cause	
Hyperoxaluria	Primary	Orthophosphate and pyridoxine	
	Enteric	Ca? Fluid Citrate Magnesium Oxalate restrict	Hypercalciuria
HUCN		Allopurinol	Hepatic dysfunction Hypersensitivity Gout Xanthine stones
		K citrate Purine restrict?	
Hypocitraturia	Chronic diarrhea	K citrate (liquid)	
	Thiazide	K citrate	
	Idiopathic	K citrate	
	Distal RTA	K citrate	
Hyperuricosuria	Gout	K citrate to pH 6.5–7.0	Hyperkalemia
		Na citrate	Ca stones
		Allopurinol	
	Other hyperuricemia	Allopurinol	
	Normouricemic	Treat cause	

Table 12.11 (continued)

Table 12.11: continued

Condition	*Therapy*	*Problems*
Normouricosuria	Fluid	
	Alkaline	
Cysteine	Fluid	
	Alkali	Ca phosphate stones
	Penicillamine	Gastrointestinal
		Anosmia (Zn deficiency)
		Dermatologic
		Hypersensitivity
		Hematologic
		Renal function
		Pyridoxine deficiency
	MPG	Less than above
Infection	Surgery	
	Hemiacidrin or Suby G	Hypermagnesemia
		Sepsis
	AHA	Gastrointestinal, etc.
Low volume	Fluid	
Hypomagnesiuria	Magnesium citrate	

This algorithm is limited in that it does not diagnose resorptive hypercalciuria caused by normocalcemic hyperparathyroidism. In a laboratory setting, this could be done by measuring urine cAMP levels (a reflection of PTH effect) after calcium loading; in renal hypercalciuria, these should partially normalize, while in primary hyperparathyroidism they remain elevated. More simply, the diagnosis of renal hypercalciuria would likely be made; therapy would then consist of thiazides to reduce renal excretion of calcium. If the true etiology is resorptive, hypercalcemia will ensue, allowing the correct diagnosis to be made by follow-up serum calcium measurement.

PRINCIPLES OF MEDICAL THERAPY

Stone recurrence rate is variously reported at 5% (with medical therapy) to 80% over a lifetime; in other studies rates reported are 5 to 7% per patient-year. There is a significant "stone clinic effect" in patients treated only with fluids and dietary changes. In one study, the 5-year stone recurrence rate decreased from 50 to 27%. Specific metabolic intervention may further reduce the stone recurrence rate to about 15%.

Some authors recommend thiazides for all stone-forming patients. This approach obviates the need for the extensive evaluation. However, specific therapy allows improved efficacy, avoids unnecessary medications, and reduces the risk that therapy will worsen the lithogenic state. One universally appropriate recommendation is to increase fluid intake. This reduces the concentration product of all stone constituents and decreases the likelihood of precipitation. A urine output of at least 2000 ml/day is recommended, which usually requires an oral intake of approximately 3000 ml/day or more if fluid losses are unusual. Fluid intake must be spread throughout the day and night. Selective drug therapy, derived from the known pathophysiology of stone formation, is summarized in Table 12.11.

Absorptive Hypercalciuria

Therapy is directed at reducing either the systemic calcium load or urine calcium excretion. Dietary calcium should be limited to less than 600 mg/day, and exogenous calcium supplementation should be eliminated.

Sodium cellulose phosphate (2.5 g t.i.d. with meals), a nonabsorbable ion exchange resin, binds calcium in the gut lumen and reduces its absorption. This may result in increased oxalate absorption, since less complexes with the lowered free calcium. Sodium cellulose phosphate may also cause hypomagnesemia by binding magnesium in the gut lumen. These potential drawbacks are avoided by adding magnesium citrate (10 mEq b.i.d.), which provides the added bonus of citrate supplementation. Oxalate restriction is necessary to prevent increased oxalate absorption. Sodium cellulose phosphate is reserved for patients with marked hypercalciuria (urine calcium > 350 mg/day) who are not at increased risk for bone disease.

Thiazide diuretics (hydrochlorothiazide 50 mg b.i.d., chlorthalidone 50 mg qd, or trichlormethiazide 2 mg b.i.d.) reduce urinary calcium. This treatment, though not specific therapy in absorptive hypercalciuria, is widely used. Thiazides increase fractional calcium reabsorption by the distal nephron and cause extracellurlar volume depletion, which promotes sodium and therefore calcium reabsorption in the loop of Henle. Bone densitometry demonstrates increased calcium deposition in the skeleton.

Because of the sodium-linked calcium transport in the proximal tubule and loop of Henle, sodium restriction reduces urine calcium by promoting sodium reabsorption. A high sodium excretion counteracts the beneficial effect of thiazides in decreasing calcium excretion. Sodium intake should be limited to 100 mEq/day. Diuretics that increase sodium excretion proximal to the ascending limb of the loop of Henle (e.g., furosemide) are contraindicated in hypercalciuria. The long-term efficacy of thiazides may be limited by an escape phenomenon in which the bone deposition ability is reduced, again re-equilibrating to increased calcium excretion. Lithogenic efficacy may also be reduced by an accompanying decrease in citrate excretion, attributed to hypokalemia and intracellular acidosis. Tubular reabsorption of uric acid is also sodium-linked, so the volume depletion caused by thiazides promotes hyperuricemia. The potassium-sparing diuretic triamterene, commonly added to thiazides, should not be used as it can form stones itself; amiloride is an acceptable alternative.

The less severe absorptive hypercalciuria, type II, can be corrected by dietary calcium restriction to 400 mg/day, combined with sodium restriction. Again, the sodium must be limited to 100 mEq/day.

Renal Hypercalciuria

Thiazides are direct, selective therapy for renal hypercalciuria, and there does not appear to be an escape phenomenon up to ten years of therapy.

Resorptive Hypercalciuria (Primary Hyperparathyroidism)

Treatment of resorptive hypercalciuria is surgical. Thiazides are specifically contraindicated because of the risk of worsening hypercalcemia by reducing urinary calcium excretion.

Renal Phosphate Leak

Orthophosphate (0.5 g of phosphorous t.i.d. to q.i.d. as neutral salts) reduces hypophosphatemia and blocks the stimulus for 1,25-$(OH)_2D$ formation. Neutral phosphate salts are preferred for renal phosphate leak, as alkaline salts raise urine pH, predisposing to calcium phosphate precipitation, while acid salts may cause hypocitraturia. Dosage is adjusted to produce urine phosphate excretion of 1900 to 2000 mg/day.

Excess Vitamin D

No good medical therapy is available for excess vitamin D because vitamin D's direct effect on bone resorption (discussed above) may lead to bone disease if calcium intake is blocked by sodium cellulose phosphate.

Hyperoxaluria

Primary hyperoxaluria is difficult to treat. Orthophosphates increase levels of pyrophosphate and citrate inhibitors. Pyridoxine 100 mg b.i.d. may decrease oxalate formation from precursors. Treatment of enteric hyperoxaluria requires dietary oxalate restriction, which is difficult to maintain, and a high fluid intake. Additional treatment with citrate (potassium citrate 15 mEq t.i.d. to q.i.d.) contributes inhibitor activity as well as counteracting the metabolic acidosis that may be present from diarrheal bicarbonate losses. In diarrheal states, the liquid formulation of potassium citrate is preferred, to ensure complete absorption. Calcium restriction is inappropriate, as it reduces intraluminal oxalate complexing and increases oxalate bioavailability.

Hyperuricosuric Calcium Nephrolithiasis

Hyperuricosuria resulting in nucleation of calcium oxalate stones can be effectively treated with allopurinol (300 mg qd). Allopurinol inhibits hypoxanthine and xanthine oxidases, resulting in the excretion of more soluble precursors. Urine uric acid falls to below 600 mg/day, and serum uric acid drops by 2 mg/dl. Calcium oxalate stone formation can be inhibited by the addition of potassium citrate.

Hypocitraturia

The beneficial effects of potassium citrate in hypocitraturia include reduction of calcium ionic activity, inhibition of crystallization, and elevation of urine pH, which increases uric acid solubility. On the usual dose of liquid potassium citrate (15 mEq q.i.d.), the urine citrate rises about 400 mg/day and urine pH by about 0.5 units. Treatment of distal RTA requires larger doses, while treatment of isolated idiopathic hypocitraturia requires half the dose. A potential drawback of potassium citrate therapy is potassium accumulation in patients with renal insufficiency.

Hyperuricosuric Urate Nephrolithiasis

The mainstay of therapy of hyperuricosuria associated with uric acid stone formation is alkalinization of the urine to pH 6.7 to 7. While any alkali can do this, potassium citrate is preferable; citrate provides an inhibitory action, and potassium obviates the risk of sodium loading predisposing to hypercalciuria. Rarely, if the hyperuricosuria is marked or is associated with hyperuricemia (i.e., gout), allopurinol is added (300 mg qd).

Cysteinuria

Therapy for cystinuria is directed at reducing the supersaturation of cysteine in the urine. Conservative measures include fluid loading to reduce the concentration of cysteine, dietary methionine restriction to reduce the biosynthetic contribution to cysteine supplies, and alkali therapy. Alkalinization is controversial, as cysteine's solubility does not significantly increase until the pH reaches 7.5, which is the highest obtainable with oral alkalinization. With higher pH, the risk of calcium phosphate precipitation also increases. If alkalinization is used, the usual dosage is potassium citrate, 15 to 20 mEq b.i.d. to q.i.d.

More specific therapy includes D-penicillamine or alpha-mercaptopropionylglycine (alpha-MPG; tiopronin). These compounds form sulfhydryl linkages with cysteine, resulting in more soluble hybrid complexes. Penicillamine's use is limited by multisystem toxicities, which require cessation of therapy in 50% of patients. Alpha-MPG appears to be better tolerated and is now preferred. After surgery, residual stone fragments may be dissolved with direct percutaneous irrigation with alkalinizing agents such as sodium bicarbonate or tromethamine-E (THAM-E), an organic amine buffer.

Infection Stones

The cornerstone of therapy for infection stones is complete surgical removal (open surgery, percutaneous procedures, and ESWL) and elimination of the urea-splitting bacteria trapped in the stones. If bacteriologically active residua are present, renal irrigations should be considered, for example, 10% hemiacidrin (Renacidin), which contains an acidic solution of citric acid and magnesium. It is theorized that the magnesium substitutes for calcium from the stone, the resulting magnesium complex being soluble in the other components of the solution. The two significant risks of hemiacidrin irrigation are hypermagnesemia and urosepsis. Of note in this regard was the FDA's former ban on hemiacidrin renal irrigation following four deaths; these were subsequently felt to be due to sepsis, and hemiacidrin is now approved for renal use. Serum magnesium levels must be monitored, and suppressive antibiotics should be administered during irrigation. The irrigation setup must have a pressure limit of 30 cm H_2O, and the irrigations should be stopped if infection or hypermagnesemia develop.

Recent ESWL literature suggests that complete elimination of stone material may not be necessary, as some residual fragments have been documented not to recur either radiologically or bacteriologically. When remaining fragments cause infection persistence, ESWL may increase the surface area, allowing chemodissolution or antibiotic sterilization. Systemically administered urease inhibitors such as acetohydroxamic acid (AHA) have been used, but major toxicities preclude their widespread use.

Hypomagnesiuria

Hypomagnesiuria can be treated with magnesium citrate (10 mEq b.i.d. to q.i.d.). Diarrhea is common, and is particularly troublesome in patients with enteric hyperoxaluria. Magnesium supplementation has been recommended for its inhibitor effect even in the presence of normal urine magnesium, but there is little evidence to support this usage.

SUGGESTED READINGS

Broadus NE, Burtis WJ, et al. Concerning the pathogenesis of idiopathic hypercalciuria. Contrib Nephrol 1987; 58:127.

Results of a large series of metabolic workups at a single center is presented. Monograph includes clinical as well as research aspects of metabolic stone evaluation.

Burns JR, Finlayson B. Strategies for the medical management of patients with urinary stone disease. Monogr Urol 1981; 2(4):106.

Early guide to metabolic evaluation from the University of Florida group. Includes guides to the assessment of stone-forming activity and strategies for medical treatment.

Coe FL, Parks JH, Asplin JR. The pathogenesis and treatment of kidney stones. N Engl J Med 1992; 327:1141.

Thorough review of the pathogenesis of stone formation with emphasis on crystal formation and inhibition. The principles of medical treatment are clearly enunciated.

Hosking DH, Erickson SB, Van den Berg CJ, Wilson DM, Smith LH. The stone clinic effect in patients with idiopathic calcium urolithiasis. J Urol 1983; 130:1115.

The stone clinic effect is described. The important role of adequate hydration during treatment is emphasized.

Goldwasser B, Weinerth JL, Carson CC. Calcium stone disease: an overview. J Urol 1986; 135:1.

Review article on metabolic evaluation of calcium stones, including an algorithm for evaluation.

Gregory JG. Hyperoxaluria and stone disease in the gastrointestinal bypass patient. Urol Clin North Am 1981; 8(2):331.

Report of a large experience with enteric hyperoxaluria. Pathophysiologic mechanisms are detailed and animal studies reviewed. All aspects of enteric hyperoxaluria are included in this discussion.

Herring LC. Observations on the analysis of ten thousand urinary calculi. J Urol 1962; 88(4):545.

Extensive series of stone composition analyses. Classic paper in the stone literature.

Menon M, Krishnan CS. Evaluation and medical management of the patient with calcium stone disease. Urol Clin North Am 1983; 10(4): 595.

Metabolic evaluation of calcium stones is carefully outlined and integrated into the urologic management of urolithiasis.

Uribarri J, Man SO, Carroll HJ. The first kidney stone. Ann Int Med 1989; 11:1006.

Assessment of the controversy regarding the metabolic evaluation of first-time stone formers. Efficacy and benefits are discussed. Guidelines for medical evaluation are presented.

Singer A, Das S. Cystinuria: a review of pathophysiology and management. J Urol 1989; 142:669.

Comprehensive, updated review of cystinuria and cystine lithiasis. Pathophysiology and treatment are emphasized.

Lerner SP, Gleeson MJ, Griffith DP. Infection stones. J Urol 1989; 141(2): 753.

Emphasis on the urologic aspects of infection stone disease. Role of urease enzyme described and the efficacy of various treatment modalities presented.

Williams HE. Oxalic acid and the hyperoxaluric syndromes. Kidney Int 1978; 13:410.

Strong biochemical and metabolic emphasis. Recommended reading for urologist seeking an understanding of the fundamentals of oxalic acid synthesis, oxalate absorption, and stone formation.

CHAPTER 13

Renal and Adrenal Causes of Hypertension

R. Ernest Sosa

Of the estimated 50 million patients in the United States who have hypertension, between 5 and 10% have surgically curable, or secondary, hypertension. Urologic evaluation aims to identify and treat those renal and adrenal conditions that cause hypertension and are reversible by operative procedures. This avoids lifelong medical therapy and reduces the mortality and morbidity associated with end-organ damage to the kidneys, heart, and brain.

The goal of urologic evaluation is the rapid, cost-effective, and minimally invasive identification of the causes of secondary hypertension. A clear understanding of the pathophysiology of the kidneys and adrenals that leads to hypertension and the use of modern radiologic imaging techniques allow for precise diagnosis in most patients with secondary hypertension.

PRIMARY VERSUS SECONDARY HYPERTENSION

Hypertension is usually defined as a blood pressure that consistently exceeds 140/90 mm Hg on three occasions when obtained at least 1 week apart. Proper measurement of blood pressure requires a nonstressful environment, a qualified observer, and a properly functioning sphygmomanometer with an appropriately sized cuff. Some elderly patients have pseudohypertension due to sclerotic, poorly compliant arteries, which require high cuff occlusion pressures. "White coat" hypertension occurs in patients who have normal blood pressures at home but elevated levels in the doctor's office.

Hypertension is classified into primary and secondary categories. Secondary causes have well defined etiologies and mechanisms of hypertension (Table 13.1). Primary hypertension, on the other hand, is less well understood, much more prevalent than secondary hypertension, and has strong genetic/familial tendencies. Complications of hypertension result from the increased levels of systemic blood pressure and accelerated atherosclerosis, which leads to coronary artery disease, cardiac failure, and peripheral vascular disease.

Nondrug treatment is useful in patients with mild hypertension. Weight loss, salt restriction, exercise, and reduced stress contribute to a lowering of blood pressure. Drug treatment includes beta blockers, diuretics, and vasodilators. More recently, there is an increasing reliance on calcium channel blockers, converting enzyme inhibitors, and alpha$_1$-antagonists.

Disorders responsible for secondary hypertension include chronic renal disease, renovascular disease, pheochromocytoma, Cushing's syndrome, and primary aldosteronism. Patients with these conditions either do not respond to typical antihypertensive drug therapy or become refractory to treatment after initial control of their blood pressure. Variable renal diseases, renal trauma, glomerulonephritis, pyelonephritis, urinary-tract infection, severe childhood vesicoureteral reflux, and diabetes mellitus can cause renal parenchymal damage and secondary hypertension. Labile hypertension associated with vasomotor instability, headaches, sweating, and palpitation occur with pheochromocytomas. A family history of multiple endocrine adenomatosis (types I and II), neurofibromatosis, and von Recklinghausen's disease raises the possibility of pheochromocytoma. Uncontrolled, malignant hypertension, or acceleration of previously well controlled hypertension, suggests a renovascular etiology, particularly in young patients. Polyuria, polydipsia, and muscle weakness, especially in young women with mild hypertension, are typical of primary hyperaldosteronism.

The presence of hypertensive retinopathy, abdominal vascular bruits, carotid bruits, diminished lower extremity pulses, and other signs of generalized atherosclerotic vascular disease also suggests renovascular hypertension. Patients with Cushing's syndrome usually have external stigmata,

Table 13.1: Common Causes of Secondary Hypertension

Renovascular disease
Pheochromocytoma
Glucocorticoid excess (Cushing's syndrome)
Primary hyperaldosteronism
Renal parenchymal disease
Coarctation of the aorta

for example, truncal obesity, skin striae, purpura, moon face, and buffalo humps. The clinical clues to the various causes of secondary hypertension are summarized in Table 13.2.

Essential laboratory tests in suspected cases of secondary hypertension include a complete blood count, urinalysis, urine culture, fasting blood sugar, chest x-ray, electrocardiogram, serum electrolytes, and renal function studies. Depending on the suspected cause, further diagnostic tests are indicated. The history and physical findings may suggest the cause of the secondary hypertension; however, specific biochemical and radiographic studies are necessary for definitive diagnosis.

Table 13.2: Clues to Suspected Secondary Hypertension

Renovascular Disease

Abrupt onset of moderate/severe hypertension
"Malignant" hypertension
Acceleration of hypertension in spite of established blood pressure control
Flank/abdominal/carotid bruits
Rare in blacks
Decline in renal function after initiation of antihypertensive therapy

Primary Hyperaldosteronism

Young females
Fatigue, muscle weakness
Hypokalemia
Mild to moderate hypertension
Polydipsia, polyuria

Cushing's Syndrome

Women aged 20–40 years
Truncal obesity, buffalo hump, moon facies
Skin striae, easy bruising
Hirsutism
Muscle weakness
Osteoporosis

Pheochromocytoma

Sustained but fluctuating hypertension
Episodic headaches, tachycardia, diaphoresis, palpitations
Association with multiple endocrine neoplasia syndromes (types II, III)
Familial tendency

HYPERTENSION OF RENAL ORIGIN

In the early nineteenth century, Bright (1836) first noted the association between renal disease and hypertension. Several decades later, Tigerstedt and Bergmann (1898) injected a water-soluble extract derived from the renal cortex of a healthy rabbit into a vein of a second rabbit, producing a marked and sustained hypertension. They coined the term *renin* for this extract. No further study on the association of renal disease and hypertension was carried out until Goldblatt (1934) produced a reversible elevation in systemic arterial blood pressure by placing a clamp on the main renal artery of one of two healthy kidneys. The blood pressure later returned to normal on removal of the kidney or the occluding clamp.

Taking a cue from Goldblatt's observations, clinicians began to perform nephrectomies in hypertensive patients with either small or hydronephrotic kidneys. Unfortunately, in many patients the hypertension did not improve. In 1956, Homer Smith critically reviewed the world's literature and reported a disappointing 26% cure rate of hypertension by nephrectomy. It became clear that unilateral renal disease coexists with hypertension more often than it is causally related to it. Stricter and more reliable guidelines were necessary to justify the removal of morphologically abnormal kidneys in hypertensive patients.

The advent of arteriography shifted the focus of surgical cure of hypertension to patients with renovascular disease. In 1974, the National Cooperative Study on renovascular hypertension reported a 51% cure rate, a 15% improvement rate, and a disappointing 34% failure rate with renal revascularization. Moreover, the morbidity and mortality rates associated with the revascularization surgery were 13% and 6%, respectively.

More reliable selection of patients for renal revascularization to cure hypertension has come about over the past decade, due in large part to a better understanding of the renin–angiotensin–aldosterone system. Renovascular disease is now regarded as the most common cause of secondary hypertension. Unilateral renal parenchymal disease is a rare cause of hypertension in adults; the exact incidence is not known. In contrast, renal vascular hypertension is potentially curable and accounts for blood pressure elevation in 5 to 10% of adult hypertensive patients.

Physiology of the Renin–Angiotensin System

The development of a variety of pharmacologic antagonists to the components of the renin–angiotensin cascade has led to a better understanding of its physiology and the elucidation of the pathophysiology of renovascular hypertension (Figure 13.1). Renin is a proteolytic enzyme formed by modified smooth-muscle cells of the afferent arteriole (juxtaglomerular

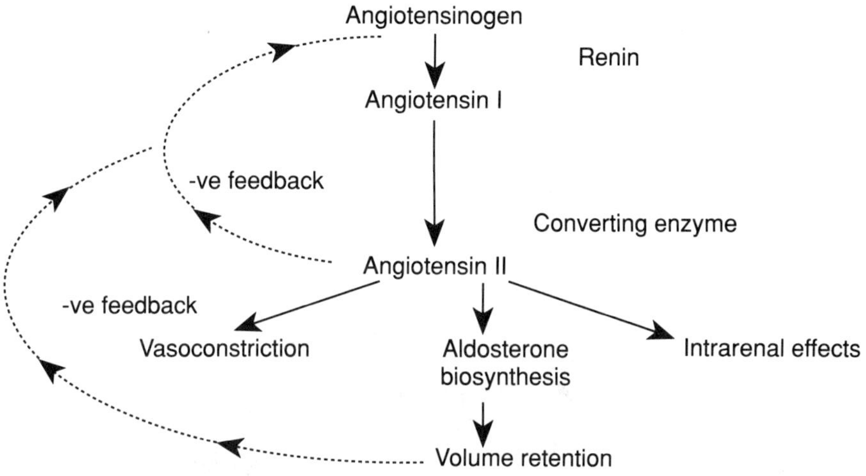

Figure 13.1: The renin–angiotensin cascade

cells), found in intimate proximity to the macula densa of the distal tubule. These microstructures are collectively known as the juxtaglomerular apparatus (Figure 13.2). Renin is released in response to (1) low glomerular perfusion pressures (baroreceptor mechanism) due to renal artery stenosis or a decrease in the mean systemic arterial pressure, (2) low chloride or sodium concentrations in the filtrate reaching the distal convoluted tubule (macula densa mechanism), and (3) adrenergic stimulation of beta$_1$-receptors in the juxtaglomerular cells. Renin is metabolized in the liver and has a half-life (T1/2) of 10 to 20 minutes. Renin splits angiotensin I (A I) off an alpha$_2$-globulin (angiotensinogen) that is produced by the liver. Angiotensin converting enzyme (ACE) cleaves a dipeptide off the inactive angiotensin I to produce active angiotensin II (A II), the protagonist of the renin–angiotensin system.

The negative feedback controls for renin release are volume retention and angiotension II (see Figure 13.1). A II regulates blood pressure and the sodium-volume balance by several mechanisms. It activates the zona glomerulosa of the adrenal gland to increase the biosynthesis of aldosterone and increase renal sodium reabsorption. A II also stimulates thirst, and it has a direct antidiuretic effect on the renal tubule. A II is a potent vasoconstrictor that is secreted in response to rapid-onset hypotension so as to restore systemic blood pressure. Angiotensin converting enzyme (ACE)—also known as kininase II—is present in plasma, vascular endothelium, and the lungs. In addition to catalyzing the conversion of angiotensin I to angiotensin II, ACE is responsible for the degradation of active renin species to inactive fragments.

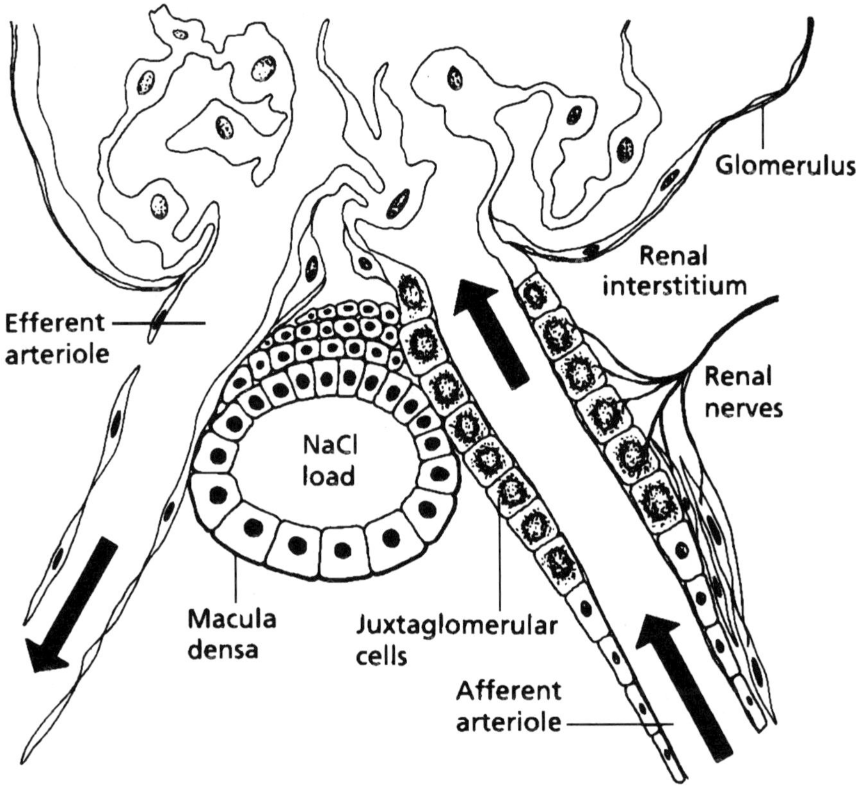

Figure 13.2: Components of juxtaglomerular apparatus. *Reproduced with permission from Webster G, Kirby R, King L, et al eds. Reconstructive Urology Vol 1. Boston: Blackwell Scientific Publications, 1993:5.*

Pathophysiology of Renal Vascular Hypertension

Our understanding of the pathophysiology of renal vascular hypertension is largely derived from work in experimental models of hypertension. In a two-kidney, one-clip, hypertensive animal model, the clipped kidney has markedly decreased perfusion pressure and blood flow. The decrease in mean renal perfusion pressure stimulates the baroreceptor mechanism, and the decrease in the filtered sodium load activates the macula densa mechanism to increase renin secretion. The contralateral normal kidney experiences an increase in mean systemic arterial blood pressure and a pressure-induced natriuresis, which serves to shut off renin secretion by totally suppressing the baroreceptor and macula densa mechanisms.

There are no pathognomonic signs for identifying patients with renal vascular hypertension. It is rare in blacks. However, certain risk factors can be identified in patients with sustained blood pressure elevations (Figure 13.3), and a high index of suspicion should be entertained if multiple risk factors are present. Marked reduction of severe hypertension or sudden decrease in glomerular filtration rates in response to treatment with converting enzyme inhibitors or calcium channel-blocking drugs are good clues to the presence of renovascular hypertension. Hypokalemia

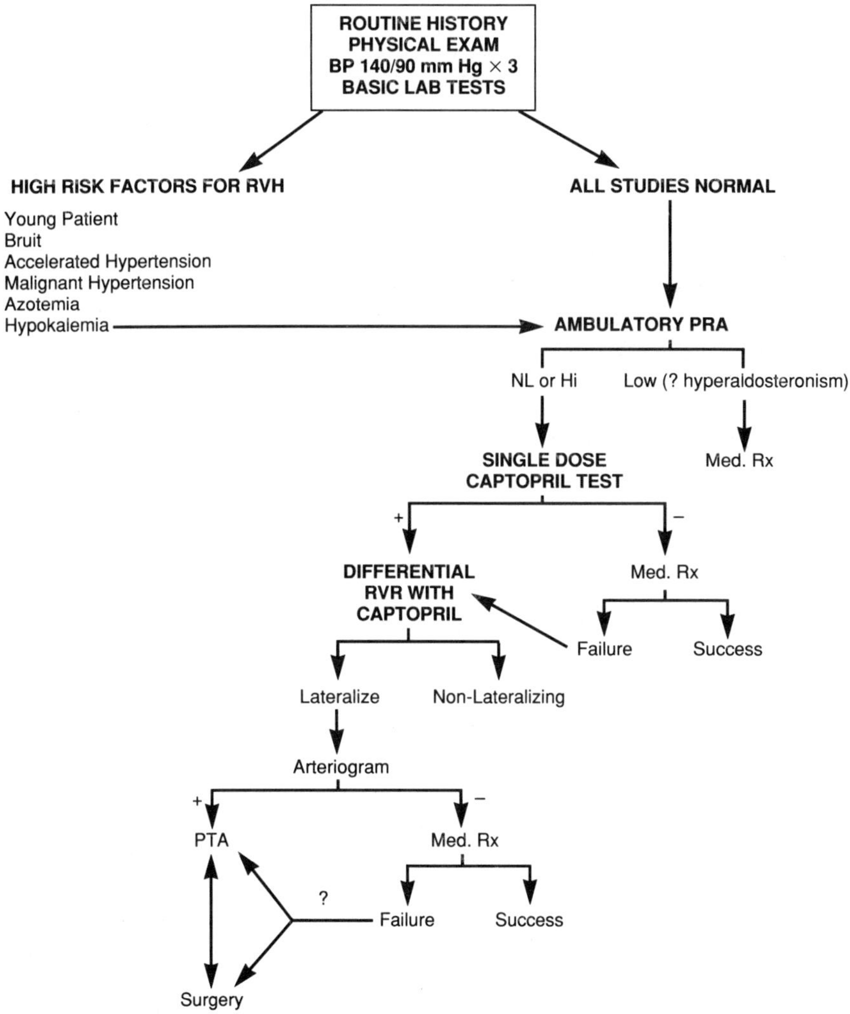

Figure 13.3: Renovascular hypertension—clinical and diagnostic algorithm

(unprovoked or in response to thiazide diuretic therapy) may reflect the increased aldosterone activity of the activated renin–angiotensin cascade in response to renal vascular disease. Young patients with renal vascular hypertension or patients with hypertension and abdominal bruits, accelerated or malignant hypertension, or azotemia associated with hypertension are at an increased risk for "high renin" hypertension.

Evaluation of patients with suspected renovascular hypertension starts with an ambulatory plasma renin activity (PRA) determination. For this test all antihypertensive medications, particularly diuretics, are discontinued. Patients with cardiac disease may continue using beta blockers. A 24-hour urine collection is obtained to establish the sodium content of the urine. Following 4 hours of ambulation, plasma renin activity is determined by sampling the peripheral venous system. Plasma renin activity level is then indexed to the 24-hour urine sodium concentration. Patients with low plasma renin activity are unlikely to have renal vascular hypertension, and they should be evaluated for hyperaldosteronism and started on medical treatment.

Eighty percent of patients with renal vascular hypertension have increased plasma renin activity. Clearly 20% of the patients with renal vascular hypertension will display a normal plasma renin activity. Moreover, 10% of patients with essential hypertension have high plasma renin activity. Therefore, measurement of plasma renin activity has limitations in its sensitivity and specificity. These false-negative (low or normal) and false-positive (elevated) PRA values somewhat limit the usefulness of PRA determination for screening. The sensitivity of PRA measurement in peripheral venous blood can be increased by the administration of captopril (an angiotensin-converting enzyme inhibitor) prior to sampling.

Renovascular hypertension should be evaluated in a stepwise fashion from the less sophisticated, less invasive, and less quantitative tests to the definitive, invasive procedures that confirm the hemodynamic significance of anatomically localized renal arterial lesions (Figure 13.3). The more definitive tests provide measurable assessment of the anatomy, pathophysiology, and potential reversibility of the hypertension.

To identify more predictively patients with renal vascular hypertension, a single-dose captopril test is performed. For this study, patients are seated and have plasma renin and blood pressure determinations. Twenty-five milligrams of captopril, a converting enzyme inhibitor, is administered by mouth, and the plasma renin activity is determined 45 minutes later. Throughout this period, the blood pressure is monitored closely to assure the patient does not become hypotensive. Patients with renal vascular hypertension will have a hyperreninemic response; that is, the final renin level will be over 12 ng/ml/hour. The increment of change will be 10 ng/ml/hour, and the percent will be at least 150%. Patients with normal or high renin essential hypertension do not exhibit a hyperreninemic response to captopril administration. Patients having a positive test proceed to localization studies in the out-patient setting. Renal-vein renins are sampled with and without captopril. Samples of venous blood are obtained from each renal vein and the superior and inferior vena cavae. Interpretation of renal vein renin activity is based on (1) renin hypersecretion by the kidney with the stenotic artery and (2) renin suppression in the normal, uninvolved kidney. A PRA ratio of over 1.5 (ratio of the PRA involved side to the PRA uninvolved kidney) strongly suggests renal arterial stenosis with a high expectation of cure of hypertension following renal revascularization.

Drugs that stimulate renin release (e.g., diuretics and angiotensin converting enzyme inhibitors) accentuate the differences between the kidneys and improve the sensitivity of the test. The ischemic kidney will show a high renin secretion, whereas the normal kidney will have its renin secretion suppressed. The addition of captopril further increases the renal-vein renin levels from the ischemic kidney. Patients with negative captopril tests are treated medically. Measurement of renin in selective samples of renal venous blood is the best method to quantitate the functional contribution of renal artery stenosis to potentially reversible hypertension. Angiographic contrast materials alter renin release, and renal venous PRA sampling should therefore be done before angiography. Following successful revascularization of an ischemic kidney, the hypersecretion of renin returns to normal levels and the contralateral normal kidney begins to secrete renin at expected, normal levels.

The major causes of renal vascular hypertension are atherosclerotic renal arterial disease and the various types of fibromuscular dysplasia (Table 13.3). These account for over 95% of cases of renal vascular hypertension. Aneurysms of the renal artery, dissection, or arteritis rarely cause renovascular hypertension. Renal atherosclerosis accounts for approximately two-thirds of all patients with renal vascular hypertension and is more common in males. The atheroma typically involves the proximal third of the renal artery, is usually eccentric, and is frequently bilateral. Fibromuscular dysplasia accounts for one-third of renovascular hypertension and commonly occurs in young (<40 years) women. The most common type of fibromuscular dysplasia is medial fibromuscular dysplasia, which results in the angiographic pattern of a "string of beads" affecting the distal renal artery, and which is often bilateral (Figure 13.4). The other types of fibromuscular dysplasia (perimedial, intimal, etc.) are less common but frequently associated with progressive renal arterial disease and thrombosis (occlusion of the artery).

Table 13.3: Renovascular Hypertension

Atherosclerotic Disease
Patients >50 years, usually white males
Heavy smoking history
Clinical evidence of widespread vascular disease
Affects proximal arterial segment
Frequently bilateral
Best treated surgically (bypass graft, endarterectomy)
Fibromuscular Dysplasia
Patients <40 years
Female preponderance
Distal segments of renal artery
Percutaneous transluminal angioplasty effective

Because of a high false-negative rate (20 to 30%), the intravenous urogram (IVU) is too insensitive to be used as a screening test for renovascular disease. The following findings on an excretory urogram done

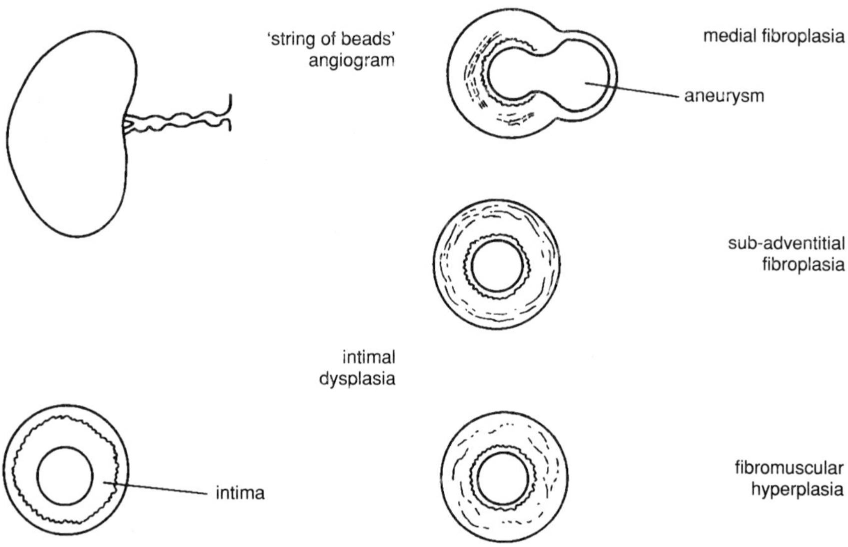

Figure 13.4: Renal arterial dysplasia may give a "string of beads" appearance and may take several histological forms: intimal dysplasia, medial fibroplasia, subadventitial fibroplasia, or fibromuscular hyperplasia. *Reproduced with permission from Blandy J. Lecture Notes on Urology, 4th ed. Oxford: Blackwell Scientific Publications, 1991: 115.*

for other indications may suggest renal vascular disease: renal asymmetry, delayed pyelogram with contrast hyperconcentration, and collateral blood vessels (notching of the pelvis or ureter). The vascular anatomy of the kidneys can be visualized radiographically by selective renal angiography or intravenous/intra-arterial digital substraction angiography. Renal artery stenosis of less than 50 to 60% of the luminal diameter is unlikely to cause reduced blood flow to the affected kidneys.

The choice of treatment in a particular patient depends on the type, extent, and location of the lesion, the risks of surgical revascularization, and the expertise of the surgeon and interventional radiologist. The risks of revascularization include the anesthetic risk and the risk of kidney infarction. Blood pressure is surgically cured or improved in up to 60 or 80% of patients with atherosclerotic renovascular hypertension. Percutaneous angioplasty, though safer, carries the risks of dissection or thrombosis, failure to improve renal blood flow, and the likelihood of restenosis. In general, localized, discrete lesions (e.g., fibromuscular dysplasia) are best treated by percutaneous transluminal angioplasty. The more diffuse lesions of atheromatous renal artery disease are more amenable to surgical revascularization (Table 13.3).

UNILATERAL RENAL PARENCHYMAL DISEASE AND HYPERTENSION

Approximately 90% of hypertensive patients with unilateral renal parenchymal disease can be expected to have low or normal plasma renin activity. Sodium and volume retention play a primary etiologic role in hypertension associated with compromised renal function. Thorough evaluation of these patients requires correction of urinary-tract obstruction and infection (Figure 13.5). Differential and total renal function should be determined by standard clearance methods or by excretory pyelography or nuclear imaging, as possible. Assessment of differential renal function is imperative in considerations for nephrectomy as an attempt to cure the hypertension.

For purposes of this discussion, renal parenchymal diseases associated with hypertension are divided into two sections. Conditions that usually do not require surgical intervention are discussed first. The second section considers renal parenchymal diseases that almost always require surgical management.

Renal Parenchymal Diseases Not Requiring Surgery

Reflux nephropathy is defined as renal parenchymal scarring associated with vesicoureteral reflux. Approximately 10 to 12% of children with reflux nephropathy who have undergone successful ureterovesical reim-

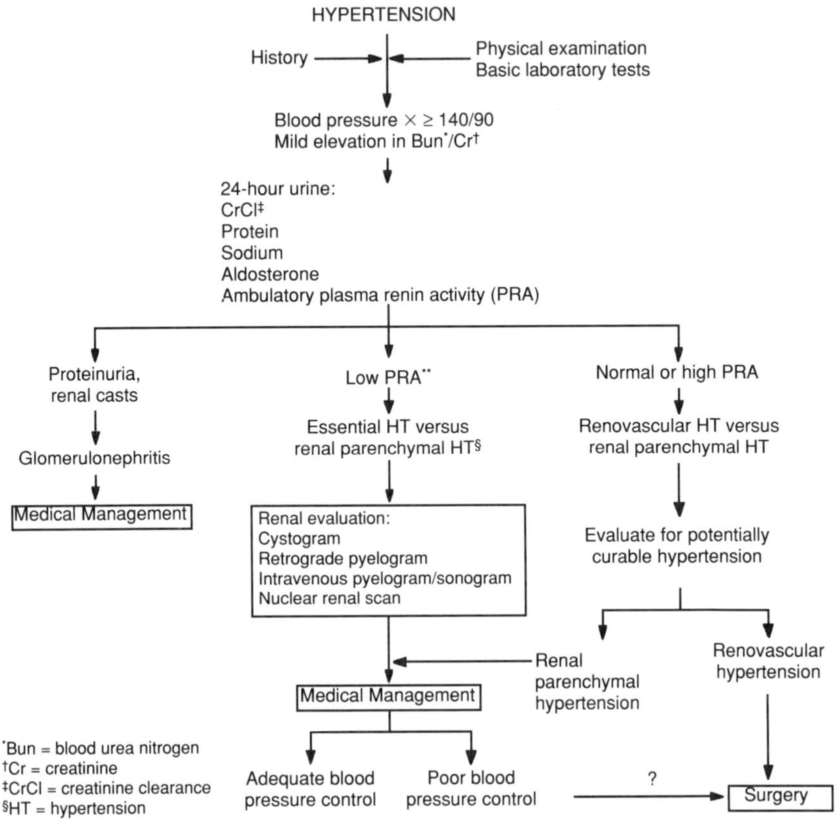

Figure 13.5: Renal parenchymal hypertension—clinical and diagnostic algorithm

plantation become hypertensive by late adolescence or early adulthood. Retrospective analyses of prereimplant radiographs have revealed that 19% of patients with bilateral and 11% of patients with unilateral renal scarring at the time of reimplant surgery later develop hypertension in early adulthood. In contrast, patients with radiologically normal renal contours and normal renal function at the time of reimplant surgery do not become hypertensive.

The precise mechanism producing hypertension in reflux nephropathy has eluded researchers. Lateralization of renin production to the diseased kidney has been documented in unilateral as well as bilateral asymmetrical reflux nephropathy. However, young patients with reflux nephropathy who are not hypertensive have also been shown to have increased plasma renin activity. The roles of the hormonal systems involved in the regulation of blood pressure, such as the sympathetic nervous system and vasopressin and calcium metabolism, are not well defined.

The slow onset of hypertension in patients with reflux nephropathy dictates careful, long-term follow-up after ureteral implantation, including periodic determinations of blood pressure, renal function, and size. Blood pressure increases should be controlled medically. The urine should be checked for the presence of infection, blood cells, casts, and protein. A number of patients with reflux nephropathy suffer progressive deterioration in renal function that is hastened by uncontrolled hypertension and infection.

Ask-Upmark Kidney

Ask-Upmark described a rare form of segmental renal hypoplasia (affecting one or both kidneys), associated with hypertension in children and young adults. The involved kidney tends to be small with globular contours. Radiographically, deep grooves on the cortical surface are present overlying dilated calyces. The adjacent renal tissue appears to be well preserved. Histologically, the hypoplastic areas are devoid of glomeruli and manifest thickened, stenosed vessels, and an increased number of juxtaglomerular cells near the damaged vessels. An increased renin content in these JG cells has been demonstrated by immunofluorescence and peroxidase/antiperoxidase techniques. Histologically, the inflammatory cell infiltrates that characterize the appearance of interstitial nephritis in reflux nephropathy are absent. This condition afflicts females twice as often as males and may be associated with radiation nephritis.

Therapeutic doses of radiation delivered to the kidney within treatment portals can produce renal injury that may progress to renal insufficiency and hypertension. Radiation injures the glomeruli, renal tubules, and intrarenal vessels. Hypertension may be a late manifestation of radiation nephritis, presenting as a result of salt and water retention induced by renal insufficiency.

Page Kidney

Page (1939) produced a renin-dependent model of hypertension by wrapping a dog kidney in cellophane. The hypertension could be reversed by removing the cellophane wrap or the kidney. The clinical equivalent of this hypertensive model is that of a kidney compressed by a subcapsular or perirenal process causing renal ischemia and unilateral hypersecretion of renin. Etiologies for the perinephric processes include blunt trauma, percutaneous nephrostomy tube placement, closed renal biopsy, anticoagulant overdose, and tumor hemorrhage. In the majority of patients with benign causes of subcapsular bleeding, removal of the offending factors and medical management of the hypertension often lead to a reduction of the blood pressure.

The treatment of hypertension in patients with unilateral renal parenchymal disease is primarily pharmacological. Patients with low plasma renin activity respond favorably to calcium channel blockers or diuretics. In normal or high renin hypertension, beta blockers decrease renin secretion and converting enzyme inhibitors prevent the formation of angiotensin II. The former drugs have a depressor effect that is synergistic with the effects of calcium channel blockers. Most hypertensive patients with unilateral renal parenchymal disease can be adequately managed in this manner. A sterile, unobstructed urinary tract complements the medical management of hypertension and decreases the progression of renal disease.

Nephrectomy should be avoided if the blood pressure can be controlled with antihypertensive medications and if the glomerular filtration rate in the uninvolved kidney is sufficient to ensure the patient's survival. Historically, only a small percentage of hypertensive patients have been helped by unilateral nephrectomy. In renal parenchymal disease, a decrease in the number of functioning nephrons occurs, with significant compromise of sodium and water excreting capacity. Moreover, renal disease tends to be progressive in nature and may initially afflict the contralateral kidney in a subclinical manner. Removal of the diseased kidney may gain a transient lowering of the blood pressure, only to have the parenchymal disease process unmasked in the contralateral "normal" kidney. Therefore, every attempt should be made to preserve total renal mass. Nephrectomy is justified only if medical management proves unsatisfactory, if split renal function studies indicate that the glomerular filtration rate of the diseased kidney is less than 10 ml/min with adequate contralateral function, and if the criteria for identifying curable renal vascular hypertension are strictly satisfied.

Renal Parenchymal Diseases That May Require Surgical Treatment

Acute unilateral ureteral obstructing can produce a renin profile that mimics the pattern seen in patients with unilateral renovascular hypertension. Removal of the obstruction factor returns peripheral plasma renin activity levels to normal and cures the hypertension. However, less than one-third of patients with acute unilateral hydronephrosis are hypertensive. Regardless of the effects on blood pressure, intervention is indicated to decompress the obstructed renal unit for maximization of renal function and prevention of the known complications of urinary obstruction.

Sixty percent of children with renal tumors are hypertensive. The blood pressure elevation is generally moderate, but severe or "malignant" elevations do occur. The mechanisms of hypertension include tumor secretion of renin and compression of the renal artery or normal, adjacent renal parenchyma by the tumor. The hypertensive state is eliminated by eradication of the tumor.

Another renal neoplasm found in young patients is the reninoma—a renin-secreting juxtaglomerular tumor. These rare tumors have been reported in patients ranging in age from 7 to 69 years. Reninomas produce large amounts of renin and systemic blood pressure elevation. Diagnosis relies on the documentation of increased peripheral plasma renin activity indexed to a 24-hour urinary sodium test and lateralization of renin secretion to the side of the tumor, reminiscent of the pattern seen in unilateral renal vascular hypertension. Arteriography, however, reveals a normal renal vasculature. Occasionally, a small subcapsular lucency is detected during the nephrogram phase. Treatment by removal of the involved kidney has been curative, although partial nephrectomy has been shown to be equally advantageous.

Up to 30% of patients with renal cell carcinoma are hypertensive at initial presentation. The incidence of renal cell carcinoma peaks in the sixth decade, which is also the time in life during which essential hypertension is most frequently found. Blood pressure returns to normal levels in approximately one-third of patients after radical nephrectomy; the remaining patients have essential hypertension. Renal cell carcinomas can produce hypertension due to their endocrine function; renin and erythropoietin can be secreted by these tumors. Erythropoietin is theorized to elevate the arterial pressure due to an associated increase in the blood's viscosity secondary to polycythemia, which increases peripheral vascular resistance. Hypertension can also be due to compression of the normal renal parenchyma by the tumor mass.

In summary, unilateral renal parenchymal diseases are rarely associated with high plasma renin activity but are characterized by a progressive loss of functioning nephrons and a diminution in sodium-volume excreting capacity, which contributes to the hypertensive state. Therapy in most cases aims at preserving nephrons by medical management of the hypertension, eradication of urinary infection, and correction of urinary obstruction. Nephrectomy is generally contraindicated if renal function has been compromised. When medical management has proved ineffective, two general indications for nephrectomy are the treatment of renal neoplasm and the removal of a nonfiltering kidney producing large amounts of renin.

ADRENAL DISORDERS THAT PRODUCE HYPERTENSION

Primary Hyperaldosteronism

Soon after the hormone electrocortin (aldosterone) was identified, Dr. Jerome Conn (1955) described a case of hypertension caused by an aldosterone-secreting adrenal adenoma. The patient exhibited hypertension, severe muscular weakness, hypokalemia, and alkalosis—signs and symptoms that still characterize the disease and alert the physician to its presence. Primary hyperaldosteronism accounts for about 1% of all cases of hypertension. Excessive aldosterone produced in the adrenal cortex results in hypertension, suppressed plasma renin activity, and hypokalemia. Most patients (about 75%) have unilateral, aldosterone-producing adrenal adenomas; the remainder have bilateral, nodular adrenal hyperplasia. Hypokalemia leads to marked muscle weakness, metabolic alkalosis, and polyuria—characteristics of primary aldosteronism. Spontaneous or provoked (by use of diuretics or salt-loading) hypokalemia should arouse the suspicion of primary aldosteronism and lead the clinician to perform specific diagnostic tests. The typical patient is a young woman with polyuria, polydipsia, muscle weakness, and mild hypertension.

Unprovoked hypokalemia is a major clue to the presence of primary hyperaldosteronism (Figure 13.6). Alert patients may realize that their muscular weakness is less severe when salt intake is restricted. In this setting with less sodium delivery to the distal nephron, the serum potassium may be normal. Thus, before the disease is excluded a patient should be saltloaded with 10 g of sodium intake daily for 1 week and serum potassium levels rechecked. A low plasma renin level and a significantly elevated aldosterone

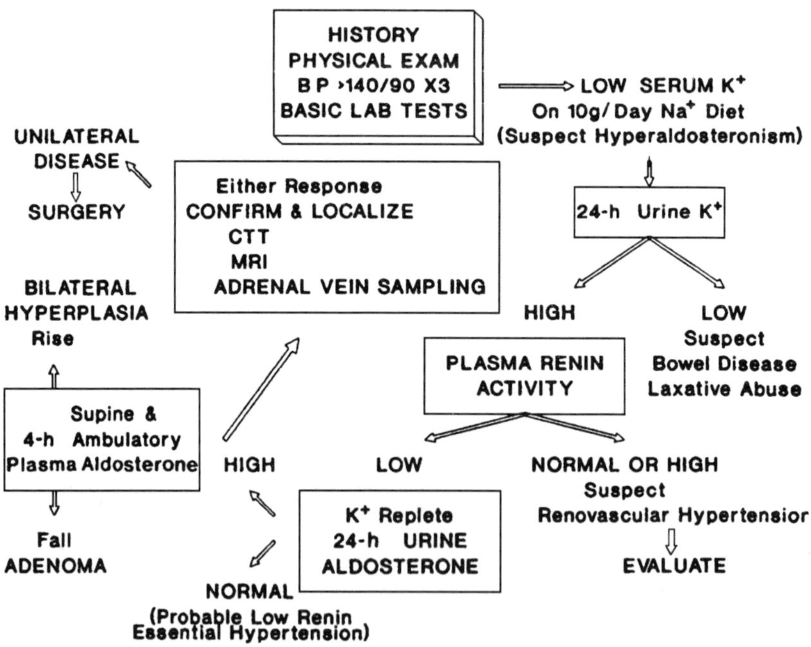

Figure 13.6: Primary hyperaldosteronism—clinical and diagnostic algorithm

level in plasma or urine are typically diagnostic. Sodium restriction probably explains reported cases of normokalemic hyperaldosteronism. Documentation of renal loss of potassium should be carried out with a 24-hour urine collection since bowel disorders associated with diarrhea can induce potassium loss, weakness, and diarrhea. When hyperaldosteronism is suspected, the renin–angiotensin–aldosterone axis is evaluated. Plasma aldosterone and plasma renin activity are measured and indexed to the 24-hour urinary sodium content. The 24-hour urinary excretion of aldosterone is equally accurate. Since potassium is a major stimulus for aldosterone secretion, the serum potassium should be normalized by oral potassium supplementation before plasma or urinary aldosterone determinations are made.

Most patients with hypokalemia and hypertension have secondary hyperaldosteronism due to renal artery stenosis or renal parenchymal disease rather than primary hyperaldosteronism due to adrenal adenoma or hyperplasia. These patients exhibit elevated plasma renin activity. In contrast, patients with primary adrenal disease resulting in elevated plasma and urinary aldosterone exhibit salt retention that is sensed by the kidney, resulting in a low plasma renin activity that does not respond to normal stimulus of sodium depletion on diuretic administration. Thus, the current criteria for the diagnosis of primary hyperaldosteronism are hypokalemia, low plasma renin activity that persists despite sodium depletion, and high plasma or urine aldosterone levels that remain unsuppressed despite sodium loading.

It is recognized that some patients exhibiting the above criteria have bilateral adrenal hyperplasia as the underlying pathologic entity. This disorder has a variety of names, including idiopathic adrenal hyperplasia, pseudoprimary hyperaldosteronism, or simply bilateral hyperplasia, and is composed of a family of subtypes. The hypertension in these patients is not cured by adrenalectomy, and the etiology of the disease is unknown, although a central stimulatory hormone is suspected. The two entities must be differentiated before surgical exploration is recommended. Once primary aldosteronism is confirmed biochemically, the variety caused by a solitary adrenal adenoma should be distinguished from that caused by multinodular, bilateral adrenal hyperplasia. Plasma aldosterone levels determined in the supine and upright positions (after 4 hours of ambulation) can be diagnostic. Most patients (70%) with aldosterone-producing adenomas fail to show the expected rise in plasma aldosterone that occurs in normal patients and patients with bilateral hyperplasia after a 4-hour ambulation period. In fact, there is often a paradoxical fall in plasma aldosterone level despite a small rise in plasma renin activity in patients with adenomas.

The localization tests used in suspected cases of hyperaldosteronism include adrenal vein sampling for aldosterone levels, computerized axial tomography, and magnetic resonance imaging. Venous sampling confirms the biological activity of the adenoma. The major difficulty is engaging and sampling the short right adrenal vein. Plasma cortisol levels should always be obtained to confirm proper catheter placement within the adrenal veins.

Once a patient has been diagnosed as having an adenoma, spironolactone is given to normalize serum potassium levels, and the adenoma is surgically removed. Lesions on the right are approached through a modified posterior 11th or 12th rib incision, and those on the left through a standard 11th rib flank incision. Patients with bilateral hyperplasia are treated primarily with spironolactone, although a few undergo unilateral adrenalectomy if the adrenal vein sampling shows marked asymmetry with predominant aldosterone production on one side.

Cushing's Syndrome

The clinical stigmata of hypercortisolism found on history and physical examination remain the cornerstone for the diagnosis of Cushing's syndrome. Hypertension is only one of the many clinical features of Cushing's syndrome, the clinical picture that results from the excessive production of cortisol, regardless of the underlying cause. Cushing's disease denotes the cases of Cushing's syndrome caused by the overproduction of ACTH in the pituitary gland. Most cases of Cushing's syndrome (about 85%) represent secondary hypercortisolism, in which adrenal hyperplasia results from overstimulation by the excessive production of ACTH from pituitary microadenomas. The first step in diagnosis is verification of the clinical impression. Normal yet obese subjects exhibit a diurnal variation in plasma cortisol levels. The normal morning rise in plasma cortisol is suppressed by dexamethasone 1 mg given orally the preceding night (Figure 13.7). Patients with Cushing's syndrome have elevated evening plasma cortisol levels, and they fail to suppress in response to dexamethasone administration.

Cushing's syndrome results from adrenal glucocorticoid excess due to adrenal, bilateral hyperplasia (Cushing's disease), adrenal carcinoma, and rarely, ectopic adrenocorticotropic hormone (ACTH) production by tumors of the lung, bronchi, thymus, kidney, or pancreas. The diagnosis of Cushing's is established by the demonstration of excessive cortisol secretion, loss of the normal diurnal variation in cortisol secretion, and loss of the normal feedback over the pituitary gland. All of these groups are identified by the screening tests mentioned above. The next step in evaluation is the high-dose dexamethasone suppression test: dexamethasone 2 mg orally q.i.d. Patients with Cushing's disease (pituitary adenomas) show suppressed morning plasma cortisol levels. The cortisol level of patients with adrenal adenoma, carcinoma, or ectopic ACTH-producing tumors is not suppressed by high-dose dexamethasone administra-

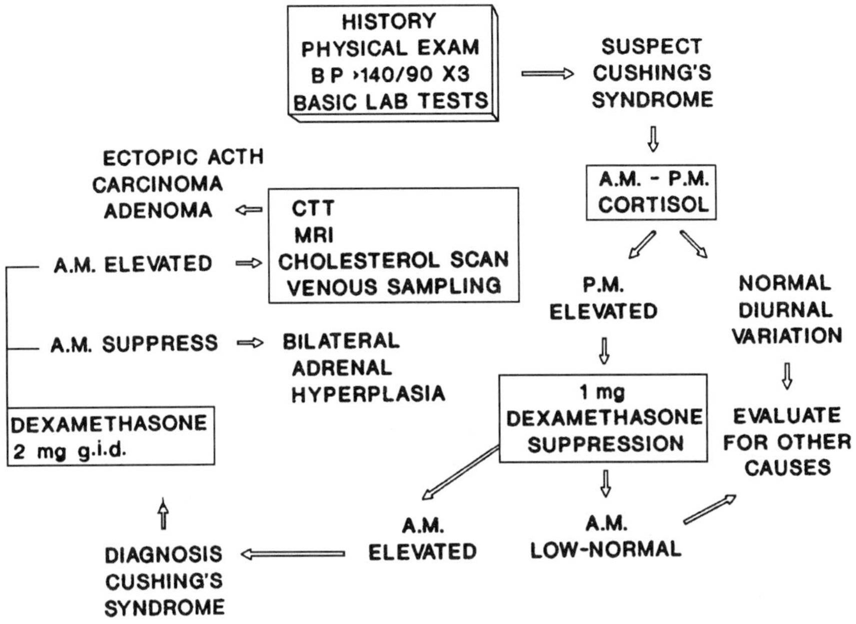

Figure 13.7: Cushing's syndrome—diagnostic approach

tion. In patients with Cushing's disease further evaluation is directed to the hypothalamic–pituitary axis to determine etiology of the abnormally increased ACTH production. Cushing's disease is best localized by computed tomography and treated by surgical excision (transphenoid resection) or pituitary irradiation.

The other causes of Cushing's syndrome represent primary hypercortisolism, in which a primary disorder of the adrenal cortex elaborates excessive cortisol. Adrenal adenoma is the cause in 10% of cases and adenocarcinoma in 5%. The typical Cushing's syndrome patient is a young to middle-aged woman who is obese, hirsute, and hypertensive. Plasma ACTH level differentiates adrenal hyperplasia from adrenal tumors. The normal range for plasma ACTH is 20 to 100 pg/ml. A higher value indicates adrenal hyperplasia; a lower level suggests adrenal tumor. The highest levels are found in ectopic ACTH syndromes. The high-dose dexamethasone suppression test does not reliably separate ACTH-dependent pituitary Cushing's disease from ectopic ACTH Cushing's syndrome. A new investigational test—the corticotrophin-releasing hormone (CRH) stimulation test—can be used in the outpatient setting. CRH stimulation causes an elevation of ACTH and cortisol in patients with ACTH-dependent Cushing's disease, whereas patients with ectopic ACTH production have no rise. Dexamethasone suppression also causes a drop in urinary free cortisol and 17-hydroxycorticosteroids. ACTH-dependent Cushing's disease can be confidently diagnosed (>90% of patients) if urine cortisol suppression is over 90% and 17-hydroxycorticosteroid excretion falls by over 65%. Recently, inferior petrosal sinus blood sampling has been suggested as a definitive test of ACTH-dependent Cushing's disease.

Localization of adrenal adenomas or carcinomas is best carried out by CT, MRI, or iodocholesterol scanning. The CT scan is highly accurate and is widely employed. However, MRI may be very helpful in differentiating adenomas from other lesions such as metastatic deposits, some primary carcinomas, and pheochromocytomas, and may be used during pregnancy to avoid the risk of irradiation.

Once a primary adrenal lesion has been diagnosed, surgical adrenalectomy is recommended. Following adrenalectomy, all patients with Cushing's syndrome require steroid replacement until the suppressed contralateral gland regains steroid production, usually ascertained by exogenous ACTH administration. Cushing's syndrome caused by the ectopic production of ACTH is best managed by surgical excision, provided the responsible tumor is localized. Bilateral total adrenalectomy is indicated in patients with pituitary tumors or ectopic carcinoma in whom the source of excess ACTH cannot be removed.

Pheochromocytoma

Although pheochromocytomas are uncommon tumors that account for less than 0.5% of all hypertension, all hypertensive patients should be screened for pheochromocytoma because of the high morbidity associated with this disease. This tumor, which leads to the excessive secretion of catecholamines from neurosecretory chromaffin cells, arises in the adrenal medulla in 90% of cases. Ten percent of pheochromocytomas are extra-adrenal (sympathetic cells along the aorta, within the organ of Zuckerkandl, within the urinary bladder), 10% are bilateral, and about 10% are malignant. The clinical features mimic several other conditions—anxiety states, psychosis, diabetes mellitus, thyrotoxicosis. A familial incidence is found in 5 to 10% of patients. Pheochromocytoma often occurs in familial multiple endocrine neoplasia (MEN) syndromes. Most notably, this tumor is associated with medullary carcinoma of the thyroid and hyperparathyroidism in MEN II or Sipple's syndrome. Pheochromocytoma is found in about 1% of patients with neurofibromatosis (von Recklinghausen's disease); it also occurs in patients with von Hippel-Lindau syndrome, acromegaly, or Addison's disease.

In patients with characteristics of severe hypertension and exacerbations associated with symptoms of catecholamine excess such as headaches, excessive sweating, palpitations with and without tachycardia, anxiety, nervousness, tremulousness, pain in the chest, abdomen, lumbar regions, or groin, plasma catecholamine levels are usually diagnostic. In contrast, one-third of patients with pheochromocytoma exhibit relatively normal blood pressure with only intermittent elevations. In these patients, urinary metabolite and catechol levels measured following a hypertensive episode can be more diagnostic than a random plasma catechol level taken when the patient is not having an attack. Moreover, since plasma catechols are extremely responsive to stress, activity, pain, and other stimuli, the occurrence of falsely elevated readings (false-positive test) in normal individuals is not uncommon. However, accurately collected and analyzed plasma or urinary catecholamine determinations will identify over 95% of patients with pheochromocytomas (Figure 13.8). The demonstration of elevated plasma or urinary levels of catecholamines (norepinephrine, epinephrine, and dopamine) or their metabolites (metanephrine, normetanephrine, and vanilmandelic acid [VMA]) is required for diagnosis (Figure

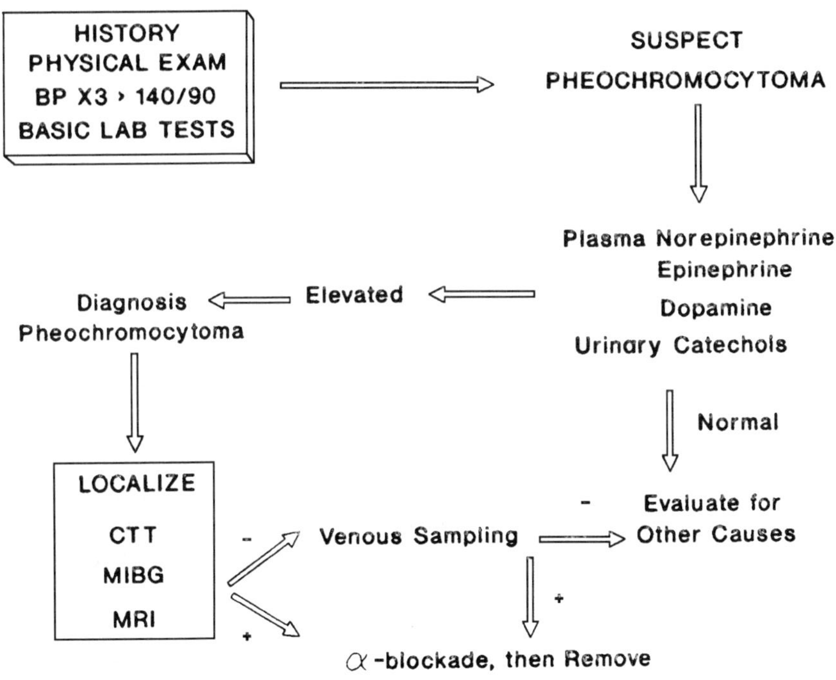

Figure 13.8: Pheochromocytoma—diagnostic and treatment algorithm

13.8). Various substances and drugs affect the urinary levels of catecholamine metabolites. Measurement of blood catecholamine levels most accurately confirms the diagnosis of pheochromocytoma. Family members of patients with pheochromocytoma or multiple endocrine adenomatosis should be screened for pheochromocytoma.

The clonidine suppression test is useful to suppress the borderline elevations of catecholamines associated with anxiety. Plasma catecholamine levels are obtained prior to and 180 minutes after the oral administration of 0.3 mg of clonidine. Plasma catecholamine levels fall to within a clearly normal range in patients with essential hypertension but do not change in patients with pheochromocytoma.

Once the biochemical diagnosis of pheochromocytoma has been ascertained, tumor localization is mandatory (Figure 13.8). Ninety percent of pheochromocytomas are localized within the adrenal, 10% are extra-adrenal, and 10% are multiple. The patients likely to have multiple lesions are children, those with a family history of the disease, and those with the multiple endocrine adenopathy type-III syndrome. Fortunately, excellent techniques are available for localization. CT scan and indobenzylguanidine scan (MIBG) are extremely useful in identifying adrenal and extra-adrenal pheochromocytomas. Another useful test is magnetic resonance imaging. Taken together, these studies allow for the precise localization of pheochromocytoma, especially as the tumor relates to vascular structures. Occasionally, selective adrenal venous sampling for biochemical localization is needed to identify small or extra-adrenal lesions. If all localization studies indicate a solitary lesion, contralateral adrenal and para-aortic exploration via transabdominal approach is not required. Unless the patient is in a high-risk group for multiple lesions, a standard flank or thoracoabdominal approach is employed in most patients.

Surgical excision is the preferred treatment of pheochromocytoma. The use of adrenergic blockage preoperatively reduces the surgical risks. Prior to surgery, patients are prepared with phenoxybenzamine 20 to 60 mg/day for alpha blockade. The tyrosine hydroxylase inhibitor alpha-methyltyrosine (Demsa) is occasionally used at a dose of less than 2 g/day in conjunction with alpha blockade to reduce catechol production as well as receptor blockade. Alpha blockage controls the blood pressure and expands the circulating blood volume. Since most patients with pheochromocytoma have constricted vascular spaces, low blood volume, and high hematocrits, plasma expansion with blood transfusions is often used preoperatively. A skilled anesthesiologist who is prepared to control the wide fluctuations in blood pressure and cardiac rhythm that often result from intraoperative manipulation of the tumor by the surgeon is required during operative therapy. The tumor is approached via an anterior, transperitoneal incision when extra-adrenal, multiple, or bilateral adrenal tumors are suspected. Malignant pheochromocytomas are unresponsive to irradiation or chemotherapy. After surgical excision, recurrent hypertension usually signifies metastases. This recurrent hypertension usually can be controlled pharmacologically, especially by use of alphamethyltyrosine, a competitive inhibitor of catecholamine synthesis.

In summary, accurate endocrine assays and radiographic techniques are currently available for the diagnosis and localization of adrenal lesions that secrete hormones causing hypertension. Although these adrenal lesions are unusual, they should always be suspected in the hypertensive patient because of the potentially high morbidity associated with these pathologies and the real possibility of permanent cure by surgical excision.

SUGGESTED READINGS

Goldblatt H, Lynch J, Hanzal RF. Studies on experimental hypertension. I. The production of persistent elevation of systolic blood pressure by means of renal ischemia. J Exp Med 1934; 59:347.

Original experimental model of the "Goldblatt kidney" demonstrating the relationship between renal ischemia and systemic hypertension.

Riehle RA Jr, Vaughan ED Jr. Renin participation in hypertension associated with unilateral hydronephrosis. J Urol 1981; 126:243.

Description of the interrelationship between hydronephrosis, renin production, and hypertension.

Savage J, Shah V, Dillon MJ, Williams DI. Renin and blood pressure in children with renal scarring and vesicoureteral reflux. Lancet 1978; I:441.

Careful documentation of the effects of reflux, reflux nephropathy, and renal scarring on plasma renin activity and the development of hypertension in children.

Sealey JE, Beuhler FR, Laragh JH. The physiology of renin secretion in essential hypertension: estimation of renin secretion rate and renal plasma flow from peripheral and renal vein renin levels. Am J Med 1973; 55:391.

Clear exposition of the physiology of renin secretion in patients with hypertension.

Smith H. Unilateral nephrectomy in hypertensive disease. J Urol 1956; 6:685.

Early report on the role of nephrectomy in patients with hypertension.

Vaughan ED Jr, Beuhler FR, Laragh JH. Hypertension and unilateral parenchymal renal disease: evidence for abnormal vasoconstriction–volume interaction. JAMA 1975; 233:1775.

Pathophysiologic changes in hypertensive patients with unilateral kidney disease are clearly described. Includes a sophisticated discussion of blood volume and vasoconstrictor status of these patients.

Weinberger MH, Grim CE, Hollfield JW, et al. Primary aldosteronism: diagnosis, localization, and treatment. Ann Intern Med 1979; 90:386.

Excellent overview of the clinical, diagnostic, and therapeutic aspects of Conn's syndrome.

Cryer, PE. Pheochromocytoma. West J Med 1992; 156:399.

Up-to-date review of pheochromocytoma. Includes description of the physiology of the sympathochromaffin system and the biologic activity of the compounds produced by the adrenal medulla.

Stein PP, Black HR. A simplified diagnostic approach to pheochromocytoma: a review of the literature and report of one institution's experience. Medicine (Baltimore) 1991; 70:46.

Reports a large, single institutional experience with pheochromocytoma. A logical, simplified diagnostic algorithm, based on pathophysiology, is described.

Sos TA, Pickering TG, Sniderman K, et al. Percutaneous transluminal renal angioplasty in renovascular hypertension due to atheroma or fibromuscular dysplasia. N Engl J Med 1983; 309:274.

Early experience with transluminal angioplasty for treatment of renovascular hypertension is presented. Hypertension control is better in fibromuscular dysplasia than in atheromatous renal arterial obstruction.

Orth DN. Differential diagnosis of Cushing's syndrome. N Engl J Med 1991; 325:957.

Succinct discussion of the differential diagnosis of Cushing's syndrome. The various hormonal and suppression tests are outlined and their limitations discussed.

Sosa RE, Vaughan ED Jr. Pharmacologic probes to identify patients with renovascular hypertension. Semin Urol 1985; 3(4):317.

Outstanding review of the pharmacologic tests used in the evaluation of patients with suspected renovascular hypertension. Presented from the perspective of the practicing urologist.

Vaughan ED Jr, Case DB, Pickering TG, Sosa RE, Sos TA, Laragh JH. Clinical evaluation of renovascular hypertension and therapeutic decisions. Urol Clin North Am 1984; 11(3):393.

Describes the fundamental principles governing the evaluation of renovascular hypertension. The techniques and results of the various treatment modalities are outlined. A guide to treatment selection is also offered.

Reinig JW, Doopman JL, Dwyer AL, et al. Adrenal masses differentiated by magnetic resonance. Radiology 1986; 158:81.

Useful discussion on the role of MRI in the evaluation of adrenal masses.

CHAPTER 14

Principles of Radiation Therapy

John A. Heaney
Christopher T. Coughlin

A large proportion of urologic cancer patients receive radiation therapy at some time during the course of their disease. Because urologic cancers are highly heterogeneous in site, natural history, and biology, the urologist must have a cogent understanding of the principles of ionizing radiation and their applications to specific tumors. Patients should be counseled regarding the safety and effectiveness of radiation therapy, and referrals should be made to the most appropriate facility for consultation and treatment with the optimal modality or combination of modalities. In this chapter, the types of ionizing radiation, how they are produced, their mechanisms of action and modification, their biological effects on cells, and their interaction with normal and tumor tissues are described. Subsequently it is shown how therapy for a specific urologic tumor is based on the application of these principles.

TYPES OF RADIATION

Ionizing radiation consists of sparsely ionizing electromagnetic radiation and densely ionizing particulate radiation (Table 14.1). The majority of therapeutic radiation uses electromagnetic radiation (photons) or particulate electrons. Use of other particulate radiation is investigational.

Electromagnetic Radiation (Photons)

The electromagnetic energy spectrum ranges from low-energy, long-wavelength, and low-frequency radiowaves to high-energy, short-wavelength, and high-frequency ionizing radiation (Figure 14.1). Energy is related directly to frequency and inversely to wavelength. Therapeutically useful ionizing radiation ranges in energy between 10 KeV and 100 MeV (elec-

Table 14.1: Types of Radiation

Electromagnetic Radiation (Photons)	*Particulate Radiation*
Gamma rays	Electrons (beta particles)
X rays	Alpha particles
	Protons
	Neutrons
	Negative mesons
	Positrons

tron volt, or eV, is the unit of energy acquired by an electron accelerated through 1 volt; 1 KeV = 10^3 eV, 1 MeV = 10^6 eV), although ionization may occur at energies less than 100 eV. When high-energy radiation interacts with matter, electrons are removed from atomic or molecular orbit,

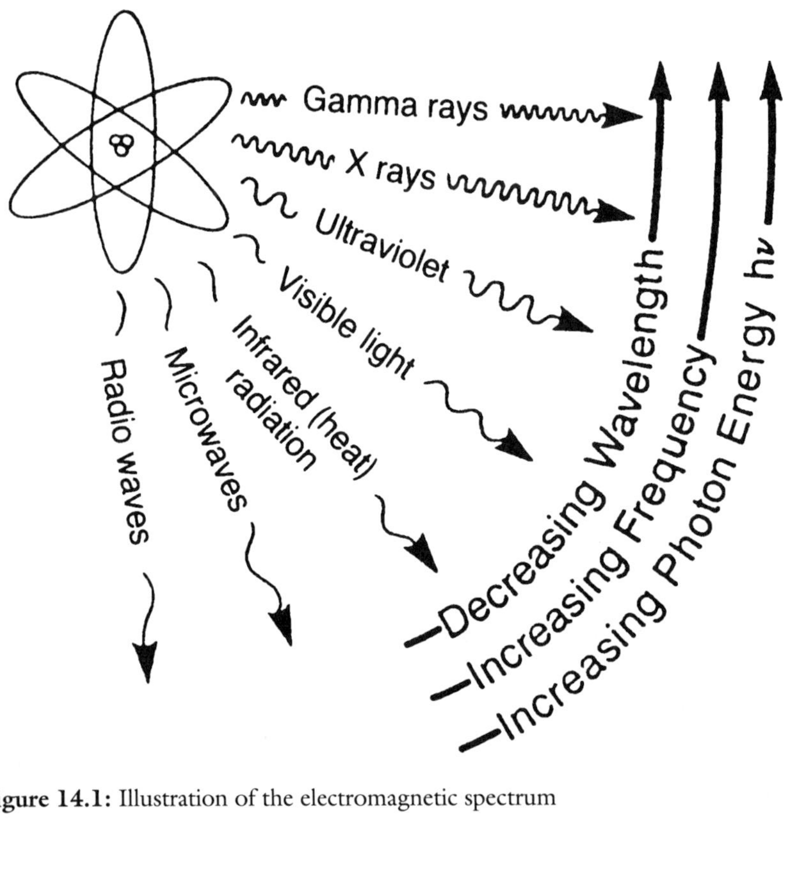

Figure 14.1: Illustration of the electromagnetic spectrum

resulting in ionization and the local release of about 33 eV per ionization in air. In practice, beams of energy greater than 24 MeV are seldom used.

X rays and gamma rays are clinically useful photon beams that differ in the ways they are produced. In *extranuclear* processes, energy is released to produce x rays when either an accelerated electron strikes a target nucleus and decelerates (bremstrahlung) or an orbital electron is removed from an atom, permitting other electrons to shift orbit (characteristic radiation), which is unique for the element involved. Gamma rays are produced by natural isotope emission. In *intranuclear* processes, energy is released during radioactive isotope decay as an unstable nucleus converts to a more stable form. Such decay decreases exponentially as a function of time.

Ionizing Particulate Radiation

Electrons (beta particles) are the ionized particles most frequently used in radiation therapy. Other ionized particles with potential therapeutic use include protons, alpha particles, neutrons, negative pi-mesons, and heavy ions. Electrons can be accelerated electrically to high energies by a linear accelerator or betatron because of their charge and low mass. Electrons may also be produced during nuclear decay, known as beta decay. The production of the other particles is an extremely expensive process that requires use of a cyclotron. The advantages and limitations of modern, high-energy radiation techniques are listed in Table 14.2.

TISSUE INTERACTION

Tissue penetration by radiation relates both to the type and energy of radiation and the characteristics of the tissue. Photons are absorbed exponentially and penetrate more deeply the higher the energy, allowing treatment at increasing depth. Electrons and other particles have a finite range and are appropriate for surface and near-surface treatment. Matter may both scatter and absorb radiation and may attenuate the intensity of

Table 14.2: Modern Radiotherapeutic Techniques

Disadvantages	*Advantages*
Expense	Skin sparing
Limited availability	Better depth-dose to tumor
	More focused beam, less scatter
	Reduced damage to normal tissues
	Biologically more destructive

an incident beam in a specific manner that depends on its absorption coefficient and thickness.

Radiation and matter interact in three ways to affect absorption. The *photoelectric effect* predominates at low energies (<35 KeV) and occurs when radiation is absorbed by an innermost orbital electron, causing the electron to be ejected from the atom. The atomic number of the absorbing material is critical, permitting the use of lead and similar materials to absorb low-energy ionizing radiation. The *Compton effect* is the most important means of tissue absorption of ionizing radiation over a wide range of energy used in radiation therapy (35 KeV to 50 MeV). It is independent of atomic number, and radiation is absorbed to a similar degree in soft tissue or bone. *Pair production* occurs in the high-energy range (>10 MeV), where radiation energy acting on a material of high atomic number is transformed into an electron and a positron.

As recognized by the Inverse Square Law, the intensity of a radiation beam is inversely proportional to the square of the distance from the source. This is an important concept when dealing with short-treatment-distance interstitial or intracavitary sources (brachytherapy) because there is rapid fall-off in dose over a short distance. Conversely, with high-energy external beam therapy at the usual long source distances of 80 to 120 cm (teletherapy), fall-off in dose with distance is relatively unimportant.

RADIATION MEASUREMENT AND SOURCES

Radiation beams emitted from external machines and radioisotope sources may be characterized by their penetrating power. The half-value layer is the thickness of an absorbent material required to reduce the beam intensity by half, and measurement is usually expressed in units of thickness of lead, copper, or aluminum. The depth of tissue at which 50% of the dose is delivered is often used as a means to characterize high-energy beams.

The most important quantitative measurement in radiation therapy is the amount of energy absorbed from a radiation beam per unit mass of absorbing material. Historically, the most commonly used unit of measurement was the rad, which is equivalent to 100 ergs of energy absorbed per gram of tissue. Currently the gray (Gy) is recognized and represents the absorption of 1 joule of energy per kilogram of tissue. Thus, 1 cGy (centigray) = 1 rad and 10 Gy = 1000 rad. The dose of internally delivered isotopes can be measured with a Geiger counter. Direct measurement of the absorbed dose is difficult and is usually extrapolated from a measurement of radiation exposure, which is the amount of ionization in air produced by a beam of radiation measured with thermoluminescent dosimeters (TLD) distributed at clinically relevant locations within the target tumor location. The roentgen, the unit of radiation exposure, is equivalent to 2.58×10^{-4} coulomb per kilogram of air. With knowledge of the exposure, the radiation energy, and the tissue absorption coefficient, the absorbed dose may be estimated. Thus, in the therapeutic energy range, one roentgen is roughly equivalent to 0.95 cGy absorbed dose in tissue.

External Beam Radiation Units

A beam of ionizing radiation may be delivered from a variety of external sources. These external beam radiation units include conventional x-ray machines, cyclotrons, radioisotope source machines (e.g., Cobalt-60 orthovoltage machines), linear accelerators, and betatrons. These machines are characterized by the penetrating power of their beam output (Table 14.3).

Superficial and orthovoltage x-ray machines are generally outdated and are used only for skin and other superficial lesions. The photons are produced by accelerating electrons emitted from a hot filament across a simple cathode-ray tube to strike a tungsten target. The penetration of the x rays depends on the voltage applied across the tube. Filters can be placed in the beam to screen out photons of lower energy. Superficial units produce x-ray energies of 30 to 125 KeV; the maximum energy of orthovoltage equipment is between 125 and 500 KeV. In general, these units produce unacceptably high skin doses and inadequate penetration for treatment of deep-seated tumors.

Cobalt-60 is a naturally occurring radioactive isotope. In its decay to ^{59}Ni it emits gamma rays with two major energies (1.117 MeV and 1.33 MeV), with an average of approximately 1.25 MeV. ^{60}Co pellets are housed in a cylinder. Because of the cylinder's large size (4×6 cm commonly), the ^{60}Co source must be housed in a bulky lead treatment head and must be tightly collimated to achieve beam sharpness. There are distinct advantages to its use over other orthovoltage machines, including skin-sparing and better beam penetration. A major disadvantage is the

Table 14.3: Energies of Photons Produced by External-Beam Radiation Units

Radiation Source	*Energy*
Superficial x rays	30 to 125 KeV
Orthovoltage x rays	125 to 500 KeV
Cobalt-60 (gamma rays)	1.25 MeV
Linear accelerators (x rays)	1 to 24 MeV
Betatrons (x rays)	20 to 45 MeV

slow dose delivery rate, which results in long treatment times that progressively lengthen as the source decays.

Linear accelerators and betatrons are used to produce supervoltage or megavoltage energies in the range of 1 to 24 MeV. In a linear accelerator, electrons are accelerated to high energies along a linear path in a wave-guide by the use of microwaves. With modern technology, the path length may be less than 2 cm. In a betatron, a changing magnetic field accelerates the electrons along a circular path. The electrons strike a tungsten target to produce x rays. The effective energy of the photons is slightly lower than the energy of the electrons from which they are produced. The maximum energy is limited by the accelerating potential of the device. The beam characteristics of the low-energy 4 MeV linear accelerator are similar to those of cobalt (1.25 MeV), but the beam edge from the accelerator is much sharper. The higher energy accelerators in the 10 to 20 MeV range and betatrons in 20 to 45 MeV range produce high-energy photons that have important advantages in treating deep-seated tumors. Electrons also may be extracted simultaneously from these machines to create a particle beam or a mixed beam.

Depth dose curves may be derived for each modality and represent the percentage of the maximum dose delivered as a function of depth within the absorbing tissue. Increased beam energy translates into increased tissue penetration and skin-sparing. Field size and the distance of the target from the source also affect dose delivery and tissue penetration.

Brachytherapy

Brachytherapy allows the delivery of high-intensity radiation within a defined volume by interstitial or intracavitary application of radioactive isotopes (Table 14.4). Isotopes (^{198}Au and ^{125}I) that are placed permanently have short half-lives (T½) and low energy in contrast to those used for temporary application (Iridium-192, Cesium-137, and Radium-226), which have long T½ and high energies. For example, T½ for ^{198}Au is 2.7 days, the tissue half-valve layer (HVL) for ^{125}I is 0.25 mm,

Table 14.4: Characteristics of Radioactive Isotopes

Isotope	*Energy (MeV)*	*Half-Life*	*Half-Value Layer*
Radium-226	0.61 to 2.43	1622 years	1.4 cm Pb
Cesium-137	0.662	33 years	0.6 cm Pb
Iridium-192	0.34	74.5 days	3 mm Pb
Iodine-125	0.028 to 0.035	60 days	0.25 mm Pb
Gold-198	0.42	2.7 days	3 mm Pb

the energy range of Iridium-192 is 300 to 612 KeV, and the energy of Cesium-137 is 660 KeV ($T\frac{1}{2}$ = 33 years) and that of Radium-226 is 2 MeV ($T\frac{1}{2}$ = 1622 years). Permanent isotopes are placed in the form of seeds, pellets, or a colloidal solution, and temporary delivery is usually achieved by afterloading through either interstitial cannulas or intracavitary applicators.

Intraoperative Radiation

Intraoperative radiation uses the electron-beam component of a linear accelerator or a dedicated orthovoltage machine. Radiation is delivered directly to a tumor volume during a surgical procedure. Normal tissue is mechanically removed from the radiation field. Single large doses of irradiation are delivered during the operative setting. In this manner tumor dose can be supplemented while sparing normal tissue. Clinical trials are in progress to optimize intraoperative and postoperative doses in selected tumor sites.

BIOLOGICAL EFFECTS OF RADIATION ON CELLS, NORMAL TISSUES, AND TUMORS

Cellular Interaction

The effects of radiation on cells are the result of a chain of chemical reactions initiated by the physical deposition of energy through ionization. Both electromagnetic and particulate radiation deposit energy to all parts of a cell. In tissue, little total energy is absorbed and relatively few molecules are ionized. For example, 4 Gy results in an energy absorption of approximately 10^{-3} calories per gram of tissue and the ionization of only 1 of 5×10^7 molecules. However, there are more than 10^{22} molecules per gram of tissue, and consequently more than 10^{15} molecules per gram will be ionized. Ionization occurs along the path of the high-speed charged particles (e.g., electrons), which are set in motion by the absorbed energy. The energy that is deposited per unit track length is described by the parameter, linear energy transfer (LET, in KeV/unit length). For most gamma rays and x rays, LET varies only slightly with the beam energies used. Neutrons and alpha particles produce more densely ionizing radiation (high LET) and are more efficient than photons, with a greater biological effect per radiation dose. This phenomenon of the efficiency of a specific radiation beam in producing a given biological response is defined by the *relative biological effect* ratio (RBE = D_{250}/D_r, where D_{250} and D_r are the doses of 250 KeV x rays and radiation (r), respectively), required to produce the same biological response. Most facilities use sparsely ionizing radiation from a linear accelerator that has an RBE = 1.

Deoxyribonucleic acid (DNA) is the most important target molecule and may either undergo direct ionization or, more commonly, be indirectly affected by energy released as a result of ionization of other target molecules (Table 14.5). Almost certainly, water is ionized into highly reactive free radicals that diffuse toward and react with the target molecules. The discrete damage to DNA includes loss or change of a base, hydrogen bond breakage between strands, dimerization, and crosslinkage, all of which may lead to a change in molecular structure and function. Many intracellular and extracellular factors may modify the nature and extent of molecular damage resulting from radiation. These factors include temperature, pH, oxygen concentration (often relating to tissue vascularity), and target molecule concentration. The roles of oxygen and tissue blood supply and radiation protective or enhancing chemicals are particularly important in determining radiation damage by altering the number and type of free radicals produced (see below).

Radiation has different functional effects on the tissues of various organs depending on intrinsic cellular reproductive activity (Table 14.6). Loss of function may occur as a result of interphase death in tissues where cells have little ability to divide, such as in adult nerve and cartilage. Large doses of radiation are required to cause interphase death in such tissues, with the exception of lymphocytes, which may die after receiving only 1 cGy. Interphase death produces delayed effects and complications of irradiation. In contrast, reproductive death is produced in tissues capable of rapid cell division and turnover, and this loss of reproductive ability results in a cell's inability to produce progeny capable of sustained reproduction in later generations.

Cell survival curves describe a cell's ability to survive a reproductive death at increasing radiation doses. Cell survival curves have characteristic shapes for mammalian cells whether they are normal or malignant. The "shoulder" of the curve represents the dose that must be absorbed (D_q) and the damage that must be accumulated to impart lethal damage. With

Table 14.5: Effectors of Radiation Injury

Direct Effects	*Indirect Effects*
Ionization	Free radicals
Photons	Atom or molecule with unpaired neutron
Ionizing particles (neutrons, protons)	Hydrogen free radical
	Hydroxyl free radical

Table 14.6: Mechanisms of Radiation Effect

Radiobiologic Targets	*Cellular Changes*
Nuclear > cytoplasmic destruction	Molecular DNA damage
Chromosomes	Mitotic cell death
Cellular DNA	Interphase cell death
	Chromosomal damage

increased dose, a direct logarithmic relationship develops between the fractional cell kill and dose, represented in a line of constant slope (LCS). Cell survival curves vary qualitatively between different cell lines in that a larger shoulder indicates a greater ability to accumulate or repair radiation damage and a steeper LCS indicates a more radiosensitive cell.

Many interacting factors influence cell kill and modify its expression in the survival curve (Table 14.7). Oxygen is required in the production of lethal free radicals. Tumors may reoxygenate as they shrink, allowing oxygen to become more available to the remaining viable cells. In addition, radiosensitizing chemicals may reduce the oxygen requirement, enhancing cell kill in the poorly oxygenated cell. The intrinsic ability of a cell to repair radiation damage has a marked influence on survival. Sublethal damage normally can be repaired by the cell but will increase the sensitivity to subsequent radiation if there has been insufficient time between treatments to allow repair. Recovery usually takes 4 to 6 hours for normal tissue and much longer for malignant tissue. Damage that would potentially be lethal under normal growth conditions may be repaired under suboptimal or perturbed conditions. The ability of a cell to

Table 14.7: Factors Affecting Tumor-Cell Radiosensitivity

Dose rate
Dose fractionation
Temperature
  Hyperthermia increases radiosensitivity
Cell differentiation, mitotic activity
  Well differentiated, highly dividing cells more radiosensitive
Cell cycle phase
  Mitotic (M) phase cells 2.5 times more radiosensitive than synthetic (S) phase cells
Oxygenation
  Hypoxia leads to lower levels of free radicals, which leads to reduced radiosensitivity

repair radiation damage depends greatly on the dose rate of the radiation. At the low dose rates of brachytherapy much repair of sublethal damage occurs; at the high dose rates of external beam radiation this repair is not possible. Thus with brachytherapy higher total doses may be given over a shorter time as less long-term damage occurs to normal tissues that are able to repair and repopulate. Cell survival also depends on the phase of the cycle in which radiation is delivered. Cells in the mitotic (M) phase are most sensitive, and those in the late nucleic acid synthesis (S) phase are least sensitive. Conceptually, there is great advantage to be gained by cell or tissue synchronization into M phase, but clinically this has not been technically possible.

Role of Oxygen and Blood Supply

As discussed above, oxygen is important in the production of radiation-induced lethal free radicals. Accordingly, hypoxic and anoxic cells are relatively resistant to low LET radiation, resulting in a cell survival curve with a larger shoulder and a flatter LCS. The addition of oxygen can enhance the effect of low LET radiation, while high LET radiation is less dependent on oxygen for its activity. In addition, radiosensitizing chemicals may reduce oxygen requirement.

The vascularity of tissues and tumors receiving irradiation influences both their susceptibility to radiation damage and their ability to repair it. Tissue and tumor oxygenation depend on blood supply, with cells further than 150 μ from capillaries being hypoxic and incapable of reproductive or other cellular function and commonly experiencing anoxic death (Figure 14.2). Tumors usually are poorly vascularized relative to normal tissues because of vessel distribution and structure. Malignant vasculature is poorly endothelialized and lacks regulatory smooth muscle. Impairment of vascularity further reduces the available oxygen. However, tumors may reoxygenate as they shrink and as oxygen becomes more available to the remaining viable cells.

Because radiation damage is most severe in tissues with rapid turnover and cell division, microvasculature to a tumor is impaired even early in a treatment course, whereas large, medium, and even small vessels in normal tissue suffer little damage. Endothelial damage in normal tissue is minimized by the rapidity of blood flow and normal repair mechanisms. In tumor vasculature, endothelial swelling, ulceration, and intramural edema result in a narrowed lumen, slow flow, and profound hypoxia; focal intravascular coagulation can also subsequently develop. Delayed vascular damage manifest by mural fibrosis subsequently leads to increasing problems, with recovery in normal tissues due to hypoxia. This effect may take several years to appear and is influenced by fraction size and

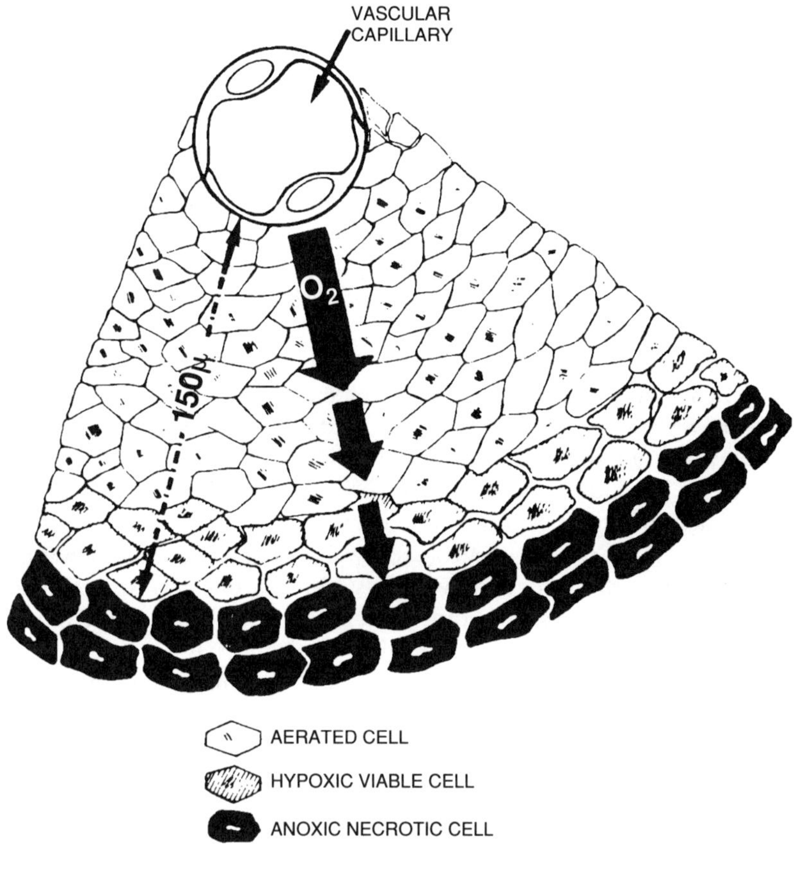

Figure 14.2: The diffusion of oxygen through tumor tissue. Up to about 150 μ from a capillary, cells are well oxygenated. Hypoxic, anoxic cells are relatively resistant to radiation.

total dose. Clinical attempts to augment vascularity during treatment is a two-edged sword in that increased blood flow and oxygenation induces increased lethal cell damage in both tumors and normal tissues, though in the latter it is offset by accelerated early postirradiation recovery. Because tumor blood vessels are poorly endowed with mural smooth muscle, pharmacological manipulation of tumor vascularity is seldom successful. Surgery in the region of a tumor bed leads to poorly vascularized scar tissue and greatly decreased oxygen delivery to residual tumor cells, which relatively increases radioresistance.

Changes in Tissue and Organ Structure and Function

In general, parenchymal cells that undergo radiation-induced injury or death exhibit a range of histological changes including cytoplasmic swelling and vacuolization, and nuclear vacuolization, pyknosis, and karyolysis. Giant multinucleated cells may develop. These cells usually undergo rapid phagocytosis. Similar changes arise in endothelial and stromal cells of blood vessels. Acute damage to capillaries leads to dilation and increased permeability, producing histologic changes recognized as tissue edema and inflammation. Chronic vascular damage is manifest by vascular narrowing and occlusion, and fibrosis of the vessels and adjacent tissues.

Because impairment of blood supply has a dramatic influence on parenchymal cell survival following radiation, the effect of radiation on tissues represents the additive result of damage occurring to the feeding vasculature and the tissue parenchymal cells. The actual effect in a particular tissue depends on whether the parenchymal cells are a population of static nondividing cells (nonrenewable system) or a population of dividing cells under homeostatic control (renewal system). In a nonrenewable system, such as the central nervous system, neurones, or striated muscle cells, injury to the vascular compartment is the most critical event, whereas the parenchymal cells are relatively radioresistant. The histological changes noted above are acute edema and inflammation or chronic hypovascularity, fibrosis, and a decrease in parenchymal cell numbers. Under normal conditions, renewal systems are characterized by the constant replacement of dead or migrating mature cells by new cells derived from the stem cell population. If the stem cells are killed by a dose of radiation, the mature functioning parenchymal cells will be severely depleted over time. Clearly, tissues with the most rapid turnover are affected soonest. Functional return depends on repopulation of stem and mature cells and is unique for an individual tissue.

The recovery time of various urologic and nonurologic tissues is primarily dependent on that of its epithelium on a cellular level. The organ recovery time depends on a number of technical factors combined with biological principles. The recovery period depends on field size, dose rate, dose per fraction of irradiation delivered, and total dose to that volume. Biologically it depends on the "health" of the target organ and on the "health" of the surrounding normal tissue. For example, a younger patient without underlying small-vessel disease, such as hypertension or diabetes, will recover more quickly than an older patient who has these underlying biological problems.

MODIFIERS OF RADIATION SENSITIVITY

Fractionation

Fractionation is one of the most important modifiers of inherent radiation sensitivity (Table 14.8). Radiation is a cell-killing agent that is rendered specific by its fractionation sequence and how it is delivered. The fundamental underlying biologic phenomenon involves differences in recovery rate. In clinical radiation oncology, multiple small fractions are given on a once-per-day basis. Normal tissue can recover from that injury within 2 to 6 hours; malignant tissue cannot recover that rapidly. A hallmark of malignancy is that repair mechanisms for any type of injury are abnormal. Malignant epithelial tissue may require a much longer period of time to recover from a sublethal radiation injury. If small, daily sublethal fractions are administered, normal tissue can recover between those fractions but malignant tissue cannot recover in that period of time. Fractions are usually given once per day, 5 days per week for 6 to 8 weeks, with treatments characteristically not delivered on Saturdays or Sundays. A dose ranging from 900 to 1200 cGy per week with once-per-day fractionation should be delivered to obtain maximum biologic effect for epithelial tissue. The usual dose per fraction is 180 to 200 cGy. Studies have shown that 7-day-per-week treatment gives less than optimal biologic effect.

Both acute and chronic toxicity are excessive, and the control rate of various cancers is suboptimal. Multi-institutional cooperative group trials have been initiated to assess whether multiple fractions with a 24-hour period enhance the tumor cell kill and give the same long-term side effects. While these side effects are minimal, any avoidable side-effect is encouraged. These clinical trials have shown that the intensity of multiple daily fractions, separated by 4 to 6 hours, are more demanding on patient tolerance. Acute, nonspecific side effects such as fatigue are more problematic. While the overall treatment time is shortened, in elderly patients the more intensive therapy is less readily tolerated. Larger fractions per

Table 14.8: Radiobiology of Dose Fractionation

Four Rs
Repair: allows recovery in slowly responding normal tissues
Repopulation
Redistribution: allows tumor cells to redistribute to more radiosensitive cell phases
Reoxygenation: hypoxic cells 2–3 times more radioresistant than normoxic cells

dose adversely affect normal tissue recovery. Long-term side effects such as tissue fibrosis are more severe with the larger doses per fraction.

Single daily fractions of less than 150 cGy per dose render less tumor cell kill unless very large field sizes are used or chemotherapy and biologic response modifiers are used. It is also important to remember that fraction size is closely and inversely related to field size. For example, the larger the field size, the less dose per fraction that can be administered with the same overlying biologic effects. An example of this phenomenon is that the single dose of total-body irradiation that is lethal ranges from 400 to 600 cGy. Conversely, a 1 cm^3 volume may easily tolerate 2000 cGy in a single dose. The technical components of fractionation and field size are quite complex and are under continuing investigation.

Hyperthermia

Hyperthermia is another actively investigated biologic response modifier. It is well known that heat by itself can selectively kill malignant tissue. However, the temperature range for this selective tumor cell kill is quite narrow, ranging from 42 to 45° C. Below this range very little tumor tissue is selectively inhibited, and above this range normal tissue effects begin to appear. Although hyperthermia can kill malignancy by itself, the selective cell kill is more efficient when another treatment modality is combined with the heat treatment. Radiation given in standard fractionated form dramatically enhances the effect of hyperthermia. Chemotherapy can also enhance this effect, and ongoing clinical trials study the effects of bimodality and trimodality therapy. The mechanism of tumor cell kill with hyperthermia is not well understood but appears to be complementary to the biologic effects of radiation. On a cellular level the radiation primarily affects the nucleus and DNA of a cell, whereas hyperthermia primarily affects the cell membrane. Radiation is most efficient in well oxygenated components of a tumor mass, whereas hyperthermia is most efficient in hypoxic areas within a tumor nodule (Table 14.7). On a macroscopic level these two modalities are complementary in their ability to render malignant tissue nonviable. Equipment limitations affect the specific and selective heat delivery to a tumor volume. This precision is currently possible only with interstitial or intracavitary applicators. Noninvasive heat delivery systems have been more difficult to control and measure. Temperatures vary with blood flow and must be measured directly during a hyperthermia treatment. A typical radiation treatment may last several minutes, whereas a typical hyperthermia treatment requires a minimum of 2 to 3 hours. Hyperthermia sessions can be delivered once or twice per week, a limitation based on thermal tolerance: If malignant tissue is heated more frequently than once in 72 to 96 hours, little additional cell kill is obtained.

Vascular Approaches

Many attempts have been made to modify radiation sensitivity through alteration in blood supply to a given tumor bed. Few of these approaches have proved either useful or practical. A possible area for investigation is the surgical manipulation of the vasculature during an operative procedure combined with an intraoperative dose of irradiation. While biologically attractive, this procedure would be limited by patient tolerance of extensive surgical procedures. To date, attempts to alter vascular supply to a given malignancy have proved either too cumbersome or have minimal additional efficacy.

Chemical and Biochemical Modifiers

Chemical and biochemical modifiers have been used in clinical trials in an attempt to separate the normal tissue and tumor dose response curves. If the tumor tissue could be made more radioresponsive, and the normal tissue more radioresistant, this would allow a greater therapeutic margin with improved tumor control and less normal tissue injury (Figure 14.3). Several classes of biologic response modifiers have been investigated (Table 14.9), and extensive data concerning the electron-affinic nitroimi-

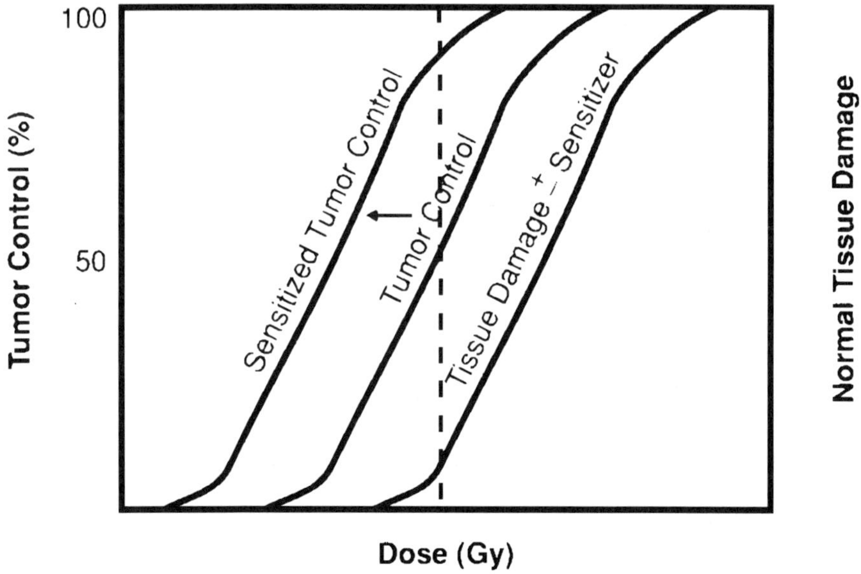

Figure 14.3: Schematic of the rationale for using sensitizers in radiotherapy. The sensitizer shifts the tumor control curve to lower radiation doses while not affecting the normal tissue complication curve.

dazoles have been accumulated. Early clinical trials using metronidazole have shown no improvement in tumor control rate or survival, primarily due to the toxicity of the compound that prevents the use in the clinic of doses required for "radiation sensitization" to appear in vitro. Analogues such as misonidazole and, most recently, etanidazole (SR-2508) have been developed in an attempt to reduce the drug toxicity. This would allow larger doses to be delivered with a goal of achieving true radiation potentiation or sensitization within the clinical setting. Misonidazole has proved to be ineffective due to neurotoxicity, and SR-2508 is now undergoing active clinical investigation.

There has been an intense interest to combine chemotherapeutic agents in a manner that will achieve radiation potentiation. This field has been fraught with biological empiricism. Few clinical trials have closely observed the pharmacology of the chemotherapeutic agent used in combination with the radiation dose delivery time. Tumor tissue drug level is more crucial than the plasma drug level. The intent is to maximize the amount of chemotherapeutic agent in the tumor itself during the time that radiation is delivered while minimizing the amount of toxic substance in normal use at that time.

The use of tissue radioprotectors also has been attempted. The most common compound used in prospectively randomized clinical trials has been WR-2721, a "free radical" scavenger (Table 14.9). The intent is to have the maximum amount of this compound in normal tissue at the time that radiation is delivered. Normal tissue would recover quickly

Table 14.9: Modifiers of Radiation Effects

Radiosensitizers
Rise in free radicals, rise in DNA damage
Metronidazole
Nitroimidazoles
Platinum
Radioprotectants
"Scavenge" free radicals, lower DNA damage
Sulphydryl-containing compounds
Hyperfractionation
Accelerated treatment
Combination modalities
Radiation plus surgery
? Predictive assays
Cell tumor characteristics, e.g., O_2, ploidy
Tumor-specific antibody

from irradiation injury, but tumor tissue would not. To date it has not been possible to administer a sufficient quantity of this agent with reliable frequency to enhance tumor control and improve survival in patients with malignancy. Attempts to coordinate this bimodality treatment with meaningful dose intensity and frequency have been achieved only in a few centers devoted specifically to intense clinical trials.

Tumor Phenotype-specific Factors

Most conventional approaches have tended to focus on a combination of tumor blood supply, tumor growth characteristics, and underlying inherent radiation sensitivity or resistance. The field of monoclonal or polyclonal antibody development to a specific malignant tissue is currently undergoing intense scientific study in controlled clinical trials. To date the problem has been that of specificity and sensitivity: an antibody that cross-reacts with any type of normal tissue would not be as useful as one that would react only with a given patient's malignancy. Once the antibody is developed, it must be delivered to the tumor cell in sufficient quantity and with sufficient cell killing agents to be effective. Radioactive isotopes that recently have been used are Iodine-131, Yttrium-90, and Strontium-89, with other isotopes used less frequently. The ideal isotope would stay irreversibly bound to the antibody and would emit a very dense flux of irradiation for a very short distance. It would also be useful for the isotope to have a rather short half-life so that the patient would not be radioactive for long periods of time. A half-life of only a few minutes or several hours would be too short to be practical in a large clinical trial because of the time needed to combine the isotope with the antibody, deliver it to the site of application, and properly evaluate its distribution in tumor and in normal tissue. An isotope with a half-life of several days would be preferable; an isotope with a half-life of months to years would be too toxic for routine clinical use. Chemical killing agents could be attached to a monoclonal antibody; ricin and other potent cell killing agents have been used.

RADIATION TREATMENT OF COMMON UROLOGICAL MALIGNANCIES

Moderately radiosensitive epithelial cancers (adenocarcinoma, transitional cell, or squamous cell carcinomas) commonly arise in the kidney, ureter, bladder, prostate, and penis (Table 14.10). The more radiosensitive germ cell tumors arise in the testis, and the less radiosensitive sarcomas infrequently involve the genitourinary tract.

Table 14.10: Radiosensitivity of Genitourinary Cancers

Prostate	6500–7000 cGy
Penis	6000 cGy
Testis	
Seminoma	3000 cGy
Embryonal cell	4000–5000 cGy
Bladder	6500 cGy

Kidney

Epithelial cancers of the kidney have been considered relatively radioresistant because the normal surrounding tissue is more sensitive to the radiation effects than is the cancer itself. Structures such as small intestine, large intestine, pancreas, and liver do not tolerate the doses necessary to eradicate clinically detectable malignancy in the kidney. Successful radiation of these structures may improve with better diagnostic procedures that can define the tumor volume more clearly. The use of surgically placed radio-opaque clips dramatically improves the targeting ability for radiation treatments and allows higher doses to be directed to smaller fields. If a small field can be reliably and repeatedly reproduced, a relatively high dose of fractionated external-beam radiation may be delivered in a tolerable fashion. Techniques to isolate a tumor bed surgically in the upper abdomen to permit several weeks of fractionated external-beam radiation have not been successful. Ideally, after removal of the majority of the tumor, a device would be implanted to isolate normal tissue in centimeter increments. This would allow reliable, theoretically reproducible radiation treatments to be delivered over several weeks, and at the same time allow the patient to recover from the surgical procedure. The device or material would ideally be reabsorbed by the patient over months to years. A number of synthetic polymers are available, but none has successfully met these requirements.

Metastases from kidney cancers can be treated depending on the site of metastasis and the need for palliation. For example, a metastasis to the liver would not be amenable to useful nontoxic radiation, whereas a metastasis to the forearm would be readily amenable to radiation control. A few radiation fractions of substantial size could be uniformly administered to the forearm with little difficulty. This would not be possible in the celiac bed due to the radiation sensitivity of the normal surrounding tissues.

Ureter

Epithelial cancers of the ureter are rather uncommon. Their radiation sensitivity is that of epithelial tissue, but the normal surrounding tissues limit the dose of radiation that can be delivered. Attempts to combine surgical extirpation with subsequent radiation to the outlined tumor bed at risk appear attractive.

Bladder

Bladder cancers are primarily of epithelial origin. The large doses of external radiation administered as a sole modality required for reliable control of urothelial carcinomas in the bladder may lead to unacceptable small bowel, rectal, and long-term bladder complications. Lesser doses result in a high incidence of "infield" tumor persistence and recurrence; the latter relates to the poorly understood fundamental biological phenomenon that caused the cancer. Because bladder cancer is a "field-change" disease thought to be initiated and promoted by carcinogens in the urine, which continually bathe the urothelium, the cure of one cancer would not prevent a new occurrence. For long-term cure, the events leading to the development of a bladder cancer must be overcome at multiple stages over a long time. Trials are being initiated using vitamin A analogs to reduce the incidence of subsequent urothelial malignancies.

A large number of clinical trials have been designed to coordinate the advantages of surgery, radiation, and chemotherapy. The intent is to combine treatment modalities in a fashion that would render the patient free of malignancy while retaining bladder function and avoiding small bowel and rectal injury. This may be possible in certain clinical settings. Neoadjuvant chemotherapy allows the use of reduced-sized pelvic portals. Extensive transurethral resection diminishes the target tumor bulk, and radiosensitization with such agents as Platinol facilitates effective tumor kill at reduced dose. To reduce further injury to adjacent organs, sharply defined fields from high-energy accelerators are necessary, delivered by parallel-opposed lateral and anterior/posterior techniques. This *4-field box* technique is designed to maximize radiation dose to the bladder while offering some protection to the small bowel and posterior rectal wall.

Prostate

Most primary prostate malignancies are adenocarcinomas. The radiation dose required for optimal tumor control is directly related to tumor size. Doses close to, or in excess of, 7000 cGy may be required when disease involves the entire prostate and/or the capsule. Potential injury to the rectal, urethral, ureteral, and other adjacent epithelia prevents dose escalation to a definitely tumorcidal range in large lesions. Attempts to minimize this injury with newer radiation-field techniques have been successful. Most institutions limit the dose of radiation to the whole pelvis to 4500 to 5000 cGy over 5 weeks. This amount is delivered in an attempt to control nodal metastases within the pelvis. Reduction in the field size to include only the prostate and seminal vesicles is then carried out with either a 4-field box technique or rotational arcs. This boost volume is carried to another 2000 to 2500 cGy over 2 to 2½ weeks, so that the total dose to the prostate approximates 7000 cGy in 7 weeks. The use of particulate beam radiation, such as neutrons or protons, is investigational and does not have wide clinical utility.

Patients with advanced local disease frequently manifest distant metastatic disease. Primary external-beam radiation may fail to control bulky, locally advanced prostate cancer. If this occurs, it is unclear whether the persistent disease in the prostate is the source of subsequent metastases or an indicator of inherently aggressive established disease. Interstitial radiation and adjuvant therapy have both been used to improve local tumor control. Interstitial implantation of ^{125}I or other isotopes allows delivery to the prostate of doses in excess of 16,000 cGy over the lifetime of the isotope. Difficulty in uniform accurate placement of these seeds and short-range (several microns) radiation result in unacceptable local failure rates. Alternatively, shrinkage of the prostate by androgen ablation prior to conventional external-beam irradiation is under investigation. Most recently, clinical investigation of the radiosensitizer etanidazole has begun in patients with bulky prostatic carcinomas.

Testis

The role of radiation in the treatment of cancer of the testis has changed dramatically over the past decade. The development of sensitive tumor markers for germ cell cancers of the testis and the development of better chemotherapy combinations for these cancers has reduced the use of radiation as a primary treatment modality. Residual metastatic deposits that are unresponsive to chemotherapy can be irradiated for patient palliation.

One malignancy that still commands the attention of the radiation oncologist is pure seminoma. This germ cell cancer is so radiosensitive that cure rates, even with significant metastatic disease, remain close to 100%. Better radiological techniques for delineation of metastatic deposits have contributed to more precise field design. Dramatically improved delivery systems such as higher energy linear accelerators (6 to 22 MeV) with sharp primary and secondary collimation, allow extreme precision in dose delivery and yield exceptional cure rates with low morbidity. The sensitivity of pure seminoma cells permits the delivery of low doses of radiation to large fields with minimal morbidity. The dose necessary to cure these tumors ranges between 2000 and 3000 cGy, depending on the volume of tissue needing treatment. After proper surgical resection, radiation is delivered to the para-aortic nodes as well as the ipsilateral inguinal and iliac nodes through carefully shaped parallel-opposed fields. With known retroperitoneal metastases, para-aortic irradiation should be followed by mediastinal and supraclavicular treatment. Although the extent of radiation depends on the stage of disease, the doses necessary for tumor control are modest and few chronic side effects are encountered.

Nonseminomatous germ cell tumors are less sensitive because of the epithelial elements they contain. However, tumor eradication has been reported with higher doses in the range of 4500 to 5000 cGy over 5 weeks at the expense of increased damage to normal tissues, especially the bowel.

Penis

Carcinoma of the penis is an uncommon malignancy that tends to spread to adjacent lymph node draining areas (inguinal and iliac) late in its natural history. While amputation remains the most common treatment, radiation can be delivered to these epithelial cancers with little difficulty. The technical challenge is to irradiate a highly curved surface with a uniform dose of irradiation. This is accomplished by mold techniques and the liberal use of a bolus material that is equivalent in density to tissue, with a uniform treatment volume delivered by molding it around the penis. This will allow the dose to be absorbed as a unit and thus will allow little damage to the skin. Typically, a 4 to 6 MeV beam produced by a linear accelerator is used.

Brachytherapy is another technique frequently used for the delivery of a uniform dose over a small, tightly curved surface. A cast of the penis is made. A radioactive material is placed on the inner surface of this cast at specific locations depending on the isotope used and the geometry of the cancer. Once constructed, this device is placed around the penis once or twice per week for 1 hour until a tumorcidal dose has been delivered. A high local dose can be administered on an outpatient basis.

A more common role for radiation therapy in carcinoma of the penis is in the treatment of the inguinal and pelvic lymph nodes postamputation of the primary tumor. In this setting, 5000 cGy over 5 weeks can be delivered by a linear accelerator with a combination of photon beams to the pelvis and electron beams to the inguinal nodes. This allows a high rate of locoregional control with minimal long-term morbidity.

SUGGESTED READINGS

Deacon J, Peckham MJ, Steel GG. The radioresponsiveness of human tumors and the initial slope of the cell survival curve. Radiother Oncol 1984; 2:317.

Excellent description of how the unique initial slope of the cell survival curve relates to radioresponsiveness of individual human tumors.

Elking MM, Sutton H. Radiation response of mammalian cells grown in culture. 1: Repair of x-ray damage in surviving Chinese hamster cells. Radiat Res 1960; 13:555.

Landmark demonstration of the relationship between dose, fractionation, and the ability of a cell to repair sublethal damage.

Bush RS, Jenkin RP, Allt WE, et al. Definite evidence of hypoxic cells influencing cure in cancer therapy. Br J Cancer 1978; 37:303.

Simple study suggests that anemia, a clinical correlate of laboratory hypoxia, has an adverse effect on tumor curability by radiation therapy.

Bloomer WD, Hellman S. Normal tissue responses to radiation therapy. N Engl J Med 1975; 293:80.

Elegant demonstration of radiation effects in normal tissues. The tissues of individual organs are unique in their sensitivity to radiation injury.

Forman JD. The role of radiation therapy in the management of carcinoma of the kidney. Semin Urol 1989; 7:195.

Review of the limited role of radiation therapy in the management of renal carcinoma. There may be an adjuvant role, and palliation is often achieved in metastatic disease.

Shipley WU, Kaufman DS, Heney NH. Can chemotherapy plus transurethral tumor resection make cystectomy unnecessary for invasive bladder cancer? Oncology 1990; 4:25.

Reports of phase II and III studies of cisplatin-sensitized external-beam radiation therapy for bladder preservation in patients with invasive bladder cancer. A disease-free bladder is initially achieved in most patients, and preservation may be prolonged with adjuvant intravesical therapy.

Hanks GE, Liebel SA, Krass JM, et al. Patterns of care studies: dose response observations for local control of adenocarcinoma of the prostate. Int J Radiat Oncol Biol Phys 1985; 11:153.

Broad-based review of outcomes achieved at centers of varying size, level of academic affiliation, and population demographics. Relationship between dose, local control, and complications is emphasized.

van der Werf-Messing B. Radiotherapeutic treatment of testicular tumors. Int J Radiat Oncol 1976; 1:235.

Timeless review of experience with radiation therapy in the management of both seminoma and nonseminoma testicular germ cell tumors.

Jones WG, Fossa SD, Hamers H, van den Bogaert W. Penis cancer: a review of the Joint Radiotherapy Committee of the European Organization for Research and Treatment of Cancer (EORTC) Genitourinary and Radiotherapy Groups. J Surg Oncol 1989; 40:227.

Literature review of therapeutic modalities used in the management of penile cancer. Specifically focuses on organ sparing with new radiation therapy techniques.

Moss ST, Cox JD, eds. Radiation oncology: rationale, technique, results. St Louis: CV Mosby, 1989.

Superbly rounded textbook covering basic and clinical aspects of radiation oncology.

McNally NJ, ed. The scientific basis of modern radiotherapy. BIR Report #19. Oxford: Alden Press, 1989.

Excellent symposium updating the cellular and subcellular events involved in the response of normal and tumor tissues to radiation. The impact of fractionation, oxygenation, radiosensitizers, and radioprotectors is discussed in detail.

Withers HR. Biological basis of radiation therapy for cancer. Lancet 1992; 339: 156.

Concise overview of the mechanisms of radiation injury, modifiers of radiosensitivity, and the new approaches to radiation biology.

CHAPTER 15

Chemotherapy

Perinchery Narayan
Badrinath Konety
Prahalad Jajodia

In 1991 it was estimated that over one million cases of cancer would be detected and cancer deaths would exceed half a million cases. During the last two decades it has become increasingly obvious that the ability to cure cancer is limited by the presence of micrometastases outside the treatment field. Chemotherapy of cancer is in fact treatment of metastases!

The principle of chemotherapeutic action is the greater suppression of growth of malignant cells compared to that of normal cells. One of the first chemotherapeutic agents was nitrogen mustard, which, during World War II, was found to cause lymphoid hypoplasia and then employed to treat lymphoma.

Most chemotherapeutic agents act by inhibiting some portion of cellular DNA synthesis. All tumors are composed of large fractions of dividing cells that actively synthesize DNA. The selective toxicity of chemotherapy for tumor cells is based mostly on the quantitative difference in multiplication of tumor cells compared to that of normal cells. Certain normal cell populations have high turnover rates because of their location and function, and they therefore receive the brunt of chemotherapy toxicity. Examples of these tissues include bone marrow, gastrointestinal epithelium, and hair follicles.

TUMOR CELL BIOLOGY AND CHEMOTHERAPY

Cell Cycle Kinetics

The life cycle of normal and neoplastic cells includes a division or mitotic phase (M), a first gap phase (G_1), a DNA replication phase (S), and a second gap phase (G_2). Normal cells exit the cycle from the G_1 phase to differentiate or enter into a quiescent phase G_0 (Figure 15.1). The timing and mechanisms by which cells leave the cycling phase and enter the G_0 phase are regulated by growth factors, regulating genes, and their protein products. Chemotherapeutic agents may act during the cycling phase (cycle specific) or may be independent of this (cycle nonspecific). Some drugs are phase specific in that they are most effective during certain phases of the cell cycle (Table 15.1).

The type of drug used, its dosage, and its route of administration depend on the cell cycle phase where maximum effect is likely. For example, cycle-specific drugs may not work well in tumors with small growth fractions; S phase specific drugs are better administered by continuous infusion so as to be available when cells enter the S phase. Cycle nonspecific drugs that act on DNA lend themselves to a variety of dosage schedules and are more versatile and effective against tumors with

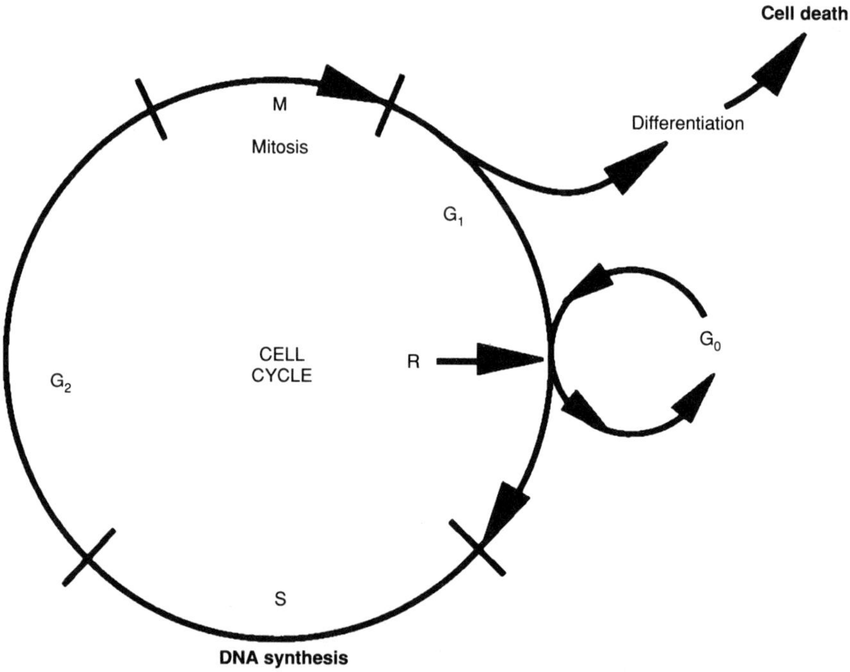

Figure 15.1: The cycle of cell division is divided into interphase and mitosis (M). Interphase can be divided into three parts: gap 1 (G_1), phase of DNA synthesis (S), and gap 2 (G_2). A point, restriction point (R), exists in G_1 and determines whether a cell can progress to S. If a cell is not triggered to DNA synthesis, it may be shunted to a resting place G_0.

Table 15.1: Phase-Specific Cytotoxic Drugs

S Phase	*M Phase*
Methotrexate	Vincristine
6-mercaptopurine	Vinblastine
5-fluorouracil	Etoposide (VP-16)

smaller growth fractions (Table 15.2). This knowledge is useful when devising better ways to improve drug delivery and concentration to selective tumor sites.

Tumor Growth Kinetics

Tumor cell kinetic studies with the L_{1210} leukemia rodent cell line reveal linear growth regardless of tumor size. Human tumors, however, have a growth curve that varies with the total volume of the tumor. As volume increases the growth fraction decreases, and this results in small tumors having a large fraction of dividing cells and large tumors having a small fraction of dividing cells. The mathematical equations describing this relation were originally described by Gompertz, a nineteenth-century mathematician, and are based on the relationship of growth and doubling time in a fetus, child, and adult (Figure 15.2). Both normal and malignant human cells grow by Gompertzian kinetics, although their "slopes of time" curves differ (Table 15.3).

Log Cell Kill and Chemotherapy

Chemotherapeutic drugs kill only a fraction of the cells exposed to them. At maximal exposure this is approximately 99.9%. This concept is termed *log cell kill* since the consistency of this killing is a first-order geometric process. A simple exposure to chemotherapeutic agent achieves, at best, 2 to 5 logs of cell kill. Since human tumors have to have at least 10^9 cells to be visible (1 cc) and most advanced tumors have cell burdens between

Table 15.2: Phase-Nonspecific Cytotoxic Drugs

Cisplatinum
Cyclophosphamide
Bleomycin
Doxorubicin
Carboplatin
Ifosfamide

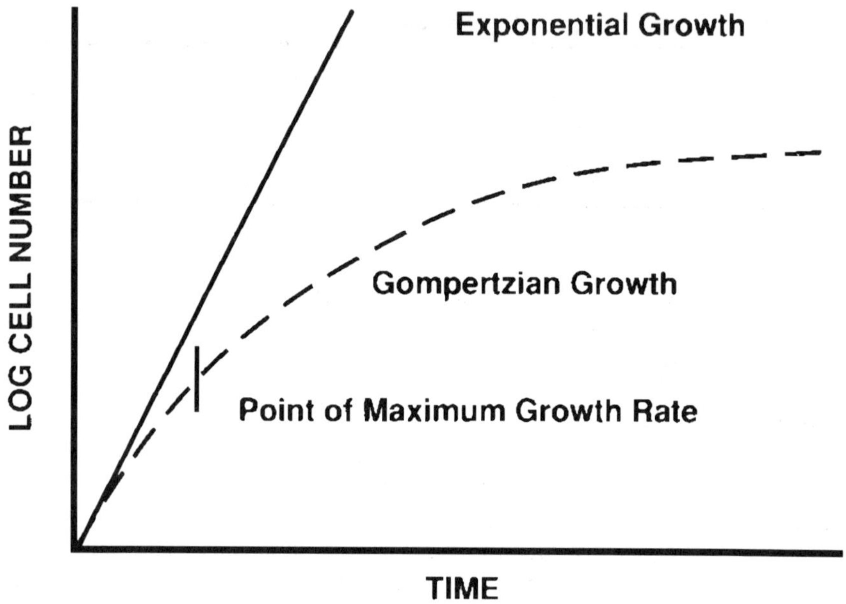

Figure 15.2: The Gompertzian growth curve

10^9 and 10^{12} cells, chemotherapy must be administered many times to affect maximal tumor cell death. This hypothesis also suggests that chemotherapy may never kill all malignant cells in patients with large tumors. The log cell kill hypothesis is nevertheless useful to determine the potential value of adjuvant chemotherapy.

Tumor Response to Chemotherapy

Tumor response to chemotherapy is a sum of the number of cells killed by therapy plus the number of new cells that grow during the same per-

Table 15.3: Basic Chemotherapy Principles

Gompertzian growth model
Growth fraction declines with increasing tumor volumes
Log kill kinetics
Possibility of cure inversely related to tumor volume
Tumor size vs. number of cells
10^9 cells = palpable tumor
10^6 cells = microscopic tumor

iod (Figure 15.3). In the Gompertzian model of human cancer cell growth, the growth fraction of cells is not exponential but decreases with larger volumes. In advanced cancer with large tumor volumes, only the small fraction of actually dividing tumor cells is killed.

When a tumor is small, its growth fraction is largest and the effect of chemotherapy is maximal. This information is only recently being applied clinically since it has been found that chemotherapy fails to cure large tumors.

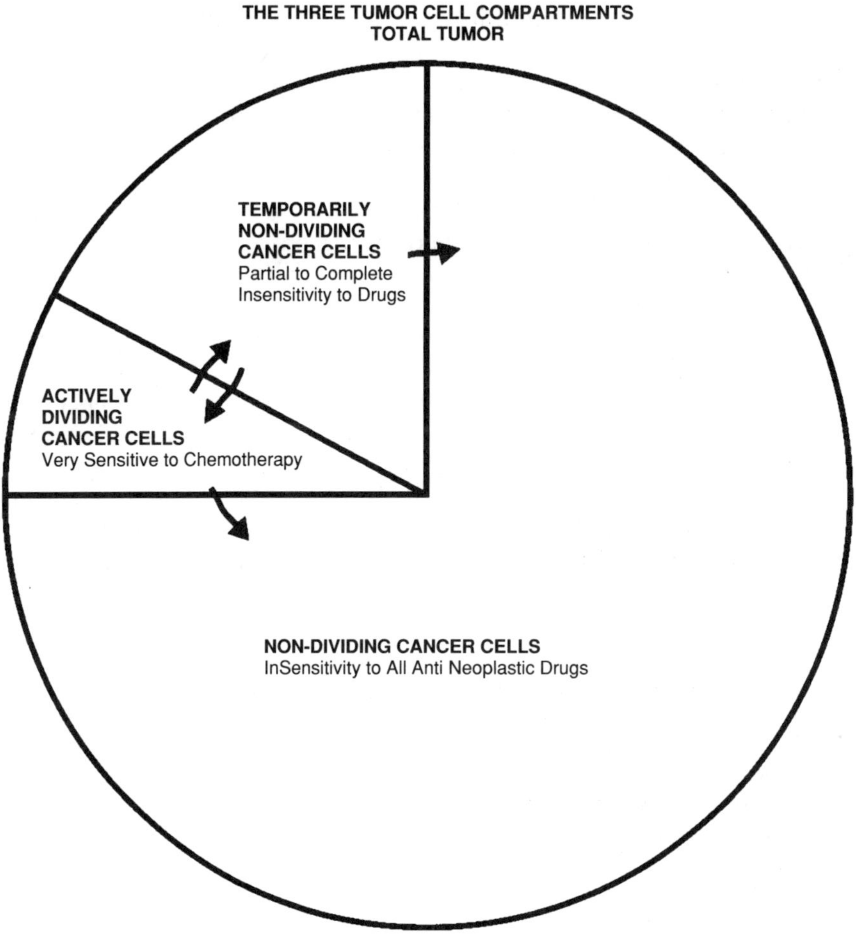

Figure 15.3: Tumor cell compartments and sensitivity to chemotherapy

Pharmacokinetics and Response

Pharmacokinetic factors that alter drug concentration over time ($C \times T$) are important in chemotherapy usage. Factors that influence $C \times T$ are drug dose, route of administration, absorption, transport, biodistribution, excretion, and interaction with other commonly used agents. The most important aspect of chemotherapy dosage is the relationship of effective concentration to duration of exposure. It is easy to understand why concentration multiplied by exposure will allow variations in drug dosage to provide the same amount of toxicity, provided duration is controlled. This relationship has made it possible to translate drug dosages developed in animals to the treatment of humans. The dosage of drugs used in animals is proportionally more per unit body weight than in humans.

Drug Resistance

Resistance to chemotherapeutic agents may be inherent or acquired by mutation. Primary mechanisms of drug resistance include decrease in uptake, transport, and activation, and alterations of target enzymes, as well as alterations in cell metabolism and repair mechanisms (Table 15.4). One documented example of genetic involvement in chemoresistance is gene amplification of an enzyme target resulting in increased copy of the target gene.

Spontaneous mutation is an inherent property of all DNA-containing cells. Malignant cells are genetically more unstable and therefore mutate more than normal cells. A mechanism similar to bacterial drug resistance has been used to explain chemoresistance. Tumor cells have an inherent capacity to mutate and probably acquire resistance to drugs at a growth level between 10^3 to 10^6. At these volumes, tumors are not clinically visible (Table 15.3). A 1-cm tumor with 10^9 cells would have at least one drug-resistant clone. Such tumors respond initially to chemotherapy but subsequently reappear as the mutant clones grow.

Table 15.4: Mechanisms of Tumor Cell Drug Resistance

Spontaneous cell mutation
Occurs at growth level 10^3 to 10^6 cells
Heterogeneous cell populations
Acquired multidrug resistance (MDR)
Expression MDR gene (P glycoprotein)
Increased DNA damage repair enzymes
Altered biochemistry of cells
Uptake, transport, activation, etc.

Clinically, tumor resistance to chemotherapy is greater than the calculated incidence. This is explained by variations in growth between parent and mutant cells. If mutant cells grow faster, more resistant clones result. Tumors with multiple mutant clones may also induce further mutations, and therefore certain tumors are totally resistant to chemotherapy regimens. Tumor dormancy, or exit of cells into the G_0 phase of the cell cycle, is another mechanism by which tumors develop resistance. This may explain the long duration between remission and recurrence in some tumors treated with chemotherapy.

Multidrug Resistance

Another type of chemotherapy resistance is acquired multidrug resistance (MDR), in which cancer cells exposed to one type of chemotherapeutic agent become resistant to several other agents that may include structurally unrelated compounds. The mechanism of MDR is believed to be decreased intracellular drug concentration related to a 170,000-KD molecular weight plasma membrane associated glycoprotein (P glycoprotein), which functions as an energy-dependent drug efflux pump. Cells with the MDR phenotype have increased expression of the MDR gene that encodes for the P glycoprotein (Table 15.4). The calcium channel blockers verapamil, quinidine, and nifedipine inhibit P glycoprotein by competitive binding, and this may be one mechanism of overcoming MDR resistance. The P glycoprotein is also present in normal colon, kidney, adrenal, and liver tissue and may be involved in normal detoxification functions. Furthermore, the differences in expression of P glycoprotein between men and women suggest possible sex hormone regulation.

Acquired mutation may also occur if chemotherapeutic agents cause DNA damage without cell death. During DNA repair, drug resistance may develop. Knowledge of this phenomenon may allow modification in selection, dosage, and schedule so as to minimize such effects. The approach to drug resistance is similar to that to antibiotic resistance. It is accomplished by use of alternative drugs initially in high-risk patients with large-volume tumors, by use of drug combinations, and, finally, by optimal dosage and duration of treatment.

Chemotherapy Dosage

Dosage response to chemotherapy is sigmoidal with threshold, lag, linear, and plateau phases. Dosage reduction in the linear phase of the dose response curve results in loss of capacity to cure the tumor before there is loss in response rate. Data from animal studies indicate that reduction in dosage during the linear phase may cause complete remission initially but results in incomplete killing of cells and eventual recurrence. In clinical practice, it is prudent *not* to reduce dosage or increase intervals between cycles just to diminish toxicity, since such changes result in diminished efficacy. Frequently, however, toxicity necessitates dose limitation despite the loss of effectiveness.

Drug dosage is determined by body surface area rather than weight. This has been questioned recently, since bone marrow toxicity is the major dose-limiting factor for chemotherapeutic agents, and bone marrow content correlates more closely with body weight than surface area. Drug dosages should indicate the dose of each drug administered per patient and the cumulative dose of each drug on a weekly basis. The critical drug dosage parameter is believed to be the relative dose intensity (RDI), or amount of drug delivered per unit time, expressed as $mg/m^2/week$. This assumes that dosage is more important than schedule and that the maximum tolerated dose is the best regimen. This hypothesis is not fully accepted by all clinicians because of other considerations that affect chemotherapy outcomes. The impact of each drug on combination chemotherapy is also important. Calculations of the impact of dose intensity during outcome are important in estimating effects of dosage reduction in adjuvant trials. Arbitrary reductions in dose intensity result in decreased remission rates, lowered threshold of effectiveness, and reduced efficacy of the combination chemotherapy.

Route of Administration and Metabolism

The choice of route of administration is geared toward facilitating maximal drug concentration at the desired site while minimizing toxicity to normal tissues. The most common routes are intravenous and oral administration. Instillation into cavities is also useful (e.g., intravesical, intraperitoneal, and intrapleural chemotherapy). Other routes of instillation, such as intrahepatic and intra-arterial, are still experimental. Toxicity is variable depending on the route of administration. Examples of lethal toxicity include neurotoxicity with intrathecal vincristine and intravenous carmustine (BCNU).

A primary requirement of successful chemotherapy is drug delivery to the tumor site. If this is not possible by intravenous or oral use, selective delivery may be required, for example, intrathecal injection to overcome the blood–brain barrier. Local drug concentrations can be augmented by delivery systems such as liposomes, microspheres, or monoclonal antibodies. The liver and kidneys are the common routes for drug excretion, and drug type and dosage are influenced by the functions of these organs. For example, doxorubicin and vincristine require dosage adjustments if there is liver damage, and the same holds true for methotrexate and cisplatinum in renal insufficiency. Production of large amounts of uric acid during leukemia therapy may also cause renal damage as a result of uric acid nephropathy.

Drug interactions may occur due to a variety of reasons, including the type of vehicle used, acid–base balance, salt content, absorption from the GI tract, cumulative toxicity on organ systems, alterations in metabolism, and excretion.

Drug Toxicity

Anorexia, nausea, and vomiting are the most common toxic effects of chemotherapy and may result in GI bleeding (Mallory-Weiss syndrome), weight loss, malaise, dehydration, and metabolic imbalances (Table 15.5). Nausea and vomiting are believed to be caused by the interaction of the drugs with central (fourth ventricle and parietal cortex) or peripheral receptors. The antiemetic agents used to treat nausea and vomiting act by binding to these receptors. Commonly used antiemetic agents include prochlorperazine (Compazine) and triethylperazine (Torcan). Combinations of agents are required in more severe situations. The side effects of antiemetic therapy include sedation, diarrhea, and extrapyramidal effects. The treatment of nausea and vomiting cannot be overemphasized. About

Table 15.5: Common Side-Effects of Chemotherapy Drugs Used in Urology

Side effect	Drugs
Myelosuppression	Alkylating agents Vinblastine, etoposide, etc. Doxorubicin, ifosfamide, carboplatin
Nausea, vomiting	All agents
Alopecia	Vincristine, bleomycin, doxorubicin, methotrexate, cyclophosphamide, 5-Fluorouracil
Hemorrhagic cystitis	Cyclophosphamide, ifosfamide
Peripheral neuropathy	Vinblastine, vincristine, etoposide, cisplatinum
Cardiomyopathy	Doxorubicin, danorubicin, cyclophosphamide
Sexual, gonadal dysfunction	Alkylating agents, cisplatinum, methotrexate, procarbazine
Pulmonary dysfunction	Methotrexate, mitomycin C, procarbazine, alkylating agents
Arachnoiditis or encephalopathy	Methotrexate, thiotepa, 5 FU
Hypersensitivity reactions	Platinum, methotrexate, etoposide (VP-16), bleomycin
Nephrotoxicity	Cisplatinum, methotrexate, mithramycin, mitomycin C
Pulmonary fibrosis	Bleomycin
“Second” malignancies	Alkylating agents, actinomycin, cisplatinum, doxorubicin, Lomustine (CCNU)

20% of patients develop anticipatory vomiting associated with chemotherapy, and they sometimes need behavioral therapy.

The side effects of gastrointestinal epithelial damage include stomatitis, esophagitis, peptic ulcer, and diarrhea; these effects are usually self-limiting. Hepatic and pancreatic toxicity occur with 5 Fluorouracil (5 FU) or 5Fluoro 2'Deoxyuridine (FUDR) hepatic infusion therapy. Hepatic veno-occlusive disease can develop with a variety of agents including cyclophosphamide and busulfan.

Drugs vary in their myelosuppressive potential and time to recovery based on type of drug, dose, schedule of administration, and patient's marrow reserve (Table 15.6). On the basis of degree of primary myelosuppressive activity, chemotherapeutic agents are divided into category I, II, or III agents as those having predominant, moderate or minimal myelosuppressive activity (Table 15.7). Apart from granulocytopenia and thrombocytopenia, these agents may also induce qualitative changes in white cell and platelet function.

The most important development in treatment of myelosuppression has been the development and use of genetically engineered granulocyte and macrophage colony stimulating factors (G-CSF and GM-CSF). Another alternative is the use of autologous bone marrow transplantation.

Immunologic Effects, Biologic Therapy, and Chemotherapy

The concept of biologic therapy is based on evidence that the immune system has a role in regulating and preventing malignant transformation in various organs (see Chapter 8). Recombinant technology has allowed the production of clinically useful quantities of various cytokines and biologic agents, and their roles in suppressing and destroying malignant cells are being explored. Current biologic therapies include alpha interferons in hairy cell leukemia and bladder cancer, intravesical Bacillus Calmette

Table 15.6: Grades of Myelosuppression*: Cell Count (1000 Cells per Microliter)

Toxicity Grade	*White Blood Cells*	*Granulocytes*	*Platelets*
0	≥4.0	≥2.0	≥100
1	3.0–3.9	1.5–1.9	75–99
2	2.0–2.9	1.0–1.4	50–74
3	1.0–1.9	0.5–0.9	25–49
4	<1.0	<0.5	<25

*As recommended for international use by Miller, et al.: Cancer 1981; 47:207.

Table 15.7: Chemotherapeutic Agents and Their Degrees of Myelosuppressive Activity

Category I: Predominant Myelosuppressive Activity
Busulfan
Vinblastine
Etoposide
Category II: Moderate Myelosuppressive Activity
Cyclophosphamide
5 FU
Methotrexate
Doxorubicin
Category III: Minimal Myelosuppressive Activity
Vincristine
Bleomycin
Cisplatinum

Guerin (BCG) vaccine in superficial bladder cancer, and interleukins in renal cancer. There is also considerable interest in use of tumor infiltrating lymphocytes and monoclonal antibodies in cancer therapy.

Chemotherapy affects all dividing cells including immune competent cells (e.g., B cells, T cells, and macrophages) with a decrease in cellular and humoral immunity. This leads to an increased likelihood of infection and inflammation during chemotherapy. The chronic effects of chemotherapy are unknown and may include an increased risk for other malignancies. Even if the role of the immune system in preventing malignancy is discounted, the risks of fatal infections is cause enough to design chemotherapy programs that minimize such effects. With the current knowledge of the increasing importance of the immune system in cancer defense, there is increasing likelihood that chemotherapeutic drugs will be used in combination with biologic agents to treat cancers (e.g., interleukin-2 with vinblastine for metastatic renal cancer).

Skin Effects

A variety of skin effects occur with chemotherapy. Effects related to administration include necrosis or sloughing due to extravasation at the site of administration. The incidence of serious extravasation is estimated to be 0.1% despite adequate precautions. Therapy in extreme cases may require skin grafting. Other skin reactions include changes in pigmentation, hair loss, photosensitive changes, and secondary hypersensitivity.

Alopecia is the most common dermatologic side effect, and it has physical and emotional impacts. It is most common with doxorubicin and cyclophosphamide but occurs with methotrexate, 5 FU, vincristine, and bleomycin (Table 15.5). Alopecia is usually reversible within a few days to weeks after therapy. Alopecia can be diminished or prevented by the application of ice packs to the scalp immediately before and for 30 minutes after administration of chemotherapy. However, there are some contraindications and limitations to this preventive therapy.

Hypersensitivity Reactions

Anaphylaxis may occur with agents such as platinum, methotrexate, etoposide (VP-16), and bleomycin (Table 15.5). Bleomycin can also cause Raynaud's phenomenon and scleroderma-like effects. These effects are more pronounced when bleomycin is used in combination with platinum and methotrexate for the treatment of testicular germ cell tumors.

Pulmonary Toxicity

Bleomycin causes a dose-related pulmonary fibrosis, which is most likely to occur when the dose exceeds 400 units (Table 15.5). This effect may be compounded when the drug is used in combination with other agents and in patients with renal dysfunction. Pulmonary dysfunction can also be caused by methotrexate, mitomycin C, procarbazine, and the alkylating agents.

Cardiac Toxicity

The dose-limiting toxicity of doxorubicin, daunorubicin, and cyclophosphamide is related to their cardiac effects (Table 15.5). Two types of cardiac damage occur with doxorubicin and daunorubicin. Acute changes include arrhythmias and a lethal myoepicarditis syndrome. Congestive heart failure occurs as a delayed effect and can be manifest up to 7 years after therapy is completed. Cardiotoxic effects of cyclophosphamide occur with higher doses of the drug (180 mg/day), and electrocardiographic abnormalities are rarely encountered.

GU Toxicity

Hemorrhagic cystitis occurs in 10% of patients treated with cyclophosphamide (Table 15.5). Renal toxicity occurs with methotrexate, mithramycin, cisplatin, and mitomycin C. Uric acid nephropathy related to treatment of leukemia and lymphoma may be diminished by use of allopurinol and hydration. Renal toxicity may be compounded by use of drugs in combination and in patients with pre-existing renal insufficiency.

Neurotoxicity

Intrathecal agents that cause arachnoiditis or encephalopathy include methotrexate, thiotepa, and 5 FU. Peripheral neuropathy is associated with the use of vinca alkaloids, cisplatin, etoposide, and procarbazine (Table 15.5). Acute cerebellar syndromes occur with 5 FU and procarbazine and cranial nerve palsies with 5 FU and cisplatinum (ototoxicity and optic nerve damage). Inappropriate antidiuretic hormone (ADH) secretion may occur with vinca alkaloids, cyclophosphamide, and cisplatinum. Alterations in smell, taste, and vision (pseudohallucinations) are associated with doxorubicin, cisplatinum, and vincristine.

Sexual and Gonadal Dysfunction

Alkylating agents, procarbazine, cisplatinum, and methotrexate may affect spermatogenesis (Table 15.5). Recovery is variable depending on functional capacity prior to therapy, the age of the patient, and the duration of therapy. Counseling and pretherapy sperm storage are desirable in selected patients. Congenital malformations may result if chemotherapeutic drugs are administered in the first trimester of pregnancy.

Second Malignancies

The potential carcinogenic potential of some chemotherapeutic agents is manifest by the delayed occurrence of lymphoid tumors in patients treated with busulfan, chlorambucil, and cyclophosphamide. Other potentially carcinogenic drugs include thiotepa, actinomycin, cisplatinum, doxorubicin, and lomustine (CCNU). The importance of this is twofold. First, in younger patients it is desirable to avoid any drug with a known propensity to cause a second malignancy. Second, the preparation, administration, and disposal of chemotherapeutic agents should be performed by trained personnel undertaking proper precautions to avoid accidental contamination of personnel or the environment.

PRETREATMENT EVALUATION AND STRATEGY FOR CHEMOTHERAPY

Prior to instituting chemotherapy, it is important to evaluate the patient completely and define a strategy for cure or palliation. The principles of evaluation include a knowledge of tumor histology; differentiation and stage of disease; prior therapy; the functional, psychologic, and socioeconomic status of the patient; and the presence and extent of comorbid conditions. Depending on the type of disease and type of therapy planned, detailed studies of individual organ systems may be required. Pretreatment evaluation should be multidisciplinary and must involve the patient's family. A realistic approach and frank discussion of the proposed therapy should include a discussion of established versus experimental therapies.

PRINCIPLES OF COMBINATION CHEMOTHERAPY

Combination chemotherapy is superior to single-agent therapy because it allows (1) maximal cell killing within tolerated dose ranges and (2) killing of resistant cell clones with reduced chances of recurrence. Guidelines for selection of multidrug combination chemotherapy include (1) the use of drugs that when used alone produce partial or complete remission of the specific tumor; (2) the use of agents with no overlapping toxicity so as to allow maximal dosage; (3) dosage adjustment to obtain maximal cytotoxicity; (4) the duration between cycles should be the shortest possible to allow normal tissue recovery and minimize the development of resistant clones; and (5) the selection of drugs with different mechanisms of action so as to prevent the development of resistance (Table 15.8).

Intermittent high-dosage therapy allows maximum cell kill while allowing periods for normal tissue recovery. The use of agents that work within specific areas of tumor cell growth cycle kinetics further improves the chances of maximal cell kill and reduces the incidence of drug resistance. Combination regimen cycles are usually administered 3 to 4 weeks apart because of the bone marrow storage capacity. Bone marrow stores replace lost peripheral blood cells for up to 8 to 10 days, and therefore leukopenia and thrombocytopenia are not evident until 8 to 10 days after therapy. The blood count nadir is reached by 14 to 18 days. Recovery begins around 21 days and is maximal by 28 days.

A second treatment given on day 8, after initial treatment on day 1, does not worsen bone marrow toxicity because the stem cells are in a quiescent state after the first dose. A second treatment on day 8, even in the presence of leukopenia, is not additive in toxicity. The highest risk of infection occurs when granulocyte counts fall below 500/ml and platelet

Table 15.8: Principles of Multidrug Combination Chemotherapy

Minimal overlapping toxicity
Maximal cell kill with tolerable toxicity
Decreased chance of tumor cell resistance
Administered cyclically at constant intervals
Shortest time between cycles (usually 28 days) to allow recovery of bone marrow
Individual drugs induce complete remissions in some patients
Use optimum doses of drugs

counts below 20,000/ml. This suppression usually lasts for 4 to 5 days, and most patients do not need supportive therapy. This knowledge has led to the commonly used method of giving cyclic combination therapy; that is, the most effective drugs are administered on days 1 and 8, and this is repeated after day 28. Bone marrow transplant is an alternative that allows the use of maximal chemotherapy, especially in younger patients.

PRIMARY CHEMOTHERAPY

Primary chemotherapy is the use of chemotherapy as initial treatment. The term *neoadjuvant* is a misnomer. Based on the Goldie-Coldman hypothesis, primary chemotherapy is more likely to be beneficial if used in the early treatment of small tumors because visible tumors (10^9 cells) will already have resistant cell clones. However, because of the lack of nontoxic agents and because primary therapy by surgical excision may be easier on the patient, the use of chemotherapy subsequent to surgery may also be reasonable because the tumor volume is reduced. Timing of such adjuvant therapy is critical because of the Gompertzian growth curve of human cancers. If chemotherapy is delayed, the resultant rapid growth of the residual cells may result in patient death prior to effective intervention. This has not been fully appreciated by many patients, and some clinicians and patients continue to succumb to rapidly progressing cancer after debulking procedures because effective chemotherapy is delayed for one reason or another.

Primary chemotherapy also downsizes tumors. Surgical/radiation therapy is then easier to administer and more effective. However, the large tumor volume obviates the favorable influence of tumor proliferation kinetics and ability to counter metastatic clones. The toxicity of chemotherapy may also restrict radiation or surgical therapy or even delay such therapy. Additionally, a subset of patients who may be cured by local therapy (surgical or radiation) alone may be subjected to the systemic toxicity of chemotherapy if primary chemotherapy is used for all patients.

ADJUVANT CHEMOTHERAPY

Any chemotherapeutic drug with therapeutic or toxicologic advantages over current therapies is a candidate for testing in an adjuvant setting. The major issues of toxicity, dosage, and schedules are addressed during phases I through IV clinical trials. The issues of adjuvant therapy are related to timing in relation to primary therapy, duration, and the ratio of risk to benefit with regard to quality of life and survival.

Because of the prior emphasis of the National Cancer Institute

(NCI) in using murine leukemia as the major initial screening tumor model, many of the currently available drugs discovered through this process have most activity against hematologic malignancies. The NCI has recently opted for an approach with emphasis on solid tumor models using cell cultures and xenograft; this should increase the yield of drugs with better activity against solid tumors. Other avenues that have been pursued on the basis of recent knowledge are the use of newer regimens and combinations for adjuvant therapy even if the agents lack effectiveness in advanced disease. The effectiveness of 5 FU and Levamisole in adjuvant therapy for colon cancer is an example of this approach. Neither 5 FU nor Levamisole is of great benefit in metastatic cancer, but they clearly have demonstrated utility in the adjuvant setting. Newer forms of therapy, such as tumor infiltrating lymphocytes, suppressors of drug resistance, and use of agents that act as antagonists to growth factors and trigger programmed cell death, are being explored in the adjuvant setting.

Even cancers that exhibit excellent initial responses to chemotherapy, such as those of the breast and ovary, have poor results with adjuvant therapy. The theory that micrometastases are likely to have lesser numbers of drug-resistant clones because of their smaller size has not been borne out by recent experience. Alternative explanations, such as MDR resistance and existence of cells with differing potentials for growth and metastases, are being tested.

PRINCIPLES OF EVALUATION OF CLINICAL RESPONSE

Complete response (CR) is defined as relapse-free survival from the time all treatment is discontinued. Since many tumors do not show a high CR rate to chemotherapy, an alternative definition of CR rate is the fraction of patients who have progression-free intervals of a certain duration based on the natural history of the disease.

Partial response (PR) rate is defined as the fraction of patients who demonstrate a 50% or greater reduction in measurable tumor mass. Although PR rates are not of much clinical benefit, they provide a means of assessing efficacy of newer agents undergoing clinical trials.

In vitro tests to determine chemosensitivity of tumors have not been clinically useful. Such tests include clonogenic assays, short-term cultures, and biochemical assays. Because of the technical difficulties in performing these assays and the lack of consistency in results, these tests remain experimental.

PRINCIPLES OF CANCER DRUG DEVELOPMENT

The first step in the process of cancer drug development is mass screening using rodent models and human tumor cell lines grown in athymic mice. The colorimetric assay provides reliable information on growth inhibition of tumor cells by potential compounds. The NCI, which has the largest such program, tests approximately 10,000 compounds annually. Compounds are selected from existing plant, marine, and biological sources either randomly or on the basis of their known functions. Compounds are also identified from molecular biology studies (e.g., oncogene products and antisense RNA). A potential problem with use of animal models and cell lines for screening is that agents effective in humans but ineffective in in vitro or rodent models can be missed. However, most of the current chemotherapy regimens have been developed using murine and in vitro cell models.

Following screening, the following test sequence occurs prior to general clinical application: preclinical toxicity testing, clinical safety testing, clinical efficacy testing, and, finally, approval for clinical use. This process is regulated by the Food and Drug Administration (FDA). Preclinical safety testing is performed in mice, and the reproducible lethal dose in 10% of animals is the basis for initial human dosage formulations. Translations of dosage across species is made by reference to standards determining ratios of weight to body surface area of different species and humans. One advantage of the surface-area technique over the weight technique is the avoidance of separate calculations for pediatric patients.

Steps of Clinical Trials for Anticancer Agents

Phase I trials are done on small groups of patients (20 to 30) so as to delineate a maximum tolerated dose without prohibitive toxicity. Dosage is determined on the basis of established techniques and information from preclinical trials. Phase II trials determine response rates and activity of a drug on several tumor types. Data from murine transplantable tumors often do not translate into similar activity in clinical studies. In phase II testing patients with advanced disease, maximum performance status, and minimal prior chemotherapy are usually included. Patients who have failed one chemotherapeutic regimen are eligible. If there is no response in 14 patients, there is a 95% possibility that the drug is ineffective. One or two responses indicate that the trial should expand to 30 patients, since this would constitute a 15 to 20% response rate. Partial responses of 5 to 10% are normal because of observer variation and therefore tantamount to no clinical efficacy. However, a complete response even in the range of only 5 to 10% deserves additional study. Phase II trials should use varying doses and treatment schedules. Phase III and phase IV trials require larger numbers of patients tested in a randomized, controlled manner and in comparison to standard regimens.

Despite all of these systematic approaches, some currently useful drugs were discovered serendipitously. For example, cisplatinum was almost missed by the usual techniques employed in identifying useful chemotherapeutic agents.

CHEMOTHERAPY OF GENITOURINARY CANCERS

Testis Cancer

Among GU cancers, testicular cancer has been the most responsive to chemotherapy, and bladder cancer has been somewhat less so (Table 15.9). Germ cell tumors are important because they affect young men. The combination of surgery and platinum-based chemotherapy has resulted in the cure of virtually all patients with early-stage disease and 70% of patients with metastatic disease. The main first-line combination therapy is cisplatinum, vinblastine, and bleomycin (PVB). Approximately 25 to 30% of patients fail PVB therapy. In patients resistant to PVB therapy, etoposide (VP-16), alone or in combination with platinum and cyclophosphamide, along with autologous bone marrow transplantation is an effective salvage therapy in 60% of patients. Etoposide is an epipodophyllotoxin. Etoposide alone produces 25 to 30% CR and PR rates, but this response is not durable. Because of the effectiveness of etoposide in combination therapy, the standard PVB regimen was compared to a newer PEB (etoposide substituted for vinblastine) regimen in a large randomized trial; this revealed a better survival rate with PEB than PVB (83% versus 74%). In some centers, PEB is now the standard first-line regimen for metastatic testicular cancer. For patients failing initial cisplatinum therapy and subsequent salvage therapy, the only other effective agent is ifosfamide, an oxazophosphorine derived from cyclophosphamide. As single-agent therapy, ifosfamide has an impressive 66% response rate, but this is of short duration. Ifosfamide and etoposide have synergy with cisplatinum. For salvage therapy, ifosfamide in combination with cisplatinum and vinblastine or etoposide produces a durable response in 40 to 50% of patients. The role of ifosfamide for first-line therapy remains to be completely defined.

Myelosuppression is the main toxicity of etoposide, resulting in mild leukopenia in 60 to 90% of patients. Other toxic manifestations include nausea and vomiting, alopecia, anorexia, diarrhea, stomatitis, and hepatic

Table 15.9: Chemotherapy Combinations Used to Treat GU Cancers and Response Rates

Cancer Site	*Combination Regimen*	*Response Rates (CR + PR)*	*Median Survival*
Bladder Cancer	Cisplatinum + methotrexate (MP)	45%	10 mo.
	Cisplatinum + methotrexate + vinblastine (CMV)	56%	44/29[b] mo.
	Cisplatinum + methotrexate + vinblastine + doxorubicin (MVAC)[a]	65–70%	11 mo.
	Cisplatinum + methotrexate + vinblastine + epirubicin (MVEC)	70%	—
Renal Cancer, Testicular Cancer	High-dose methotrexate CF + vinblastine + bleomycin	26%	25.5 mo.
	Cisplatinum + methotrexate + bleomycin (MPB)	74%	
	Bleomycin + etoposide + cisplatinum (BEP)	83%	
	High-dose cisplatinum + vinblastine + bleomycin (VPB)	63%[c]	
	Low-dose cisplatinum + vinblastine + bleomycin (VPB)	43%[c]	
	Vinblastine + ifosfamide + cisplatinum (CIV)	36%	34 mo.
Prostate Cancer	Doxorubicin + mitomycin + 5 Fluorouracil (DMF)	48%	12 mo.
	Estradiol + nitrogen mustard (estramustine)	30%	11 mo.[d]
	Doxorubicin + cyclophosphamide	15–32%	5–8[d]
	Cyclophosphamide + prednisolone	8%	6[d]

[a]Lower response rates seen in nonrandomized studies by Sternberg, et al.
[b]Median survival for complete responders/median survival for partial responders
[c]Complete response only
[d]Duration of response

dysfunction. Peripheral neuropathy and neuromuscular toxicity occur with etoposide but are considerably less frequent than with other drugs. Allergic reactions and vasomotor hypersensitivity are other well documented side effects of etoposide.

Ifosfamide toxicity is usually manifested as hematuria because of the urothelial damage caused by acrolein and chloroacetic acid, metabolites of the parent drug. Other toxic effects include renal insufficiency, nausea, vomiting, and myelosuppression. The urothelial toxicity of ifosfamide can be prevented by concomitant administration of protective agents such as 2 mercaptoethylsulfonate sodium (Mesna) and N-acetylcysteine.

Bladder Cancer

Chemotherapy has been most successful in the treatment of superficial bladder cancer (Table 15.9). Bladder cancer is superficial in 50 to 60% of patients at the time of initial diagnosis. The easy accessibility of the superficial bladder cancers via endoscopy or catheterization has made it possible to use local instillation of antineoplastic agents. Intravesical chemotherapy provides high drug concentrations at the tumor site and is used for local control of existing lesions as well as the prevention of recurrence and progression. Initial trials of intravesical chemotherapy were conducted with thiotepa, but other agents have equal or greater effectiveness. Intravesical drugs used to treat superficial bladder cancer include thiotepa, doxorubicin, mitomycin C, alpha interferons and Bacillus Calmette-Guerin (BCG). These agents are instilled via a catheter into an empty bladder, retained for 1 to 2 hours, and then evacuated. Most are administered weekly for approximately 6 weeks and may be maintained at monthly intervals in patients requiring prolonged therapy. BCG has proven to be superior to the other agents in most trials. Complications of BCG include local irritation, malaise, a flu-like syndrome, bladder contractures (rarely), and a tuberculosis-like syndrome. If the tuberculosis-like syndrome develops, therapy with iso nicotinic acid hydrazide (INH) is administered for 6 months. All intravesical agents are contraindicated when there is hematuria, urinary infection, or intraurethral trauma. BCG is contraindicated in patients with active TB and in immunosuppressed individuals. Some intravesical agents (e.g., thiotepa) cause myelosuppression. Local irritation manifests as hematuria, dysuria, frequency, and urgency. Allergic responses resulting in palmar and genital rashes may also occur.

Of patients with bladder cancer, 25 to 40% present with muscle infiltrative disease. Conventional therapy with radical cystectomy is initially effective in most patients. However, the 5-year disease-free survival is only 50% with surgery alone. This has led to the use of chemotherapeutic agents for primary therapy (neoadjuvant therapy) in attempts to improve survival and preserve the bladder. Neoadjuvant trials in bladder cancer are still experimental, and the regimens are similar to those used to treat metastatic bladder cancer. Initial trials with cisplatinum, methotrexate, vinblastine (CMV) or platinum, methotrexate, vinblastine and doxorubicin (MVAC) have shown complete responses in 17 to 20% of patients and tumor downstaging in an additional 50%.

Chemotherapy with CMV or MVAC is currently used for the treatment of metastatic bladder cancer. Apart from doxorubicin, the two regimens also differ in their platinum dosage, which is higher in the CMV regimen than in the MVAC regimen. The CMV regimen gives a CR in 28% of patients and a PR in 28%. With MVAC, the CR is 36%, and the overall response rate (CR+PR) is about 72%.

A major problem among patients who achieve a remission is that 10 to 20% will develop CNS metastasis, almost half of them during systemic remission. Modification of therapy to treat spinal and CNS metastasis is currently being explored. Other combinations that have shown promise for metastatic bladder cancer include cisplatin and doxorubicin (CA); cisplatin, doxorubicin, and cyclophosphamide (CISCA); cisplatin and methotrexate (MP); and cisplatin and methotrexate, vinblastine, epirubicin (M-VEC).

All combination regimens use cyclic administration of the individual agents in a sequential order. Toxicity is high, and dose reduction is necessary in most patients. The concomitant use of granulocyte colony stimulating factor (GCSF) is helpful in reducing the hemopoietic toxicity of these agents. Strategies to circumvent resistance to these drugs are being developed (e.g., concurrent use of hydroxyurea and cytosine arabinoside with cisplatin to inhibit DNA repair, and use of buthionine sulfoximide).

The use of newer alternative drugs is being explored in clinical trials. One study reports a total response of 63% with the less toxic analogues carboplatinum and mitoxantrone substituted for cisplatinum and doxorubicin in the MVAC regimen. A PR of 30% in patients with advanced bladder cancer who were refractory to other chemotherapy has been reported with 5 FU and alpha interferon. Methods to prevent the development of multiple-drug resistance (MDR) include reversal of MDR gene expression by calcium channel blockers, the use of antibodies against MDR gene products, and progestational agents.

Renal Cancer

Attempts aimed at control or treatment of metastatic renal cancer with chemotherapy have been unsuccessful. Vinblastine and the nitrosourea (CCNU) have been the most successful, but response rates are only between 10 to 20% (Table 15.9). Other drugs that could be applied are hydroxyurea and ifosfamide. There appears to be no significant advantage for using a combination of agents in lieu of a single agent for chemotherapy of renal cancers. The use of high-dose methotrexate with citrovorum factor rescue holds initial promise. Biologic therapy seems to hold more promise in renal than in other GU cancers (see Chapter 8).

Prostate Cancer

Chemotherapy for prostate cancer has shown marginal effectiveness in prolonging patient survival. Most agents have been administered to patients with advanced hormone-resistant disease, and response criteria have been inconsistent. Initial studies indicate response rates of 6 to 7% and disease stabilization in a further 15% of patients (Table 15.9). Cyclophosphamide, 5-Fluorouracil, methotrexate, cisplatin, and semustine (Methyl CCNU) have been used as single-agent therapy for stabilization of progressive disease. Subjective response and survival have been better than with hormonal therapy alone. Another treatment strategy is the administration of chemotherapeutic agents and hormones in combination, for example, estramustine (Estradiol and nitrogen mustard) and prednimustine (Prednisolone and Chlorambucil) for newly diagnosed tumors. Though toxicity is lower with these combinations, objective improvement is rare. These drugs cause less feminization than diethylstilbestrol. Doxorubicin is another agent of some utility in prostate cancer. Combination treatment with doxorubicin, mitomycin C and 5 FU gave an objective response of 48% lasting 47 weeks. A recent innovative trial of chemotherapy for prostate cancer utilizes suramin, an anti-growth factor with adrenolytic properties and the capacity to inhibit intracellular enzymes. Preliminary trials in metastatic, hormone-refractory tumors have not yielded optimistic results, but further investigation with refinements in administration technique and dosage could result in better outcomes.

Penile Cancer

Chemotherapy for penile cancers is commonly administered in patients with advanced disease. Primary therapy in such cases is usually with 5-Fluorouracil, methotrexate, or bleomycin, and can be followed by surgery or radiotherapy. These agents have induced some remissions. Single-agent cisplatin therapy, effective against other epidermoid tumors, results in a partial response (PR) rate of 15% for 1 to 3 months. In the absence of strong supportive evidence for the use of chemotherapy, conventional therapy with surgery or radiation is the mainstay in the management of men with penile cancers.

Urethral Cancer

Treatment of urethral cancers with antineoplastic agents is not yet widespread. Cisplatin-based combination regimens have shown promise for transitional cell cancers, and the topical administration of these agents is an interesting possibility. Chemotherapy is an adjunct to surgery or irradiation in patients with urethral cancer.

FUTURE DIRECTIONS

Because of the lack of extensive clinical experience with the chemotherapy of genitourinary cancers and the paucity of long-term, randomized controlled clinical trials, reliable recommendations for chemotherapeutic strategies against GU cancers, with the exception of testicular tumors, cannot be made. The issues regarding this subject can be expected to be clarified as data from ongoing clinical trials become available and current experience is tempered by acquisition of newer knowledge.

Current experimental approaches to improve the effectiveness of chemotherapy focus on (1) the synthesis of newer, more efficient, and less toxic analogues of parent drugs, for example, carboplatin (parent drug is cisplatinum); (2) the use of compounds to counter specific toxic manifestations (e.g., leucovorin rescue for methotrexate, mesna with ifosfamide; and (3) the replenishment or augmentation of organ reserves that bear the brunt of the toxicity (e.g., bone marrow transplants). Biologic response modifiers such as cytokines and interferons are also being used to alter the tumor–host relationship and improve therapeutic benefits. With the exception of alpha interferon (hairy cell leukemia and bladder cancer) none of the other agents used for this purpose has been successful. A subclass of chemotherapeutic agents that holds promise for the future includes the differentiating agents (e.g., retinoic acid cytosine arabinoside [Ara-C], butyric acid, vitamin D_3, and others) which are being used in attempts to induce maturation of tumor cells into nonmalignant phenotypes. Gene modulation is another area of research with promising possibilities. Finally, agents such as Warfarin and Razoxane are being investigated as antimetastatic agents, and this is another potential area for future research.

SUGGESTED READINGS

Skipper HE, Perry S. Cancer Res 1970; 30:1883.

Critical review of tumor cell growth, kinetics, and concepts of Gompertzian model of growth.

Morrow GR, Morrell C. Behavioral treatment for the anticipatory nausea and vomiting induced by cancer chemotherapy. N Engl J Med 1982; 307 (24):1476.

Study showing usefulness of systematic desensitization for an antiemetic effect in cancer patients.

Bauer KA. Pulmonary complications associated with combination chemotherapy programs containing bleomycin. Am J Med 1983; 74:557.

Discussion of bleomycin-associated pulmonary complications, which are greater in patients receiving bleomycin as a component of combination chemotherapy regimens than in those receiving bleomycin alone.

Stillwell TJ, Benson RC Jr. Cyclophosphamide-induced hemorrhagic cystitis: a review of 100 patients. Cancer 1988; 61(3):451.

Critical review of cyclophosphamide-induced hemorrhagic cystitis in 100 patients. Recent advances in uroprotective agents may decrease the bladder toxicity of cyclophosphamide therapy.

Williams SD, Birch R, Einhorn L, et al. Treatment of disseminated germ-cell tumors with cisplatin, bleomycin, and either vinblastine or etoposide. N Engl J Med 1987; 316:1435.

Critical clinical trial demonstrating role of platinum, bleomycin VP-16 combination over CVB in initial therapy for metastatic testes cancer.

Lamm DOL, Stogdill VD, Stogdill BV, et al. Complications of BCG immunotherapy in 1278 patients with bladder cancer. J Urol 1986; 135: 272.

Concise overview of complications of BCG immunotherapy in 1278 patients with bladder cancer. Most of the severe irritative side effects and subsequent systemic complications can be prevented with prophylactic isoniazid.

Whitmore WF Jr, Yagoda A. Chemotherapy in the management of bladder tumors. Drugs 1989; 38(2):301.

Critical review of various chemotherapeutic agents for superficial and metastatic bladder cancer. Special emphasis on combination therapies and their development for use in metastatic cancer.

Logothetis CJ, Dexeus FH, Finn L, et al. A prospective randomized trial comparing MVAC and CISCA chemotherapy for patients with metastatic urothelial tumors. J Clin Oncol 1990; 8:1050.

A randomized clinical trial demonstrating superiority of MVAC over CISCA for treatment of metastatic transitional cell cancer.

Hainsworth JD, Williams SD, Einhorn LH, Birch R, Greco FA. Successful treatment of resistant germinal neoplasms with VP-16 and cisplatin: results of a Southeastern Cancer Study Group trial. J Clin Oncol 1985; 3:666.

Study on successful use of VP-16 in treatment of metastatic testis cancer not responding to standard platinum-based chemotherapy protocols.

Samson MK, Rivkin SE, Jones SE, et al. Dose-response and dose-survival advantage for high- versus low-dose cisplatin combined with vinblastine and bleomycin in disseminated testicular cancer. Cancer 1984; 53:1029.

Comparison of high-dose versus low-dose platinum-based combination chemotherapy for metastatic testis cancer demonstrating both an improved response and survival benefit to high-dose platinum.

Eisenberg MA, Abrams JS. Chemotherapy for prostatic carcinoma. Semin Urol 1988; 4:303.

Comprehensive overview of current concepts in treatment of advanced prostatic cancer with chemotherapy.

CHAPTER 16

Flow Cytometry in Urologic Oncology

Colin P. Dinney
Robert A. Stephenson

Cytology and fine-needle-aspiration biopsy (FNAB) are widely used for the diagnosis and staging of malignant tumors, assessment of treatment responses, and selection of patients for adjuvant therapy. The application of ancillary studies such as flow cytometry, immunocytochemistry, and image cytometry has improved the accuracy of cytologic diagnosis and contributed to a better understanding of human tumor biology.

A tumor mass is composed of a heterogeneous population of cells with varying degrees of differentiation. Well differentiated tumor cells have normal cellular function and little or no growth capacity. However, cells with poor differentiation have unlimited growth potential. The degree of differentiation is an important parameter in tumor assessment. This is usually achieved by histological analysis, but flow cytometry measures tumor cell DNA content, which is a rough approximation to tumor cell differentiation (Table 16.1).

Apart from routine histology and flow cytometry, there are emerging techniques for tumor cell assessment. These include cytogenetic analysis (e.g., chromosomal karyotyping) and molecular genetics (e.g., oncogenes, tumor suppressor genes). Increased oncogene expression and tumor suppressor gene inactivation have been identified in human colonic cancers. A tumor suppression gene situated on the long arm of chromosome 13 has been identified in retinoblastoma and bladder cancer, and a Wilm's tumor suppressor gene (short arm chromosome 11) in Wilm's tumors and adrenal carcinoma. The P53 suppressor gene has also been implicated in oncogenesis in multiple organs, including the prostate. Tumor progression is believed to be a consequence of the sequential accumulation of specific genetic alterations that promote uncontrolled cell growth.

Table 16.1: Human Tumor Characteristics

Heterogeneous cell populations
Degree differentiation
"Growth fraction"
Assessment
Histology
Flow cytometry
Image cytometry
Cytogenetic study
Molecular genetics
Tumor growth
Disregulated oncogenes
Inactivated tumor suppressor genes

CELL CYCLE KINETICS

The abnormal proliferation of cells is a characteristic feature of malignancy. A knowledge of tumor cell kinetics may help to unravel the disease process and optimize treatment. Howard and Pelc described five phases in the life cycle of proliferating cells. From the G_1 (gap 1) phase cells enter the G_0 (resting) or S (DNA synthesis) phase. Chromosomes are duplicated during the S phase, from which cells enter the G_2 (gap 2) phase and progress to the M (mitosis) phase and then back into G_1. The timing of the S, G_2, and M phases is characteristically constant for a given cell type. This model of the cell cycle allows experimental and mathematical analyses of cellular populations in normal and malignant tissues (Table 16.2).

The study of cell cycle kinetics requires the labeling of newly synthesized DNA with a detectable precursor molecule (e.g., tritiated thymidine) and the use of autoradiography. Autoradiography allows the estimation of the labeling index, but time-dependent measurements, such as the cell cycle time, can be estimated only by using multiple, serial biopsy specimens. This approach is rarely feasible in clinical practice. However, the recent introduction of monoclonal antibodies to the halogenated analogues of thymidine (bromodeoxyuridine and iododeoxyuridine) allows immunohistochemical examination of DNA in proliferating cells.

The proliferative, or growth (S, G_2, M) phase, averages about 10 hours for human cells, whereas the G_1/G_0 phase is quite variable, ranging between hours and days. In a solid tumor the majority of the cells are in

Table 16.2: The Basics of Cell-Cycle Kinetics

G_0/G_1 phase	Presynthetic or gap phase Diploid DNA content in normal cells Increasing RNA content from G_0 to G_1
S phase	Proliferative DNA content between diploid and tetraploid High S phase with actively proliferating cells
G_2/M phase	Mitotic phase Tetraploid DNA content
Diploid cells	Normal DNA content Two sets of chromosomes
Aneuploid cells	Chromosomal aberrations Abnormal quantity of DNA

the G_1/G_0/death phase and therefore not easily amenable to chemotherapy or external-beam radiation. Conversely, the small number of cells in the growth phase (the growth fraction) is actively cycling and responsive to chemotherapy and other treatments. Solid tumors with large growth fractions tend to respond best to chemotherapeutic intervention.

DNA CYTOMETRY

DNA flow cytometry (FCM) of a solid tumor provides information about its genetic composition (DNA ploidy) and its rate of cellular proliferation (S-phase fraction). These properties influence metastatic potential, tumor growth rate, and, possibly, responsiveness to therapy. There are two different techniques of DNA cytometry. In flow cytometry, the tumor is disaggregated by mechanical or enzymatic methods to give a monocellular suspension. The cells are then stained with a fluorescent dye that binds to cellular DNA. In image cytometry, the cells are placed on a microscope slide either as a whole-cell preparation (e.g., touch preparation of a smear from a fine-needle aspiration) or as a cut section from paraffin-embedded tissue. The slide is stained for DNA, and an automated microscope is used to measure the nuclear content of several hundred cells. Image cytometry is useful for the measurement of cell components such as cell size, nuclear size, and DNA content. Measurements are displayed as a frequency distribution histogram in which the *x*-axis represents DNA content and the *y*-axis represents the number of cells having that DNA content. Image cytometry is slower and more labor-intensive than flow cytometry. Fewer malignant cells are measured, and the resolution of the technique is further reduced since nuclei are cut at random levels during tissue sectioning. Varying portions of nuclei are therefore included within the thickness of the section.

Flow cytometry is the more widely used of the two methods. Tens of thousands of cells are measured within minutes to give histograms that are mathematically analyzed. The reliability of FCM is limited somewhat by the need to dissociate the tumor specimen. Specimens frequently contain normal cells from adjacent nonmalignant tissue as well as the stromal, endothelial, and inflammatory components of the tumor. The DNA histogram of the tumor, therefore, reflects some of the normal components of the tumor.

DNA histograms are analyzed for DNA ploidy by locating the major peak of the histogram—the DNA content shared by most of the cells. If this is the same as normal tissues, the tumor is DNA diploid; otherwise, it is DNA aneuploid, with a DNA index that is the ratio of the tumor value to the normal value. The S-phase fraction is directly related to cellular proliferation—the higher the fraction, the more rapidly the tumor growth (Table 16.2). Estimating the S-phase fraction from the DNA histogram is difficult, however; and the results become unreliable if the preparation contains much nuclear debris or if the tumor has an aneuploid population of cells. DNA aneuploidy and high S-phase fractions are associated with tumors of high clinical stage and grade and a generally poor prognosis. DNA cytometry may be more important in low-stage tumors where DNA diploid, low S-phase tumors are unlikely to metastasize.

The usefulness of DNA cytometry in evaluating solid tumors is extensively documented in studies using either flow or image cytometry. Many of these studies are retrospective, using archival paraffin-embedded tissue blocks. Thick (50 μm) sections are cut from the block and then are dissociated to obtain isolated nuclei for either flow or image cytometry.

FCM DNA histograms are constructed from the stratification of the relative fluorescene intensity of thousands of stained nuclei. This fluorescence reflects the stoichiometric dye binding to the DNA of both proliferating and nonproliferating cells, which is detected by photomultiplier tubes. The normal DNA histogram has a dominant peak representing the majority of cells in the resting (G_0) or the inseparable cycling presynthetic (G_1) phases of the cell cycle. In a normal human cell population, both G_0 and G_1 correspond to the quantity of DNA seen in the 46 human chromosomes. A second smaller peak (G_2/M) to the right of G_0/G_1 represents cells that have twice as much DNA as those in the G_0/G_1 phases. The G_2/M peak represents cells with a double copy or tetraploid (4N) complement of chromosomes that are in the postsynthetic phase of the cell cycle preceding mitosis (G_2) or in mitosis just prior to actual division (M). Events in the fluorescence channels of the histogram between G_0/G_1 and G_2/M represent cells containing intermediate DNA levels and correspond to cells in the synthesis (S) phase of the DNA cell cycle.

DNA content is measured in relation to the DNA fluorescence of a known diploid control cell standard. This ratio of the DNA fluorescence intensities of the G_0/G_1 peaks of the test sample (tumor)/standard is defined as the *DNA index* (DI). A DI of 1 is equated with normal DNA content or a 2N chromosome count of diploid sample, whereas a DI of 2 is the same DNA content as 4N, or double the number of normal chromosomal DNA. Tumors with abnormal DNA content (aneuploidy) display visually identifiable additional G_0/G_1 peaks corresponding to tumor stemlines with DNA content different from the diploid standard. A DI greater than or less than 1 is considered abnormal, although it cannot always be equated with malignancy because some benign tumors (e.g., nevi, colonic adenomas) may exhibit chromosomal abnormalities and abnormal DNA indices.

The sensitivity of FMC DNA measurement requires a 5 to 10% quantitative DNA abnormality for detection. Cancers with near-diploid cytogenetic abnormalities will have normal or diploid DNA contents. Some tumors may have chromosomal deletions/duplications that cancel out and result in a cell with normal net DNA content. Moreover, FCM DNA analysis is a morphologically "blind" technique that requires a sufficient number of cells (approximately 5% of the cell suspension) with a marker (DNA abnormality or aneuploidy) to be detected. Malignant tumors with undetectable abnormal genomes are not uncommon. For example, FCM diploid-range tumors account for roughly 30% of breast and colon carcinomas and 50% of renal cell and prostate carcinomas.

TECHNIQUE OF FLOW CYTOMETRY

Flow Cytometry (FCM) is an objective, automated technique for measuring the DNA content of individual cells or subcellular particles (Table 16.3). Although primarily a research tool, FCM is rapidly being integrated

Table 16.3: Technique of Flow Cytometry

Preparation monodispersed cell suspension
Fluorescent dye staining
Pressurized chamber
Single cell alignment
Use of laser, photomultiplier, and computer
500–100,000 cells analyzed within minutes

into the clinical management of patients with urologic cancers. The most common clinical applications include discriminating between benign and malignant neoplasms, identifying tumor cell heterogeneity, detecting minimal residual disease following therapy, and correlating DNA ploidy and other parameters with disease progression.

The stained, disaggregated specimen is placed in a pressurized chamber that regulates its passage into a flow chamber, in which the cells are hydrodynamically aligned in single file and centered at the focus of the illumination source—usually a laser (Figure 16.1). The excitation and emission spectra of the fluorescent dye must correspond with the light source emission and photodetectors of the flow cytometer. When the dye is excited by the illumination source, it emits a fluorescent flash that is collected, measured by a photomultiplier, and recorded on a computer. Within seconds to minutes, 500,000 to 100,000 cells can be measured and analyzed by the computer programs. FCM provides both rapid and objective evaluation of cellular characteristics (particularly the DNA content) in solid tumors. The clinically significant parameters measured by FCM include DNA content (ploidy), RNA content, and the S-phase fraction. All of these parameters may have prognostic value.

Urologic tumors have been extensively studied using fresh tissue

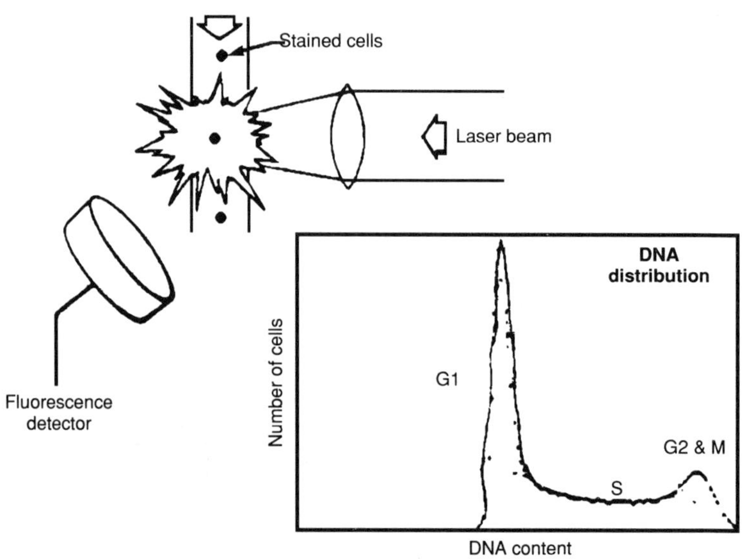

Figure 16.1: The principles of DNA distribution analysis of flow cytometry.

specimens and correlated prospectively to clinical parameters including grade and stage. Following the description of a technique for measuring DNA ploidy using paraffin-embedded tumors of archival specimens by Hedley et al. in 1983, retrospective correlations of DNA ploidy to disease progression and survival were made possible. Numerous reports using this technique have been published in the urologic literature.

Flow cytometers analyze cells on the basis of optical and electrical properties that are detected as individual cells are passed in single file through a specifically designed flow chamber. When cells are stained with a fluorescent DNA dye and excited by the instruments' laser, then the emitted fluorescent light per cell is proportional to the amount of DNA per cell. This cellular DNA information is typically expressed as a DNA histogram (DNA/cell versus number of cells) (Figure 16.2).

Neoplasia is thought to arise when a specific chromosomal aberration alters the normal DNA content of a cell. This abnormality of DNA, called aneuploidy, is thought to arise in approximately 75% of solid tumors. The degree of aneuploidy is characterized by the DNA index: the ratio of the DNA content of G_1 phase aneuploid cells to that of the diploid cells. Diploid tumors have a DNA index of 1; aneuploid tumors have a DNA index that is usually over 1 but may be less than 1.

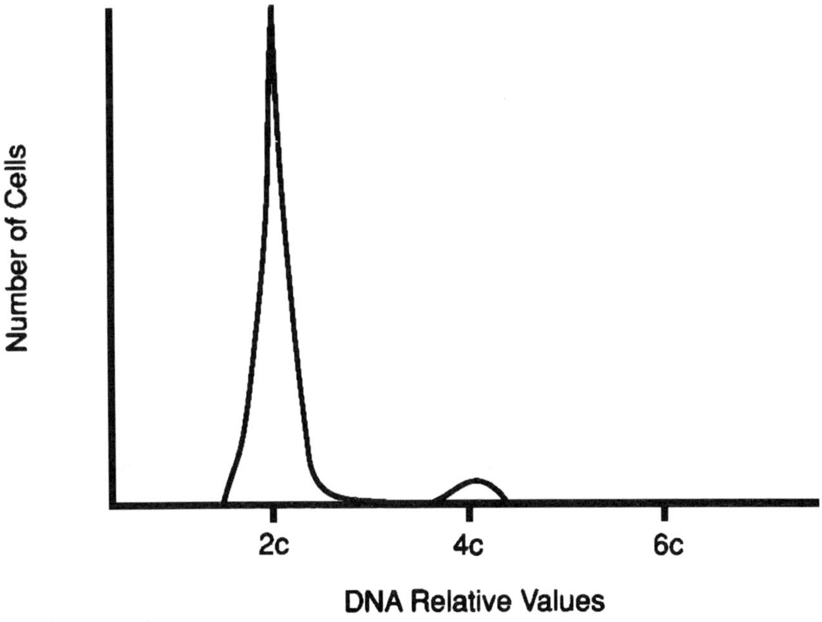

Figure 16.2: DNA histogram from a patient with no urothelial tumor or dysplasia.

Using a DNA histogram, it is possible to determine the proportion of cells within the various cell cycle phases: G_0/G_1, S, and G_2M. Two determinations commonly derived from DNA histograms are the DNA index of ploidy and the proliferation index. Tumor DNA ploidy is determined by measuring the DNA content of the tumor cells in the G_0/G_1 phase in relation to the DNA content of normal control or diploid cells. Tumors in which the DNA content is similar to that in normal controls are regarded as diploid. An aneuploid population is present if a second distinct peak of more or less cellular DNA is found in a histogram position differing from the diploid control (Figure 16.3). A tetraploid aneuploid population is typically considered to exist when a peak exceeds the normal control G_2M peak by three standard deviations. The tumor proliferative index is defined as the proportion of tumor cells in S phase. This value must be compared with the normal control population in order to detect an increased S-phase value.

A distinct aneuploid population of cells appears diagnostic for cancer. DNA aneuploidy may be present before gross or histologic changes

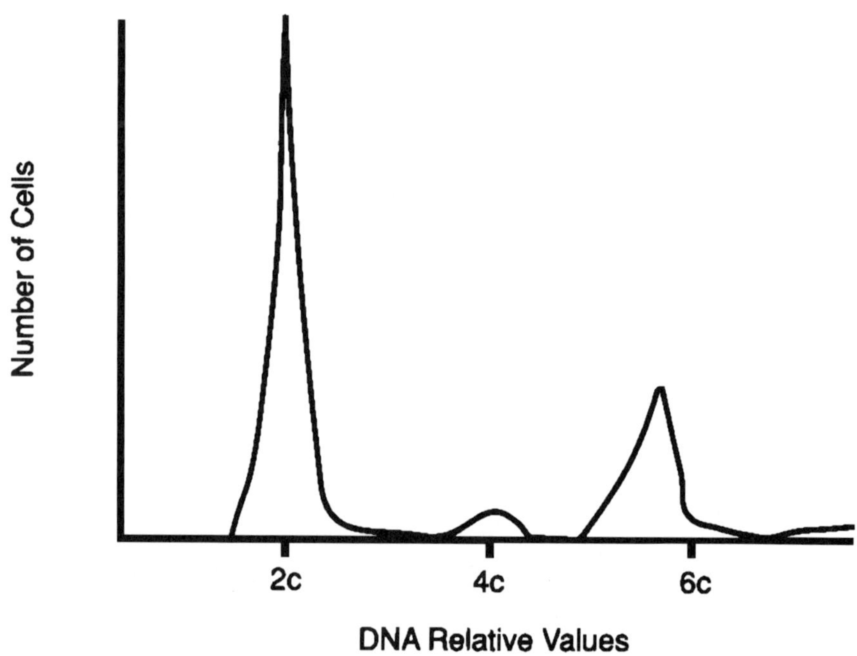

Figure 16.3: DNA histogram showing aneuploid peak (6c) in patient with invasive bladder tumor.

are appreciated. Additionally, if the primary and metastatic sites have different DNA indices, monitoring the therapeutic response of the primary tumor may not reflect the response of metastatic sites. Prospective and retrospective studies suggest that aneuploidy is a poor prognostic sign in urologic cancers.

The RNA and DNA contents of tumor cells can be measured simultaneously. The metachromatic dye acridine orange binds to double-stranded DNA and fluoresces green, whereas it binds to single-stranded RNA and fluoresces red. Use of two fluorochromes (one for RNA and the other for DNA) with similar excitation but different emission spectra is another method. RNA measurements can identify malignancy in tumors with diploid or near-diploid DNA histograms.

While FCM analysis is rapid and objective, it is not as sensitive as karyotype analysis in detecting minor chromosomal alterations. Since FCM can resolve stemline DNA content differences of only 4% or greater, more subtle change than the addition or loss of two complete chromosomes cannot be detected.

A potential application of FCM awaits the identification of tumor-specific antigens. When such antigens are isolated, complementary monoclonal antibodies can be conjugated with a fluorescent tag such as fluorescein isothiocyanate (FITC). The labeled monoclonal antibody could then be measured by FCM and provide a sensitive method for identifying malignant cells.

A major obstacle to FCM analysis of solid tumors is the need for a preparation of dispersed cells. Bladder cancer is easily disassociated and provides optimal specimens for FCM analysis, yielding abundant, well preserved urothelium in a single-cell suspension. It is, therefore, not surprising that bladder tumors have been extensively studied by FCM analysis.

PARAFFIN-EMBEDDED ARCHIVAL TISSUE

There are certain advantages to using archival paraffin-embedded tissue for flow cytometry determinations (Table 16.4). The specimen does not require immediate processing, and areas of interest can be preselected by microscopic examination. In addition, it permits the performance of retrospective studies to assess the importance of DNA ploidy in tumor behavior and patient survival. Using archival tissue has, however, a number of disadvantages. The quality of the DNA histogram tends to be inferior to that derived from a fresh specimen because of a greater amount of background debris. This results in an overestimation of the S-phase fraction of the tumor. The resolution of G_0/G_1 peaks is inferior so that aneuploid populations can occasionally be mistaken as diploid.

Table 16.4: Paraffin-Embedded Tissue for Flow Cytometry

Advantages	*Disadvantages*
Allows retrospective study	Quality of DNA histogram reduced by background debris
Correlation between ploidy, tumor behavior, and survival	Overestimates S-phase fraction
Archival tissue readily available	Technically poor preparation in 10–15%
	Paraffin block rapidly used up because of need for thick (50μm) sections

Furthermore, approximately 10 to 15% of specimens are of poor technical quality and uninterpretable.

Fluorochrome DNA staining is highly variable in paraffin-embedded tissues, so that while the stoichiometric relationship between DNA and staining is maintained, specimens cannot be compared on the basis of a single control. Because of this variability, external controls cannot be used to determine whether the G_0/G_1 peak represents the diploid population. Most studies of paraffin-embedded archival material arbitrarily define the peak of lowest channel number as 2.0 c, or diploid. This definition provides accurate classification for most specimens, but in some instances hypodiploid aneuploid lines may be erroneously classified as diploid.

Histograms of optimal quality require sections that are 50 μm thick. This rapidly consumes paraffin blocks and may preclude further studies. Notwithstanding these disadvantages, the methodology of using paraffin-embedded specimens compares favorably with methods employing fresh tissue.

FCM is a commonly used methodology to characterize human urological tumors. Early studies compared DNA ploidy with established prognostic factors, but more recent studies have attempted to define the natural history of urological neoplasms and their response to therapy. The following sections summarize current information on FCM of the common genitourinary cancers.

KIDNEY

Renal Cell Carcinoma

Renal cell carcinoma (RCC), an unpredictable neoplasm, can progress years after initial therapy. Pathological stage at presentation is the most critical predictor of clinical outcome. Tumor grade is an excellent guide to prognosis when the tumor is either well differentiated or poorly differentiated. However, most patients with renal cell tumors have moder-

Table 16.5: FCM Characteristics of Renal Cell Carcinoma

Aneuploidy 40–75%
Ploidy variance between primary and metastases 40%
Aneuploid: diploid metastases (2:1)
Solitary metastasis more common with diploid primary
? diploid metastases more likely to respond to therapy

ately well differentiated neoplasms, and prognosis cannot be confidently made on the basis of tumor grade alone. This creates a possible role for FCM in determining prognosis and, perhaps, selection of therapy for patients with renal cell carcinoma (Table 16.5).

Many studies have assessed the correlation between ploidy and tumor grade, and most report a positive correlation. Several grading systems are available, and at the extremes of grade, most correlate well with tumor behavior. The association between DNA ploidy and tumor stage is less clear. Perhaps this is because the majority of studies use Robson's classification scheme. Depending on the distribution of patients classified as Robson's stage III, a different correlation of ploidy and stage is reached. However, with the TNM system, a significant correlation between the presence of aneuploidy and high stage has been reported.

Most studies of FCM report an incidence of aneuploidy in renal cell carcinoma ranging from between 40 and 74%. Aneuploid tumors demonstrate considerable heterogeneity and contain aneuploid and diploid cell populations. The phenomenon of ploidy heterogeneity is further reflected in the significant variance (up to 40%) between the ploidy of the primary tumor and that of its metastases. An aneuploid primary may develop a diploid metastasis, and diploid primaries are capable of metastasizing. There is a higher proportion of aneuploid metastases compared to diploid metastases (ratio of about 2:1). Most metastases from diploid primaries are aneuploid.

Few diploid tumors demonstrate evidence of local invasion, as opposed to the majority of aneuploid tumors. Although distant metastasis is as common with diploid as with aneuploid primaries, there are a significant number of patients with diploid tumors who have solitary metastases as compared with the aneuploid population. This may imply that the difference in malignant behavior between diploid and aneuploid tumors may be expressed in the clinical course of patients with metastatic disease.

The most significant impact of ploidy analysis may be its ability to predict outcome. While many studies reveal that ploidy has an impact on survival, some suggest that this impact is marginal. There may be a survival advantage for patients with diploid tumors, although no clear survival advantage occurs when tumors are controlled for stage. A large retrospective study of paraffin-embedded material showed better 5- and 10-year survival rates for patients with diploid tumors compared to those with nondiploid tumors. Within any stage, recurrence was more common with aneuploid tumors. However, the indication of a higher rate of survival for patients with diploid tumors was not statistically significant. Although DNA ploidy correlates with tumor stage, grade, and disease progression in univariate analyses, multivariate analysis shows no definite survival advantage for diploid tumors when corrected for tumor (TNM) stage.

An important issue in the management of patients with renal cell carcinoma is the choice of therapy for patients with metastatic disease. Ploidy may play a role in this setting. Several studies have demonstrated that patients with metastasis from diploid primaries have prolonged survival compared to those with aneuploid primaries. The survival benefit in patients with diploid tumors is independent of tumor grade. The DNA content of the metastases also appears to influence survival, whether the metastases are solitary or multiple. Progression may be slower and survival prolonged in patients with diploid metastases, even when they are multiple. There may even be a subgroup of patients with an aneuploid primary and diploid metastasis who may have better survival rates. FCM may prove to have an important role in identifying patients with diploid metastases who might benefit from aggressive therapy. It is conceivable that ploidy status may identify patients with solitary metastases who would benefit from nephrectomy and excision of their solitary metastasis.

Renal Oncocytoma

Renal oncocytomas have low potentials for invasive or malignant metastatic behavior. Nondiploid DNA patterns have been reported in up to 50% of renal oncocytomas (39% tetraploid, 11% aneuploid). However, in the majority of patients with tetraploid/aneuploid patterns the renal oncocytomas do not progress. An abnormal DNA pattern does not appear to be a marker of disease progression. A diploid pattern nevertheless may assure lack of progression. Currently, the relative value of FCM in this variant of renal cancer is undefined and appears to be minimal.

Wilm's Tumor

Several retrospective studies describe the FCM findings in paraffin-embedded specimens from patients with Wilm's tumors. There is a progressive increase in aneuploidy and S-phase fractions between the low-risk and high-risk groups. Compared to conventional risk factors in children with Wilm's tumor, there is no statistically significant relationship between

DNA ploidy and patient survival. Although DNA ploidy may have some influence on survival, the conventional risk factors of tumor histology and stage, as defined by the National Wilm's Tumor Study Group, are more accurate predictors of survival in children with Wilm's tumors.

BLADDER TRANSITIONAL CELL CARCINOMA

The role of FCM in identifying and characterizing bladder cancer has been extensively studied. Bladder irrigation specimens provide high-quality, exfoliated cells in suspension that are of better quality than voided urine, and they provide superior cellular preservation and less background debris when analyzed by flow cytometry. The bladder is irrigated with sterile saline via an Ellik evacuator, endoscope sheath, or piston syringe. The specimen is centrifuged, and the cell pellet is resuspended in a salt solution, filtered to a concentration of 10^6 cells/ml, and stained for analysis.

Several studies have addressed the relative value of urinary cytology versus FCM in the diagnosis of bladder cancer (Table 16.6). FCM is the more sensitive discriminator, with a cancer detection rate of approximately 80% for bladder barbotage FCM. This compares to a rate of 60 to 70% for barbotaged cytology and the 60% sensitivity of voided urinary cytology. Combining FCM with cytology may well enhance cancer detection rates. The sensitivity of FCM is reduced in the presence of pyuria (>5 WBC/HPF) or extraneous squamous/inflammatory cells, especially in women.

The specificity of FCM has also been addressed. The false-positive rate of bladder wash FCM is acceptably low, usually between 1 and 2%. Unfortunately, any degree of false positivity eliminates FCM as a possible screening technique because of the low incidence of bladder cancer. Cytology, with its almost 100% specificity, is therefore a more suitable screening test for bladder cancer.

Tumor Stage and Grade

DNA ploidy has been correlated with tumor grade and stage. With few

Table 16.6: FCM Characteristics of Bladder Transitional Cell Carcinoma

Bladder barbotage FCM more sensitive than barbotage cytology
FCM specificity less than cytology
Similar ploidy patterns in primary and metastases in 50%
Metastases more common with aneuploid primaries
Multiple aneuploid cell lines in carcinoma-in-situ associated with higher rates of progression

exceptions, grade II tumors are diploid and grade III tumors aneuploid. Multiple aneuploid lines are found in a significant percentage of grade III tumors and carcinoma in situ (CIS). The frequency of DNA aneuploidy increases with tumor stage, and the proliferation index is directly related to the degree of aneuploidy and tumor stage.

Random biopsies from the macroscopically normal mucosa may reveal aneuploidy, especially in patients with aneuploid grade II and III tumors. Histopathology reveals various forms of atypia within these locations. While FCM has expanded our knowledge of the field change concept of bladder cancer, the significance of this information for patient management is currently unclear.

DNA Ploidy of Lymph Node Metastases

The flow pattern proliferation index of primary bladder tumors has been compared to that of their lymph node metastases. Nearly half the patients with hyperdiploid or triploid-tetraploid populations have lymph node metastases. The ploidy of the primary tumor and lymph nodes are similar in about 50% of patients (Table 16.6). The incidence of lymph node metastasis appears to be related to the proliferation index of the primary tumor. Patients with an S-phase fraction in excess of 20% have a high incidence of nodal metastases. Despite the correlation between ploidy and lymph node metastases, there is no evidence that flow cytometric patterns are more predictable of lymph node metastasis than tumor grade and stage.

DNA Ploidy and Superficial Bladder Cancer

Recurrence DNA ploidy is a significant factor related to tumor progression and recurrence. Recurrence rates are higher in aneuploid (nearly four times more likely) than diploid tumors. DNA ploidy analysis may therefore offer more information than tumor grade alone in predicting recurrence.

Progression Tumor ploidy and progression are also related. Progression is rare with diploid tumors, whereas aneuploid tumors progress in 30 to 60% of patients. Progression rates for patients with carcinoma in situ are related to DNA ploidy. For solitary aneuploid lines, death is uncommon. With multiple aneuploid lines, progression frequently results in death or the need for radical cystectomy.

Response to Therapy FCM has been used to assess the response of bladder cancer to intravesical therapy. FCM is more sensitive than cytology but less specific in monitoring treatment response. FCM and cytology have false-negative rates of 20 and 40%, respectively. Unfortunately, the inflammatory response and hyperplastic cellular regeneration induced by intravesical BCG (Bacillus Calmette-Guerin) affect the interpretation of FCM and cytology. Combining FCM and cytology reduces the false-negative rate to about 10%. Despite the apparent value of FCM in predicting the treatment response, it should not be used alone to monitor response. Instead, a combination of cystoscopy, FCM, and cytology is recommended. Clearly, progression would be missed in certain patients if they were followed with FCM alone.

Ploidy has also been evaluated in patients treated with neoadjuvant M-VAC (methotrexate vinblastine, adriamycin, and cisplatinum) therapy who later undergo cystectomy. The positive predictive value of FCM was 88%, with a negative predictive value of only 29%. While aneuploidy indicates that patients require additional therapy for their bladder cancer, no predictive value can be placed on a negative study. Currently, FCM has no role in monitoring patients following chemotherapy for invasive tumors. A normal FCM analysis is no guarantee of tumor eradication.

FCM ploidy determinations have been used to predict the radioresponsiveness of invasive bladder tumors. Pathological downstaging is generally associated with normalization of DNA ploidy in patients receiving external-beam radiation prior to cystectomy. Downstaging occurs more frequently in patients with diploid tumors or tumors with a single aneuploid cell line.

Cell and Tumor Markers Polyclonal or monoclonal antibodies directed against epithelial cell cytokeratins have been used in mixed cell populations, such as bladder wash and urine, to separate epithelial from nonepithelial cells. This improves sensitivity by allowing the detection of small aneuploid and tetraploid populations. Enhanced sensitivity has been reported using anticytokeratin antibodies. Tumor progression can also be assessed using multiparameter flow cytometry, with monoclonal antibodies generated against antigens expressed on bladder tumor cells. Simultaneous FCM and surface antigen detection may provide more prognostic information than FCM alone. However, the expression of these antigens is not specific enough to be useful in patient management.

TRANSITIONAL CELL CARCINOMA OF RENAL PELVIS AND URETER

In paraffin-embedded specimens from patients with transitional cell carcinoma (TCC) of the renal pelvis, ploidy pattern, grade, stage, and clinical outcome are strongly correlated. For high-stage, poorly differentiated tumors, survival correlates well with grade and stage, and the detection of aneuploidy offers no further prognostic information. For patients with low-stage, well to moderately differentiated lesions, ploidy identifies a small subgroup of aneuploid patients with a poor prognosis and worse survival outlook.

In univariate analysis, DNA ploidy is a significant predictor of disease-free survival but loses its significance when the data are subjected to multivariate analysis. DNA ploidy does not have a significant effect on overall survival rates and, at present, should not be routinely performed in patients with TCC of the upper urinary tracts.

PROSTATE CANCER

The natural history of prostate cancer is unpredictable, and the optimal therapy of patients with localized prostate cancer is controversial. Of the various clinical, biochemical, and pathological features used to predict biological activity, none has been consistently successful. Pathological stage and histological grade remain the most widely accepted predictive characteristics but suffer, in part, because of their subjectivity.

DNA ploidy analysis is a promising, objective technique for identifying the malignant potential of prostate cancer. Ideally, patients with biologically aggressive lesions with a propensity to metastasize and cause death can be identified. Numerous studies provide evidence that patients with diploid tumors have a favorable prognosis. However, the role of FCM in patient management remains unclear. Prostate cancer is characterized by variable biologic behavior, ranging from latent carcinoma to rapidly metastasizing tumor. Despite parameters such as stage and grade, accurate prediction of tumor progression in an individual patient remains relatively uncertain. FCM has been applied as a supplemental parameter for diagnosing prostate cancer and for predicting tumor progression (Table 16.7).

Stage and Grade

Most studies report a close correlation between ploidy and the grade and stage of prostate cancers. Patients with aneuploid tumors have Gleason

Table 16.7: FCM Attributes of Prostate Cancer

Aneuploidy occurs in 20–30% of glands with benign prostatic hyperplasia
Aneuploidy usually correlates with elevated PSA levels
Diploid stage A cancers unlikely to progress
DNA aneuploidy is an independent predictor of tumor progression and prognosis
Aneuploid tumors less responsive to hormonal therapy
Aneuploidy associated with higher grade and stage of tumors

scores greater than 7 more often than those with nonaneuploid tumors. The frequency of multiple aneuploid lines increases with advancing tumor stages. Most poorly differentiated tumors are aneuploid.

Although ploidy and grade or stage are closely correlated, this relationship is not invariable. Aneuploid cell lines occur in 20 to 30% of prostate glands with benign prostatic hyperplasia, and this further confuses the interpretation of tumor ploidy. These changes are due to the natural increase in DNA within benign proliferating glands, or glands affected by chronic prostatitis, rather than to neoplastic changes. The occurrence of significant DNA abnormalities in benign prostatic tissue underlines the limitations of FCM in the diagnosis of prostate cancer.

Flow Cytometry and Prostate Specific Antigen

DNA ploidy has been compared with both cellular and serum prostate specific antigen (PSA) levels. Mean intracellular PSA and prostatic acid phosphatase (PAP) values are considerably higher in diploid tumors, and this confirms earlier reports that increasing grades of malignancy are accompanied by decreasing levels of cellular PSA and PAP. About one-third of patients with diploid tumors have normal serum PSA levels, while patients with aneuploid tumors usually have PSA values greater than 4.0 ng/dl.

Ploidy and Prognosis

Early studies indicated a possible relationship between ploidy and survival. This is not unexpected since ploidy correlates with grade and stage, both important determinants of prognosis. Recent studies using paraffin-embedded tissue have substantiated the correlation between ploidy and progression, survival, and hormone sensitivity. They have searched for a significant difference in clinical behavior of diploid versus aneuploid tumors, independent of the other variables.

Prostate cancer is heterogeneous for ploidy, and ploidy disparity is noted when multiple samples from the same tumor are analyzed. The knowledge that a prostate gland can harbor multiple discrete tumors magnifies the difficulty in defining ploidy. Multiple biopsies are required if tumor ploidy is not to be underestimated.

The impact of ploidy on the natural history of conservatively treated prostate cancer has been studied. Diploid prostate cancers are less aggressive than aneuploid cancers and progress at a slower rate. Nonetheless, they do progress, with 50% of patients undergoing local progression and 3% of patients developing distant metastases within 5 years. Significant alterations in ploidy patterns have been noted in tumors treated nonsurgically.

DNA ploidy offers valuable information regarding tumor behavior of stage A cancers. Diploid cancers are unlikely to progress. If this finding is confirmed in larger studies, ploidy may well become an important variable in determining the choice of therapy for patients with stage A prostate carcinoma.

Kaplan-Meier survival curves demonstrate the significance of DNA aneuploidy as an indicator of poor prognosis. By multivariate analysis, DNA aneuploidy maintains its significance as an indicator of poor prognosis. Aneuploid stage B tumors appear to metastasize early and relentlessly, and most patients with aneuploid tumors relapse. Radical prostatectomy may not be adequate therapy for this group of patients with pathological stage B tumors (Table 16.6). DNA ploidy is also an independent predictor of tumor progression in stage C prostate cancer. Tumor progression and survival are also related to tumor ploidy in patients with stage D_1 prostate cancer.

Seminal vesicle invasion is more frequent with aneuploid tumors. The enhanced disease-free survival in patients with diploid tumors, even in the presence of seminal vesicle invasion, provides evidence that the knowledge of DNA ploidy can stratify the risk of subsequent progression, even in patients with seminal vesicle invasion.

What are the effects of immediate adjuvant hormonal therapy on tumor progression and patient survival? There is a significant likelihood of progression in patients with diploid tumors who do not receive adjuvant therapy and in those with nondiploid tumors irrespective of hormonal therapy. The influence of ploidy on the response of metastatic disease to hormonal therapy has been evaluated. In general, responders have diploid or tetraploid tumors. Nonresponders tend to be aneuploid. Some responders convert from aneuploid to diploid cell lines during the course of hormonal treatment.

The DNA ploidy of lymph node metastases in patients undergoing ^{125}I-seed implantation has been examined. Patients with diploid metastases have a significantly prolonged survival compared to patients with aneuploid metastases. Cox regression analysis has shown that DNA-ploidy status is the strongest predictor of survival.

The bulk of available evidence suggests that DNA ploidy provides valuable insights regarding tumor behavior in selected patients with prostate cancer. The fact that few patients with diploid stage A_1 prostate cancer progress suggests that prostatectomy could be postponed until these patients show evidence of local progression or a change in ploidy patterns. More data are needed to support this inference. Ploidy has an equally important impact, independent of grade, on the natural history of pathological stages B, C, and D_1 prostate cancer. It is interesting to note that tetraploidy is associated with an intermediately poor prognosis for patients with stages C and D_1 but not for patients with stages A and B prostate cancer. The presence of aneuploidy in stage B or nondiploidy for stages C and D_1 prostate cancer is associated with a poor prognosis following local therapy. Clearly, most of these patients must have unrecognized disseminated cancer such that local therapy is inadequate.

Untreated diploid prostate cancer progresses at a slower rate than aneuploid prostate cancer. Presumably, the interval in which definitive local therapy can effectively eradicate all cancer is longer in patients with diploid tumors. However, once prostate cancer is disseminated, any previous advantage associated with a diploid primary is lost. One may presume that, since cancer is heterogeneous for any of a number of variables, ploidy would not be spared. Patients with D_2 cancer most likely have both aneuploid and diploid metastases.

ADRENAL NEOPLASMS

Adrenocortical Tumors

It is often difficult histologically to distinguish adrenal adenoma from carcinoma. A number of histopathologic features have been used to predict the clinical behavior of adrenal tumors. Despite these efforts, a significant number of tumors are indeterminate by histologic examination. It has been suggested that DNA content, as measured by FCM, may distinguish between benign and malignant tumors and possibly predict clinical outcome.

Most FCM studies of adrenocortical tumors indicate a general concordance of ploidy with histologic features. Aneuploidy is more common in carcinomas than in adenomas. In one study using aneuploidy as a predictor of clinical malignancy, DNA ploidy had a false-positive rate of 43% and a false-negative rate of 3%, compared with 33% and 3%, respectively, for histopathological features. While DNA ploidy analysis is effective as a predictor of clinical outcome, it is not clearly superior to histological or pathological evaluation. The histopathology of the tumor is more sensitive and specific in predicting clinical outcome than the presence of aneuploidy. In childhood adrenocortical tumors, the situation is somewhat different. FCM may play a role in predicting the natural history of childhood adrenocortical neoplasms because the histopathological diagnosis of malignancy is not as reliable as it is in adults.

Although ploidy and the histopathological features of adrenocortical tumors are closely correlated, FCM has no advantage over the more standard techniques for predicting tumor progression. An exception may be childhood neoplasms. FCM has a role when clinical and histopathological findings are equivocal, but the diagnosis of malignancy should not be made solely on the basis of DNA-ploidy analysis.

Pheochromocytoma

The biological activity of pheochromocytoma in the absence of local invasion or metastases is difficult to predict. The results of FCM studies of pheochromocytomas are limited and conflicting regarding the significance of aneuploidy. While the number of cases reported is low and the results conflicting, one can be fairly confident that a patient with a diploid pheochromocytoma is unlikely to progress. However, up to 40% of patients with aneuploid tumors and 30% with tetraploid tumors may progress. Such high-risk patients, therefore, require careful follow-up for long periods of time.

TESTICULAR CANCER

In testicular carcinomas, FCM reveals a high incidence of aneuploidy, approaching 80 to 95%. In testis cancer, unlike other solid neoplasms, DNA ploidy is of no value in predicting survival. However, the proliferative index has been reported to be significantly increased in patients dying of their testis cancers.

FCM analysis of sperm from patients who had undergone orchiectomy as sole therapy for testis cancer reveals nuclear chromatin abnormalities in most patients. This supports existing information that patients with testis cancer often demonstrate abnormal spermatogenesis in the contralateral testicle. Testicular aspiration biopsy may also reveal carcinoma-in-situ, while FCM shows DNA aneuploidy. Since the clinical course of CIS is variable, the presence of aneuploidy may identify patients likely to develop invasive cancer. More study is needed before definitive conclusions are reached.

CONCLUSIONS

DNA-ploidy determination parallels the histologic and cytologic features of malignancy. Flow cytometry is a quantitative, reproducible method of measuring DNA content and characterizing a variety of tumor cell kinetic parameters. DNA-ploidy analysis not only complements conventional histologic and cytologic evaluations, but it is itself an independent prognostic variable in some tumor types. There is little doubt that the next several years will see continued attempts to transfer this technology from the research arena into clinical practice. The development of multiparameter FCM analysis, fluorescent dyes, and cellular probes promises to

Table 16.8: Flow Cytometry in Urology — Summary

Current applications	*Future applications*
Limited	Better definition of the biologic potential of GU cancers
Potentially useful in	Help in treatment selection
Metastatic renal cell carcinoma	Prognostic use especially in patients with metastatic disease
Prostate cancer	
Low-grade, upper tract TCC	
Mainly research tool	

enhance future applications of FCM. However, FCM is currently of limited value in the clinical management of genitourinary neoplasms.

For the most part, flow cytometry (FCM) does not add a great deal of information to that available from the more conventional techniques of tumor analysis. However, in several specific areas FCM appears to be of potential value (Table 16.8). One is in the identification of patients with metastatic renal cell carcinoma and diploid metastases. These patients may achieve an enhanced survival following removal of their primary tumor and metastases. In addition, FCM can identify a small population of patients with aneuploid, low-grade transitional cell carcinoma of the renal pelvis in whom conservative surgery may be inappropriate. Finally, FCM may help to select patients with prostate cancer who are best treated by radical prostatectomy.

While knowledge of DNA ploidy does offer some insight into the natural history of neoplasms, the existing body of knowledge does not justify the routine use of FCM in the evaluation of urological neoplasms. Refinements in flow cytometry technology hold the promise of providing better information on the growth potential and biologic behavior of GU cancers as well as the effects of therapy. Furthermore, developments in tumor cytogenetics and molecular biology hold promise for the better diagnosis of tumors and assessment of their biologic behavior and metastatic potential. Identification of oncogenes and tumor suppressor genes may allow specific tumor diagnosis as well as identification of patients at risk of developing such tumors.

SUGGESTED READINGS

Stephenson RA. Flow cytometry in genitourinary malignancies using paraffin-embedded material. Semin Urol 1988; 6:46.

General review of the use of paraffin-embedded archival material in urologic malignancies. Presented from a urologist's perspective.

Howard A, Pelc SR. Nuclear incorporation of P-32 as demonstrated by autoradiographs. Exp Cell Res 1951; 2:178.

Useful example of the application of autoradiographs for the study of cell cycle kinetics. Seminal paper describing phases of cell division.

Merkel ED, McGuire WL. Ploidy, proliferative activity and prognosis: DNA flow cytometry of solid tumors. Cancer 1990; 65:1194.

Review of the basic principles of flow cytometry of solid tumors. Includes discussion of ploidy relationship to prognosis.

Hedley DW, Friedlander ML, Taylor IW, et al. Method for analysis of cellular DNA content of paraffin-embedded pathological material using flow cytometry. J Histochem Cytochem 1983; 31:1333.

Original paper describing the methods used in paraffin-embedded flow cytometry.

Currin SM, Lee SE, Walther PJ. Flow cytometric assessment of deoxyribonucleic acid content in renal adenocarcinoma: does ploidy status enhance prognostic stratification over stage alone? J Urol 1990; 143: 458.

One of the best analyses of flow cytometry in renal cell carcinoma with particular reference to prognostication.

Rainwater LM, Farrow GM, Lieber MM. Flow cytometry of renal oncocytoma: common occurrence of deoxyribonucleic acid polyploidy and aneuploidy. J Urol 1986; 135:1167.

The most exhaustive article on flow cytometry in renal oncocytomas.

Badalament RA, Kimmel M, Gay H, et al. The sensitivity of flow cytometry compared with conventional cytology in the detection of superficial bladder carcinoma. Cancer 1987; 59:2078.

Careful analysis of the sensitivity of flow cytometry and urinary cytology for the detection of superficial bladder cancer.

Bretton PR, Herr HW, Kimmel M, Fair WR, Whitmore WR Jr, Melamed MR. Flow cytometry as a predictor of response and progression in patients with superficial bladder cancer treated with Bacillus Calmette–Guerin. J Urol 1989; 141: 1332.

Excellent discussion of the use of flow cytometry as a predictor of response and progression of bladder cancer after intravesical therapy.

Hermansen DK, Reuter VE, Whitmore WF Jr, Fair WR, Melamed MR. Flow cytometry and cytology as response indicators to M-VAC (methotrexate, vinblastine, doxorubicin and cisplatin). J Urol 1988; 140:1394.

Flow cytometry and cytology discussed as indicators of response following MVAC chemotherapy.

Benson MC, Ring K, Giella J. Flow cytometry in carcinoma of the prostate. Urol Clin North Am 1990; 17:885.

Current review of the potential utility of flow cytometry in carcinoma of the prostate.

Nativ O, Myers RP, Farrow GM, Therneau TM, Zincke H, Lieber MM. Nuclear deoxyribonucleic acid ploidy and serum prostate specific antigen in operable prostatic adenocarcinoma. J Urol 1990; 144:303.

The relationship between flow cytometry and PSA levels in a large prostatectomy series is presented.

Stephenson RA, James BC, Gay H, Fair WR, Whitmore WR Jr, Melamed MR. Flow cytometry of prostate cancer: relationship of DNA content to survival. Cancer Res 1987; 47:2504.

Presents evidence for the independent prognostic value of flow cytometry in patients with stage D_1 prostate cancer.

CHAPTER 17

Urinary Diversion

Michael O. Koch

The study of urinary diversion through intestinal segments represents a unique area of urologic physiology. Most abnormalities encountered following reconstruction of the urinary tract with intestinal segments are easily understood and predictable in light of the known physiology of bowel. The elucidation of the pathophysiology of metabolic abnormalities associated with urinary diversion has seen great strides over the last decade, though fundamental questions remain.

The normal lower urinary tract functions primarily for storage and elimination of bodily waste products. The relatively tight junctions between urothelial cells allows these waste products to be stored unchanged in the bladder until they are eliminated. The bladder is normally capable of storing urine at low intravesical pressures (<5 cm H_2O) until its capacity is reached, at which point the detrusor contracts and generates the necessary force to expel these wastes from the body.

In contrast, the intestine functions primarily as an absorptive organ and continually propulses and mixes its contents. When intestinal segments are used for urinary-tract reconstruction, these absorptive and propulsive functions can exert untoward effects on the general well being of the patient and on the upper urinary tract. This chapter reviews the known physiology of intestine as it applies to urinary diversion so as to elucidate the pathophysiology of the problems (Table 17.1) encountered in this specialized area of urology.

MECHANICAL PHYSIOLOGY

Intestinal motility varies throughout the intestinal tract. Small intestinal contractions are phasic and propagate in an oral to aboral direction so as

Table 17.1: Problems with Bowel Segments

Infection
Mucus production
Metaplasia
Carcinoma
Electrolyte abnormalities
Leakage/rupture

to propel intestinal chyme. These phasic contractions are called *migrating motility complexes*. The neurophysiologic mechanisms that control these migrating motility complexes are unclear; however, the presence of intraluminal contents and/or luminal distention are clearly stimulatory, so that these migrating motility complexes vary in the fed and fasted states.

Colonic motility differs from small-intestinal motility patterns and varies from proximal to distal colonic segments (Table 17.2). While all portions of the colon do exhibit some component of forward peristalsis, the right colon is characterized by *antiperistaltic* patterns. The right colon serves mainly a storage and mixing function. Intestinal contents are repeatedly pushed back toward the ileocecal valve from the proximal end of the transverse colon. The transverse and descending colon is characterized more by slow tonic contractions, which separate the feces into globular masses. Finally, the sigmoid colon is characterized by slow, strong contractions, which constrict the colon and move slowly caudad.

In addition to the patterns mentioned above, the entire colon exhibits a pattern of mass movement in which all previous peristaltic patterns cease while an entire segment, as much as one-third of the length of the colon, contracts. This pattern of contraction is unique to the colon and is thought to be the main mechanism responsible for the caudal propulsion of colonic contents. As in the small intestine, large-intestinal motility is dependent on a number of incompletely understood neural and humoral factors. Clearly, phenomena such as the gastrocolic reflex exist, although their mechanisms are ill defined. Distention is clearly stimulatory.

Table 17.2: Functional Properties of Bowel Segments

Peristalsis
Mass contraction
Caudal propulsion
Nonstorage (Except ? ascending colon)
Absorptive surface

With the possible exception of the ascending colon, the intestine normally does not function as a storage organ. Consequently, normal intraluminal pressures in the intestine exceed those pressures seen in the healthy lower urinary tract. Normal small intestinal pressures range from 5 to 50 cm H_2O. Large-intestinal pressures start in a similar range and then increase as one proceeds distally, reaching levels as high as several hundred centimeters of water in the rectosigmoid colon.

The ileocecal valve represents a specialized area of the intestine. This area actually consists of a portion of ileum that protrudes into the cecum and is surrounded by colonic musculature. The purpose of this segment of intestine is unclear. While the ileocecal junction is generally purported to prevent reflux of colonic contents into the ileum, reflux is generally not a problem when this area is surgically removed. Normal ileal peristalsis may in fact be enough to prevent reflux. The term valve is actually a misnomer in that this area functions more as an intestinal sphincter. With distention of the terminal ileum, ileocecal valve pressures decrease, while pressures in this same region increase with distention of ascending colon. This zone of increased pressure is generally 4 cm in length and exceeds colonic pressure by 20 mm Hg. The pressure this "valve" can generate is limited, however, as some reflux into the ileum occurs in up to 90% of patients having barium enemas. Colonic pressures frequently exceed 90 cm H_2O during barium-enema examinations.

URINARY CONDUITS

The ileal conduit was first reported in 1949, and there is an abundance of long-term follow-up data relative to this surgical procedure. The more recently described jejunal and colon conduits have sufficient follow-up information available for comparisons with ileal conduits. The most common complications of conduit diversion include stomal complications (15 to 45%), stricture at the ureterointestinal anastomotic junction (4 to 22%), and deterioration of the upper urinary tract (10 to 60%). In general, a properly functioning conduit has minimal pressures within it, and any pressures that are generated are not transmitted to the renal pelvis. However, when a conduit is placed in an antiperistaltic fashion, upper-tract deterioration will result. This is perhaps less important with the large intestine, in which mass contractions, not peristalsis, predominate. It is, however, prudent to orient all urinary conduits in an isoperistaltic fashion.

There is considerable controversy as to the importance of a nonrefluxing ureterointestinal anastomosis in a urinary conduit. In general, colonic segments lend themselves more readily to the creation of a nonrefluxing ureterointestinal anastomosis because of the thicker intestinal musculature. The seminal work in the area demonstrated that in dogs, only 7% of nonrefluxing colon conduits demonstrated pyelonephritic scarring at 3 months, while 83% of refluxing anastomoses demonstrated scarring. Most clinical series comparing refluxing and nonrefluxing urinary conduits have found some benefit with the latter. With prolonged follow-up, up to 80% of refluxing colon conduits demonstrate some evidence of radiographic renal deterioration, as opposed to only 20% of nonrefluxing systems.

The reason for this advantage with nonrefluxing systems is unclear. A successful nonrefluxing anastomosis does not appear to prevent upper-tract bacterial colonization. In the absence of other mitigating circumstances (e.g., stomal stenosis, ureterointestinal strictures), a refluxing ileal conduit in the adult constitutes adequate management. The degree of radiographic changes in the upper tracts is not clinically significant in the majority of patients. In the young adult or child with long life-expectancy, the available data suggest that a nonrefluxing system is advantageous. With continent urinary reservoirs, intraluminal pressures are frequently greater than conduit diversions, and this increases the need for nonrefluxing ureterointestinal anastomoses.

CONTINENT DIVERSIONS

Reservoir Function

The intestinal tract is used in many clinical settings to reconstruct the reservoir function of the normal bladder. These include continent cutaneous diversions, augmentation cystoplasties, and orthotopic intestinal bladders. Principles common to all of these procedures are bowel detubularization, creation of a nonrefluxing anastomosis, and the need for continence mechanisms (Figure 17.1).

Detubularization is the process whereby the normal tubular configuration of the bowel is disrupted so that the intestine is reconfigured

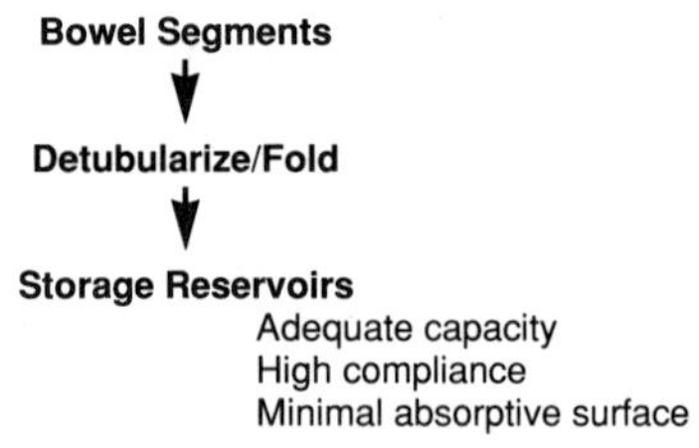

Figure 17.1: Creation of urinary reservoirs

into the most spherical configuration possible. Generally, this involves opening the intestine along its length and folding it in a Heineke-Mikulicz fashion, once or twice. The clinical importance of this technique in fashioning a urinary reservoir from intestine is accepted for small- and large-intestinal segments and all forms of continent urinary diversions. The mechanical and physiologic principles underlying this technique are geometric considerations, pressure–tension relationships, and disruption of peristalsis.

Geometric considerations are of utmost importance in the construction of high-compliance urinary reservoirs. The goal in constructing a urinary reservoir from intestine is the creation of a reservoir with adequate capacity and compliance using the shortest segment of intestine with the least absorptive surface area. The ratio of reservoir volume to surface area is maximized with more spherical configurations of bowel. For an intestinal segment whose length significantly exceeds its diameter, a single folding and closure in a Heineke-Mikulicz fashion results in a doubling of volume (Figure 17.2).

The relationship between reservoir pressure and anatomical configuration is expressed by Laplace's law: Pressure multiplied by radius is proportional to wall tension. The intestinal wall is capable of generating a

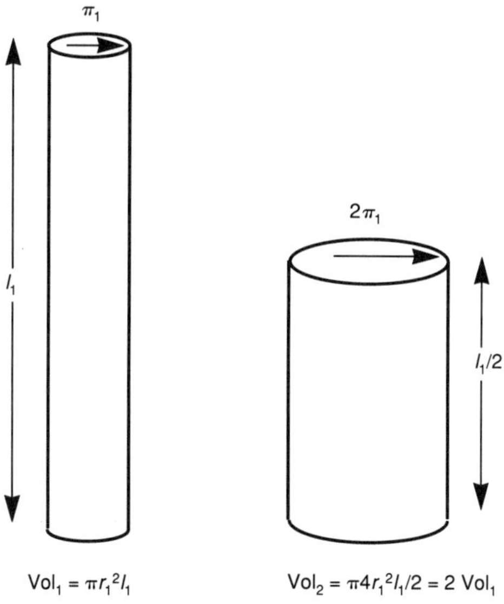

Figure 17.2: The volume of a cylinder with a radius r_1 and length l_1 is $r_1^2\ l_1$. If the cylinder is refashioned so that the radius in doubled ($2r_1$) and the length halved ($l_1/2$), the volume is doubled.

maximal wall tension that is an intrinsic function of the intestinal muscle cell and not a function of the configuration of the intestinal segment. When the radius of the urinary reservoir is doubled by a single folding of the intestinal segment, there is a corresponding 50% reduction in the maximal pressure generated by the intestinal reservoir.

The final rationale behind the detubularization of intestinal segments is its effect on intestinal peristalsis. Detubularization of an intestinal segment is thought to result in a disordering of intestinal peristalsis such that peristaltic contractions cancel each other. This phenomenon remains to be demonstrated experimentally or clinically. Observations in the dog, in the acute phase, suggest that detubularization results in a complete disordering of the migratory motility complexes rather than peristaltic wave cancellation. There is minimal support for the concept of peristaltic cancellation in the large intestine, where mass contractions rather than true peristaltic activity predominate.

Urinary reservoirs all demonstrate viscoelastic activity. Put more simply, this means that the pressure generated by the intestinal reservoir is dependent not only on the volume present in the reservoir but also on the rate at which the reservoir is filled. Furthermore, accommodation occurs so that over a period of time a urinary reservoir is capable of storing large volumes of urine at the same or lower intraluminal pressures.

Regardless of the mechanisms involved, all large-capacity reservoirs are created from spherical detubularized intestinal segments with low intraluminal pressures and high compliance. The pressure in most urinary reservoirs is usually between 10 and 40 cm H_2O, and the best clinical results are obtained with the lowest pressure reservoirs. Intestinal reservoir pressures generally exceed normal detrusor pressures, and it therefore seems advisable to construct these reservoirs using a nonrefluxing method for ureterointestinal anastomosis.

Continence Mechanisms

There are two primary continence mechanisms in cutaneous urinary reservoirs: nipple valves and the ileocecal valve (Table 17.3). Other pro-

Table 17.3: Continence Mechanisms in Urinary Diversion

Urethra, e.g., Camey
Nipple valves, e.g., Kock
Ileocecal valves, e.g., Indiana pouch
Anal sphincter, e.g., ureterosigmoidostomy
Prosthetic sphincters

cedures that are used less commonly (such as the Benchekroun and Mitrofanoff) are not discussed here.

Nipple valves were first used with ileocecal augmentation cystoplasty in which the ileocecal valve was intussuscepted and then reinforced using a variety of techniques. This particular valve was generally constructed to prevent reflux into the upper urinary tract, and unfortunately all of these procedures suffered from a tendency for this nipple valve to lose its intussusception over time with loss of its valvular effect. The largest experience with nipple valves is with the Kock pouch, in which the nipple valve acts as an anticontinence as well as antireflux mechanism. The nipple valves have accounted for the greatest portion of long-term complications with the Kock pouch.

Nipple valves lend themselves to urodynamic study. Increasing intraluminal pressures are accompanied by an equivalent and parallel increase in pressure in the efferent limb. Efferent-limb pressure is never exceeded, so that even at high reservoir pressures leakage should not occur. The same forces that cause nipple occlusion, however, also exert a force on the nipple, which, over the long term, causes eversion. The majority of modifications to the Kock pouch procedure have been directed at prevention of this problem. Using a combination of stapling techniques and polyglycolic acid mesh reinforcement, the risk of nipple erosion can be minimized. The technical difficulties encountered in fashioning these nipples have limited the widespread use of the Kock pouch for urinary diversion.

Because of its valvular effect, the ileocecal valve has been used extensively in urinary-tract reconstruction. The ileocecal valve, by itself, can provide an adequate sphincter mechanism to provide continence in most patients. The Gilchrist bladder, first reported in 1950, in fact, relied on this mechanism to achieve continence in 90% of patients. As discussed earlier, the ileocecal valve actually functions as a sphincter rather than as a valve, and at high pressures its sphincter function may be overcome. Recent procedures have modified this continence mechanism by an imbrication or tapering of the ileum. This serves two purposes: (1) the elimination of redundant mucosal folds, which then facilitates catheterization of the stoma, and (2) provision of a resistance mechanism because of pure mucosal resistance to flow and the antiperistaltic orientation. Postoperative "pouch-o-grams" frequently reveal efflux of contrast through the ileocecal valve and into the efferent limb. It is uncommon, however, to have leakage in such patients.

The ideal continence mechanism may not, in fact, be completely continent. Continent urinary reservoirs can and have been reported to rupture. When intrareservoir pressures exceed a certain level, it may be better for incontinence to occur than for pressures to continue to rise against a totally competent continence mechanism. The ileocecal valve functions in this manner.

METABOLIC ABNORMALITIES

Basic Physiology

The majority of metabolic abnormalities associated with urinary diversion through intestinal segments are predictable based upon known processes of intestinal solute and water transport. Transport of water and solutes is not homogeneous throughout the intestinal tract. The tight junctions that connect epithelial cells are "tightest" in the colon but are progressively "leakier" in the more proximal segments of the intestinal tract. Thus, paracellular movement of solutes and water plays a major role in the jejunum and ileum and a less important one in the colon. Luminal contents in the upper gastrointestinal tract, particularly the jejunum, rapidly equilibrate to isotonicity with serum. In contrast, the colon is less permeable to the diffusion of solutes and water and can maintain significant osmotic gradients (Table 17.4).

A characteristic feature of absorptive intestinal cells is the Na^+–K^+–ATPase enzyme system, which is limited (95%) to the basolateral membrane and maintains low intracellular sodium concentrations. Electrolyte transport mechanisms are similar throughout the intestinal tract, although different intestinal segments exhibit significant quantitative variability. Sodium enters into the cell via an exchange port with hydrogen ion and through conductance channels, where it is absorbed in an uncoupled state (electrogenic transport). Sodium is also absorbed via a number of other incompletely defined mechanisms (Figure 17.3). Electrogenic sodium transport, particularly in the colon, is stimulated by mineralocorticoids, so that during periods of salt depletion, the colon can reduce luminal sodium concentrations to less than 5 mM/l. The sodium/hydrogen ion exchanger in the ileum and colon is indirectly linked to another exchanger, which absorbs chloride in exchange for bicarbonate. This process is dependent on the presence of carbonic anhydrase. The net effect of sodium/hydro-

Table 17.4: Bowel Physiology

"Tight" epithelial junctions in colon
"Leakier" junctions in jejunum, ileum
Lack of chloride/bicarbonate exchange in jejunum
Jejunum avidly absorbs bicarbonate
Vitamin D, vitamin B_{12}, bile salt absorption in terminal ileum

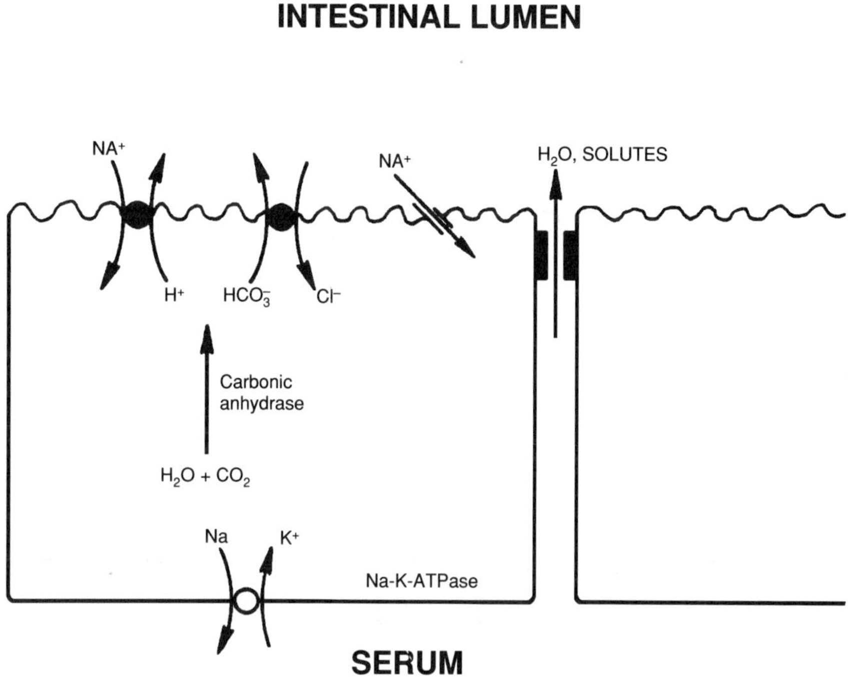

Figure 17.3: Ileal and colonic electrolyte and water transport mechanisms

gen ion exchange indirectly coupled to chloride/bicarbonate exchange is neutral sodium chloride absorption.

Electrolyte and water movement in the jejunum is markedly different from that in the ileum and colon because there is no chloride/bicarbonate exchanger (Figure 17.4). Instead, chloride is absorbed via the paracellular pathway in response to favorable electrochemical gradients. A major function of the intact jejunum is the reabsorption of bicarbonate from the duodenal and pancreatic secretions. Consequently, the jejunum avidly absorbs bicarbonate even against significant concentration gradients. The primary mechanism for bicarbonate absorption is thought to be luminal acidification with hydrogen ions secreted via the sodium/hydrogen ion exchanger, which then titrates luminal bicarbonate and generates H_2O and CO_2, which then passively diffuse according to their gradients. The net result of this is neutral sodium bicarbonate absorption.

In the intestine potassium moves passively along electrochemical gradients. Specific potassium conductance channels have been described. In the colon, net absorption generally occurs when luminal concentrations exceed 30 mm/l, whereas secretion occurs at levels below this value.

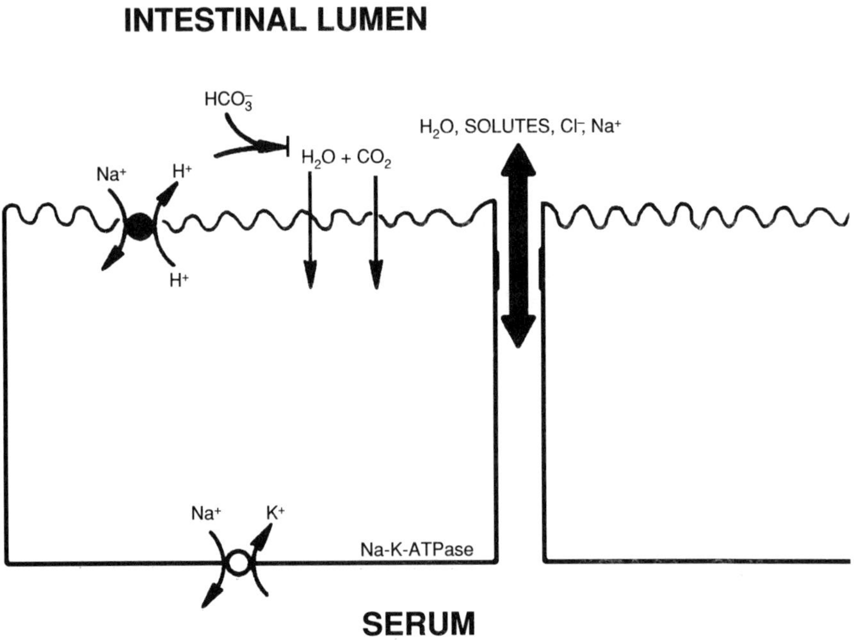

Figure 17.4: Jejunal electrolyte and water transport mechanisms. Note absence of

The intact normal intestine has a number of other functions that may impact on urinary diversion. The entire small intestine exhibits substrate-facilitated sodium transport whereby nutrients such as glucose and amino acids are absorbed coupled to sodium. The terminal ileum is the primary site for vitamin D, vitamin B_{12}, and bile salts absorption (Table 17.4). Urinary diversions that use large segments of terminal ileum may result in metabolic abnormalities as a result of the defective absorption of these substances.

METABOLIC ALTERATIONS AFTER URINARY DIVERSION

Hyperchloremic Metabolic Acidosis

Both ileal and colonic urinary diversions have been associated with the development of hyperchloremic metabolic acidosis. The frequency and the severity of this acidosis depend on the amount of intestinal surface area exposed, urine retention time within the bowel segment, and underlying renal function.

Hyperchloremic metabolic acidosis was first reported in patients with bilateral ureterosigmoidostomy. Patients presented with voluminous diarrhea, dehydration, lethargy, and fatigue, especially during episodes of clinical pyelonephritis. The first major series of patients with this problem was reported in 1950, and the complication occurs in approximately 80% of patients following ureterosigmoidostomy. During the 1950s, a number of theories was advanced to explain the cause of this syndrome. Theories included selective chloride absorption in excess of sodium leading to intracellular dehydration and acidosis, colonic bicarbonate secretion into the urine, a renal acidifying defect, and absorption of excreted urinary ammonium by the colon. However, none of these provides a definitive explanation of this syndrome.

Recent studies have provided additional insights into this problem (Table 17.5). It is now clear that both bicarbonate secretion and ammonium absorption contribute to the acidosis of urinary diversion. The degree of bicarbonate secretion or ammonium absorption is dependent on the electrolyte composition of the urine and the volume and acid–base status of the patient. At urinary electrolyte compositions similar to that in patients with chronic acidosis, ammonium absorption contributes approximately 80% of the acidosis attributable to urinary diversion. Bicarbonate secretion occurs via the chloride/bicarbonate exchanger in the ileum and colon. The mechanism of ammonium absorption is not known. Preliminary investigations have shown that ammonium is absorbed as an ionized species, that its absorption is inversely related to net sodium movement, and that it is not absorbed via the known sodium transport mechanisms.

It has been suggested that urease-producing bacteria may contribute to this syndrome. No clinical or experimental data support this concept. Bacterial urease does not generate any net acid; rather, it converts one hydrogen ion and one urea molecule into two ammonium and one bicarbonate molecules. Thus, no additional acid is generated. Urease does generate large concentrations of ammonium in the urine, however. In the presence of hepatic and/or renal dysfunction and infections with urease-producing bacteria, ammoniagenic encephalopathy can and does occur following urinary diversion.

Table 17.5: Metabolic Complications of Urinary Diversion

Hyperchloremic Metabolic Acidosis	*Jejunal Conduit Syndrome*
Ureterosigmoidostomy > ileal/colonic conduits + pouches	Occurs in 25–40% patients
Ammonium absorption	Sodium chloride, water secreted into conduit
Bicarbonate secretion	Volume depletion, acidosis
Treatment	Treatment
Bicarbonate/citrate supplements	NaCl oral supplements
Risk hypokalemia	

While hyperchloremic metabolic acidosis is most frequently associated with ureterosigmoidostomy, it also occurs in most forms of ileal and colonic urinary diversions, albeit with lower frequency. Hyperchloremic metabolic acidosis has been associated with ileal conduits (1.7 to 29%), colon conduits (0 to 11.5%), augmentation ileocecal cystoplasty (19 to 50%), Kock pouches (0 to 13%), ileocecal pouches (5 to 50%), and rectosigmoid bladders (86%). The wide variability in reported incidences is attributable to differences in the levels of acidosis considered clinically significant, the amount of bowel used in the diversion, and underlying renal function and renal tubular acidosis.

The majority of patients with normal renal function do not manifest clinically significant metabolic acidosis following urinary diversion. However, more subtle changes are detectable, even in patients with normal renal function. With an acute acid challenge, the normal renal response is increased urinary excretion of titratable acid (e.g., phosphates and sulfates). As this acute acid challenge becomes chronic, the kidney must adapt or the body becomes depleted of these titratable acid buffers that come from bone. The kidney does this by generating ammonia from glutamine in the distal renal tubular cell. Ammonia then ion-traps hydrogen in the distal tubular lumen, and acid is excreted in this fashion. The presence of an ileal or colonic segment in the urinary tract negates the ability of the patient to excrete urinary acid as ammonium, so that ammonium is recirculated until a new steady state is established.

Careful metabolic study of patients with continent ileocolonic diversions has demonstrated a number of metabolic changes following urinary diversion. Patients demonstrate mild azotemia and an increase in the BUN/creatinine ratio. This is due to free-water loss through the intestinal segment into the urine and the reabsorption of urinary urea. Most patients with diversions demonstrate a mild hyperchloremic acidosis of minimal clinical significance. In response to ammonium chloride loading, these patients are slightly more prone to manifest hyperchloremic acidosis and are unable to effectively acidify their urine.

The management of patients with clinically significant hyperchloremic acidosis centers on the correction of the base deficit. This is accomplished by oral supplementation with bicarbonate or citrate salts. Generally, 1 to 2 mEq/kg body weight of alkali is required per day. Profound hypokalemia frequently arises with correction of the acidosis in these patients, and a sudden death syndrome has been reported in this setting (vide infra). Careful monitoring of serum potassium and potassium supplementation is mandatory. Some patients may be difficult to manage with alkali supplementation because of gastrointestinal intolerance or sodium retention. Inhibitors of cyclic AMP and adenyl cyclase have been reported of benefit in these patients, although their mechanism of action is not known. Simple measures to reduce mucosal contact time, such as the insertion of a rectal tube in ureterosigmoidostomy patients, or an indwelling catheter in an intestinal reservoir, are also beneficial.

Much has been written about patient selection guidelines for the various forms of urinary diversion. Unfortunately, renal function is only crudely evaluated by routine serum creatinine and creatinine clearance studies. Intestinal urinary diversion has an antagonistic effect on the renal excretion of solutes such as urea and potassium, on renal concentrating ability and maintenance of volume status, and on urinary acidification. Accurate assessment of these renal parameters is clinically cumbersome, and the clinician has to rely on crude measures of renal function. This is further complicated by the wide variation in mucosal surface areas and urine retention times with the various types of urinary diversion. The most widely cited cutoff of minimal renal function for patients undergoing diversion is a serum creatinine level of 2 mg/dl or a creatinine clearance of 50 ml/min. These values are based on clinical experience rather than strict scientific evaluation. A patient with pre-existing chronic metabolic acidosis is clearly at increased risk, and in these patients a nonretentive form of urinary diversion should be considered.

Jejunal Conduit Syndrome

Urinary diversion through jejunal segments is associated with a unique syndrome characterized by hyponatremia, hypochloremia, hyperkalemia, azotemia, and volume depletion (Table 17.5). Acidosis is the general rule, but alkalosis may also develop. This syndrome arises in 25 to 40% of patients and is thought to be due to the jejunal secretion of large amounts of sodium chloride and water into the urine. The highly permeable nature of jejunal mucosa effectively negates the ability of the kidney to excrete a hypertonic urine and to conserve salt. This syndrome is exacerbated by parenteral hyperalimentation.

Clinicians who recommend this form of urinary diversion generally advocate oral sodium chloride supplementation. Treatment of acidosis in these patients may be complicated because of the function of the jejunal segment. Whereas a normal kidney will excrete any bicarbonate in excess of that needed to maintain normal acid–base balance, any excreted bicarbonate is avidly reabsorbed by the jejunal segment. Thus, patients with jejunal conduits are prone to develop alkalosis with alkali replacement therapy.

Jejunal segments, particularly proximal segments, should be used only as a last resort in urinary diversion; and when they are used, the shortest possible segment should be employed.

Potassium Depletion

Hypokalemia and total body potassium depletion have been reported after bilateral ureterosigmoidostomy. While this has generally been attributed to potassium secretion by the intestinal segment into the urine, most experimental models of urinary diversion have demonstrated potassium reabsorption. A more plausible hypothesis is that the chronic acidosis of urinary diversion leads to renal potassium wastage. In addition, chronic sodium and volume loss leads to a secondary hyperaldosteronism, which further exacerbates the hypokalemia.

Severe manifestations of the hypokalemia of urinary diversion can develop. Flaccid paralysis and a clinical syndrome mimicking the Guillain-Barré syndrome have been reported. Interestingly, total body potassium depletion has been reported with urinary diversions with colon, but not with ileal, segments. While it is possible that this difference is due to anatomical considerations, it is also likely due to inherent differences between ileum and colon. Experimental evidence in the rat suggests that potassium is readily absorbed from the urine by ileum but not significantly transported by colon. This potassium reabsorption would blunt any of the potassium wasting mechanisms previously described.

Vitamin Deficiency States

A number of vitamin deficiencies are possible with urinary diversions that employ large segments of terminal ileum (Table 17.6). Vitamin B_{12} and vitamin D are absorbed primarily in this section of the intestine. Few studies have carefully examined patients for abnormalities of these vitamins. In several reports, patients with urinary diversions using ileocecal segments have developed vitamin B_{12} deficiency. Patients who have un-

Table 17.6: Disturbed Bile, Fatty Acid and Vitamin Absorption

Altered enterohepatic circulation bile salts
- Diarrhea, steatorrhea
- ? increased gallstones

Fatty acid malabsorption
- Chelates calcium
- Increased absorption oxalates
- Renal oxalate stones

Liposoluble vitamin (A, D, E, K, B_{12}) absorption
- All absorbed in terminal ileum
- B_{12} deficiency = anemia
- K deficiency = bleeding
- D deficiency = osteoporosis, osteomalacia

dergone resection of the ileocecal valve may be particularly prone to this problem. Absence of the ileocecal valve allows bacterial overgrowth in the terminal ileum and consequently bacterial metabolism of vitamin B_{12}. Patients who receive radiotherapy to the pelvis also appear to be particularly prone to this problem.

Vitamin B_{12} cannot be synthesized by the human body and must be supplied in the diet. A healthy person has sufficient vitamin B_{12} stores for 3 to 6 years, and therefore a significant period of time has to elapse before a deficiency state develops. Chronic vitamin B_{12} deficiency results in megaloblastic anemia and multiple neurologic sequelae. Unfortunately, while the anemia is reversible with the exogenous administration of the vitamin, the neurologic sequelae may be permanent and even progressive.

Patients with urinary diversions that use large segments of terminal ileum or with resection of the ileocecal valve should have a complete yearly blood count with red cell indices. An alternative is to supplement all of these patients with parenteral vitamin B_{12} on a periodic basis.

Bile Salt and Fat Malabsorption

Dietary fat is normally emulsified in the presence of bile salts in the proximal small intestine. After suitable micellar suspension, fats and fat-soluble vitamins (A, D, E, and K) are absorbed in the small intestine. Bile salts are then reabsorbed in the terminal ileum into the portal circulation and then extracted by the liver. With extensive distal ileal resection, bile salt can be depleted, thereby predisposing the patient to fat malabsorption, diarrhea, and depletion of the fat-soluble vitamins (Table 17.6). Chronic diarrheal states secondary to fat malabsorption are seen after urinary diversion with ileocecal segments in up to 10% of patients. An increased incidence in biliary stone disease has not been found in these patients.

Drug Metabolism

A number of reports have appeared of altered drug metabolism following urinary diversion. Theoretically, any drug excreted into the urine in an active form is susceptible to reabsorption and consequently a prolonged half-life. Increased methotrexate toxicity and dilantin toxicity have both been attributed to urinary diversion in some patients.

Osteomalacia

The potential for the development of osteomalacia after urinary diversion has been recognized since the nineteenth century. Most reports have been associated with ureterosigmoidostomy and chronic metabolic acidosis; however, osteomalacia has also been reported with urinary diversions using ileal segments. While the chronic acidosis of urinary diversion is clearly of major significance in the development of this problem, other factors may also be operative.

Experimental studies have demonstrated changes in bone mineral content in the absence of any overt acidosis. Reabsorption of urinary sulfate has been proposed to occur, and this exerts an adverse effect on bone mineral metabolism. Diversions that involve the ileocecal valve can lead to malabsorption of vitamin D (vide supra), and this may also account for the changes seen. Fat malabsorption from altered bile salt metabolism also leads to calcium saponification with fats in the small intestine and a negative calcium balance. In any case, osteomalacia does appear to be a clinical problem following urinary diversion; and it deserves careful attention, particularly in groups at high risk, such as growing children and postmenopausal women.

NEOPLASIA

There are abundant reports of colon carcinomas following ureterosigmoidostomy (Table 17.7). The estimated lifetime risk for the development of colon carcinomas in these patients is 180 to 7000 times that of the normal population. When large numbers of ureterosigmoidostomy patents are screened by colonoscopy, up to 40% have tumors, although many of these are tubovillous adenomas, with some also showing transitional cell features. The mean lag time between ureterosigmoidostomy and the development of adenocarcinomas is 26 years, although one case has been reported 53 years after urinary diversion. These patients typically present with hematochezia and/or ureteral obstruction. Interestingly, 17% of the cases of adenocarcinomas following ureterosigmoidostomy have been reported in patients that have had their ureterosigmoidostomy taken down and have occurred at the site of the ureteral stump.

A number of research studies have investigated the pathogenesis of this problem (Table 17.7). The seminal work studying this problem used

Table 17.7: Neoplasia Risk in Bowel Segments

Ureterosigmoidostomy	*Causes Neoplasia*
180–7000 times cancer risk compared to normals	Mixing fecal and urinary streams
Long lag time: 20+ years	Bacterial conversion of amines to N-nitrosamine
40% patients have tumors (adenomas, carcinomas) by colonoscopy	Other mechanisms
	In ileal conduits, augmentation cystoplasty, colon conduits

a rat model in which the dome of the bladder was anastomosed to the sigmoid colon. A high percentage of these animals develop malignancies at the site of the anastomosis. In the original studies, proximal fecal diversion or urinary bypass completely abrogated this carcinogenic effect. More recent studies have shown that the interposition of an ileal segment between the bladder and sigmoid colon also negates the carcinogenic effect. These findings suggested that an interaction between the feces and urine was pathogenically significant, and numerous reports appeared suggesting that fecal bacteria were converting endogenous amines to N-nitrosamine, a known colonic carcinogen. Indeed, animal and human studies have confirmed high N-nitrosamine levels in the fecal-urine mixture after urinary diversion. These studies also suggested that there must be a juxtaposition of urothelium and colonic epithelium at the site where urine and feces were mixing.

While the general significance of mixing of urine and feces has found widespread acceptance, recent studies have questioned this hypothesis. First, agents that block the formation of N-nitrosamines have not had an inhibitory effect on the development of carcinomas in the experimental model. Perhaps more significantly, there are increasing reports of carcinomas occurring after colon conduit diversions, ileocecocystoplasty, and, more recently, urinary diversions that use only ileal segments.

Clearly, patients with ureterosigmoidostomy are at greatest risk for the development of cancer. Yearly colonoscopic examination should be instituted shortly after urinary diversion. Any ureterosigmoidostomy patient with hematochezia or a new onset of ureteral obstruction should be carefully evaluated for the presence of an anastomotic malignancy. Patients that are found to have multiple or recurrent polyps that develop after ureterosigmoidostomy appear to be at the highest risk, and consideration should be given to converting them to an alternative form of urinary diversion.

There are many similarities between the development of carcinomas following other forms of urinary diversion and ureterosigmoidostomy. The mean interval between urinary diversion and the development of malignancy in the published reports is 18 years, with a mean patient age of 31 years. Unfortunately, the prognosis is frequently grim due to the advanced stage of disease at presentation. While the exact risk is unknown, it appears clear that these are not simply random events, as the frequency with which they are seen exceeds the general age-matched population by at least several fold. Particularly notable are the multiple reports of carcinomas seen with pure ileal diversions with ileal tumors being exceedingly rare in the general population. The pathogenesis of tumors in augmentation cystoplasty patients is unknown but assumed to be similar to the ureterosigmoidostomy population with the one notable difference of an absence of mixing of fecal and urinary streams. Until a more accurate assessment of risk and predisposing factors is available for these patients, it is prudent to routinely screen all patients radiographically and with urinary cytologies and to perform periodic endoscopic evaluation.

SUGGESTED READINGS

Richie JP, Skinner DG. Urinary diversion: the physiological rationale for nonrefluxing colonic conduits. Br J Urol 1975; 47:269.

Experimental study comparing refluxing ileal conduits and nonrefluxing colon conduits in the dog. Refluxing renal units demonstrated a markedly increased incidence of pyelonephritic scarring.

Kock NG. Intraabdominal reservoir in patients with permanent ileostomy. Arch Surg 1969; 99:223.

Presents some of the first observations made on the concept of intestinal detubularization in intestinal tract reconstruction.

Norlen L, Trasti H. Functional behavior of the continent ileum reservoir for urinary diversion. Scand J Urol Nephrol (Suppl) 1978; 49:33.

Reviews the pressure–volume relationships of the continent ileal reservoir. Demonstrates the viscoelastic properties of this reservoir.

Lieskovsky G, Boyd SD, Skinner DG. Management of late complications of the Kock pouch form of urinary diversion. J Urol 1987; 137:1146.

Reviews the basic construction of the Kock pouch and its short- and long-term complications.

Rowland RG, Mitchell ME, Bihrle R, Kahnoski RJ, Piser JE. Indiana continent urinary diversion. J Urol 1987; 137:1136.

Reviews the basic construction of the detubularized ileocecal pouch for continent cutaneous urinary diversion.

Koch MO, McDougal WS. The pathophysiology of hyperchloremic metabolic acidosis after urinary diversion through intestinal segments. Surgery 1985; 98(3):561.

Reviews the changes in urinary excretion of electrolytes as it passes through ileal segments and suggests a mechanism for the acid–base abnormalities encountered following urinary diversion.

Koch MO, McDougal WS, Reddy PK, Lange PH. Metabolic alterations following continent urinary diversion through colonic segments. J Urol 1991; 145:270.

Examines the ability of patients with continent colonic urinary diversions to respond to acute acid loading with ammonium chloride.

Golimbu M, Morales P. Jejunal conduits: technique and complications. J Urol 1975; 113:787.

A series of patients with jejunal conduits is reviewed, and the metabolic complications are presented. A pathophysiology for this syndrome is proposed.

Husman DA, Spense HM. Current status of tumor of the bowel following uretero-sigmoidostomy: a review. J Urol 1990; 144:607.

Reviews the proposed mechanisms of neoplasia after ureterosigmoidostomy. Estimates the clinical significance of this problem, and suggests management of these patients.

CHAPTER 18

Lymphadenectomy in Genitourinary Cancers

Kevin R. Loughlin
Jerome P. Richie

The role of lymphadenectomy in the management of urologic malignancies continues to engender discussion and controversy. Although Halstead first promulgated the concept that regional lymphadenectomy could improve breast cancer survival rates, lymph node metastases are generally regarded as a manifestation of tumor dissemination rather than a barrier to tumor spread. This raises the question as to the role of lymphadenectomy in the surgical treatment of primary urologic cancers. Does regional lymphadenectomy improve patient survival by providing better locoregional control? Apart from testis cancer, there is no conclusive evidence that lymphadenectomy improves long-term survival in urologic cancers. However, it may provide some short-term survival advantages, especially in patients with microscopic nodal involvement.

Perhaps a stronger rationale for regional lymphadenectomy is that it provides accurate pathologic staging of the primary tumors. This results in better selection of treatment options (i.e., chemotherapy, radiation therapy) as adjunctive measures following surgical excision and more accurate prognostication. The predilection to metastases depends on the mechanical properties of the primary tumor of the tissue-specific preferences of the tumor cells. The first echelon or spread in genitourinary tumors is the lymphatic system. Therefore, urologic oncologists have directed much effort to the study of the impact of lymphatic metastases on the survival of patients with urologic malignancies. Despite these efforts, controversy still remains concerning the applications of lymphadenectomy in specific urologic malignancies. In this chapter, the role of lymphadenectomy in the common urologic cancers is examined and current consensus discussed (Table 18.1).

Table 18.1: Lymphadenectomy in Urologic Cancers—Considerations

Questionable increased survival
Long term
Short term
Better pathologic staging
Selection of adjunctive treatments
Radiation, chemotherapy, immunotherapy
Proven benefit in testicular cancer
Changing aspects
More limited dissections
Role in low-volume, microscopic disease
Organ-specific applications

BIOLOGY OF TUMOR METASTASES

Although the Greeks observed the lymphatic system, Gasparo Asalli, professor of anatomy and surgery in Italy, is credited with the first detailed description of the lymphatics in 1622. With the introduction of the microscope by Leeuwenhoek, knowledge and understanding of the lymphatics expanded. William Hunter described the function of the lymphatics in 1746. Starling in 1896 published evidence that lymph is formed from the blood by filtration through the capillary membrane.

Tumor metastases develop as a result of three separate mechanisms: direct spread, invasion, and vascular (hematogenous, lymphatic) spread. Direct tumor extension is uncommon in urologic malignancies, and the majority of metastases are either lymphatic (nodal) or blood-borne (pulmonary, bone, liver) (Table 18.2).

The initial step in the evolution of a metastasis is disassociation of tumor cells from the primary tumor followed by invasion of the basement membranes of vascular channels. Tumor cells then bind to matrix components (e.g., laminin, fibronectin) and then dissolve or attenuate the matrix by production of a variety of proteolytic enzymes (e.g., collagenases) (Table 18.2). The tumor cells subsequently reach the systemic circulation by invading and/or penetrating the matrix. This process is modulated by the intrinsic motility of certain tumor cells and their production of autocrine motility factors. Successful penetration of the endothelial basement membranes of blood vessels/lymphatics results in tumor cells gaining access to the systemic circulation. However, the majority of these cells are destroyed by mechanical trauma or the immune system. Surviving tumor cells may then become arrested in organ capillaries (lung, liver), where they adhere, penetrate the underlying basement membranes, and invade the organs.

Table 18.2: Biology of Tumor Metastases

Mechanisms	*Evolution of Metastasis*	*Sites of Metastasis*
Direct spread	Tumor cell dissociation	Mechanical trapping
Invasion	Matrix binding	"Seed and soil" theory
Hematogenous	Matrix dissolution/attenuation	
Lymphatic	Access to vascular spaces	
	Tumor cell motility	
	Destruction by immune system	
	Adherence to basement membrane	
	Organ penetration, invasion	

Experimental evidence in animals suggests that only a small percentage of tumor cells gaining access to the systemic circulation are capable of forming metastases. Tumor cells are initially arrested in the subcapsular sinuses of lymph nodes, from which location they may migrate via efferent sinusoids to more proximal lymph nodes or penetrate the endothelial sinus lining to gain access to the nodal parenchyma.

Lymph nodes are probably an insufficient barrier to tumor spread because of the numerous communications between lymphatics and vascular networks. Indeed, lymphatic involvement parallels bloodstream spread in certain tumors (e.g., renal cell carcinoma). Thus, in some cancers, nodal disease may be an early manifestation of disseminated, bloodborne metastases!

The patterns and progression of metastatic spread in genitourinary cancers are generally predictable and characteristic. This is the basis of all clinical and surgical staging protocols. Two theories have been postulated to explain the sites of tumor metastases: the *"seed and soil"* theory and the *mechanical* theory. In the latter, sites are determined by the passive migration of tumor cells through lymphatic/vascular channels, and this explains the common occurrence of pulmonary and liver metastases. However, multiple observations (e.g., low incidence of brain/kidney metastases, etc.) point to the "seed and soil" theory as the more appropriate model for tumor metastases. This model emphasizes the specific adherence and attraction properties of both tumor and target cells.

Optimal therapy of genitourinary tumors depends on accurate tumor staging and localization of metastases. The sites, numbers, and size of metastases impact on prognosis and, particularly, on treatment selection. Tumor staging can be accomplished by a number of imaging modalities: lymphangiography, bone scintigraphy, ultrasonography, computed tomography (CT), and magnetic resonance imaging (MRI).

However, these diagnostic imaging techniques display wide variations in sensitivity and specificity, as well as interinstitutional variation.

In general, CT scanning is probably the most widely used technique for staging of urologic cancer. It demonstrates nodal involvement, invasion of surrounding tissues by the primary tumor, and hepatic metastases. However, CT scanning cannot visualize intranodal architecture or detect micrometastases in normal-sized nodes. Lymphangiography is capable of visualizing nodal architecture and metastases in nonenlarged nodes, and this modality is sometimes used in staging testis and prostate cancer. MRI scanning is sometimes helpful in renal cell carcinoma because it distinguishes lymph nodes from vessels and provides accurate information on renal vein/inferior venal caval tumor involvement.

In certain tumors (e.g., prostate, testis) radiologic imaging is not accurate, and surgical staging by lymphadenectomy is required. In addition to staging such tumors accurately (i.e., pathologic staging), lymphadenectomy may provide therapeutic benefits, both short term and long term, to some patients. The following discussions address the roles of surgical lymphadenectomy (pathologic staging, therapeutic) in the common urologic cancers.

RENAL CANCER

The value of lymphadenectomy in the treatment of renal cell carcinoma remains uncertain. The two benefits of regional lymphadenectomy in patients with renal cell carcinoma are more accurate staging of the extent of the disease and a potential therapeutic benefit.

Central to any discussion of the role of lymphadenectomy in renal cancer is an understanding of the anatomy of the renal lymphatics. The lymphatic channels of the right kidney are divided into posterior, anterior, and middle channels. The posterior channels drain into the postcaval nodes, the interaortocaval nodes from L-1 to L-3, the upper lateral caval nodes, and occasionally into the lymphatics that pass through the diaphragm into the thoracic duct. The right anterior lymphatic vessels course upward to join the posterior lymphatics, or they may drain into the precaval or upper interaortocaval nodes. The right middle lymphatic vessels drain into the posterior and anterior lymphatic chains. The regional nodes of the right kidney are therefore composed of the lateral caval, postcaval, precaval and interaortocaval nodes.

The left renal lymphatics are composed of anterior and posterior chains. The anterior lymphatics have superior and inferior branches that drain along the aorta and interconnect with the posterior chain. The posterior lymphatics pass through the crus of the diaphragm and end in postaortic nodes at T-11, T-12, and L-1. The regional nodes of the left kidney include the upper left lateral lumbar nodes, the preaortic and postaortic lymph nodes, and nodes on the left crus of the diaphragm and along the left renal vein.

With this anatomical background as a foundation, proponents of an extended lymphadenectomy for renal cancer advocate the following. A right radical nephrectomy should include dissection of the lateral caval, precaval, postcaval, and interaortocaval nodes. The limits of the dissection should start at the right crus of the diaphragm and extend inferiorly along the vena cava to its bifurcation and laterally over the psoas muscle. A left radical nephrectomy should encompass the left lateral lumbar nodes, the left diaphragmatic nodes, and the preaortic nodes. The dissection should begin at the left crus of the diaphragm and extend inferiorly to the aortic bifurcation. Because of these anatomic considerations, a retrocaval and interaortocaval dissection is important when performing a right radical nephrectomy. Retroaortic and interaortocaval dissections are included in regional lymphadenectomy fields during left radical nephrectomy.

Despite the anatomic studies of the lymphatic drainage of the kidneys, there is variation in the lymphatic drainage of renal tumors. Detailed pathologic examination of regional lymphadenectomy specimens has shown isolated iliac node metastases in the face of negative regional nodes. Lymph node metastases have been reported in 25 to 30% of patients undergoing radical nephrectomy (Table 18.3). The fundamental question is whether a regional lymphadenectomy affords patients with renal cell carcinoma a survival advantage. At present no prospective randomized study has addressed this question. However, a number of thoughtful reviews of the available data have been written. The incidence of positive nodes increases with tumor stage, that is, up to 3 times the incidence with T_3 tumors compared to T_1 or T_2 lesions. Therefore, many patients with T_3 tumors, with or without vascular invasion (perhaps 30 to 40%) may benefit from lymphadenectomy if distant metastases are absent.

Table 18.3: Lymph Node Metastases in Renal Cancer

Equal incidence of nodal and blood-borne metastases
Variable, extensive lymphatic drainage
Cross-over lymphatic drainage
Lymph node metastases in 25–30%
Lymphadenectomy
- Beneficial in T_3 disease with micrometastasis
- Margins not clearly defined
- Changing indications in era of immunotherapy

Clinicians who routinely perform an extended lymphadenectomy report a 5-year survival rate of 40 to 50% for patients with node-positive disease. This compares with survival rates of 10 to 20% in patients not undergoing regional lymphadenectomy. The dilemma with interpretation of these data lies in the fact that in cases where lymphadenectomy is not performed, patients with low volume or microscopic nodal involvement would be erroneously staged as having node-negative disease.

Another cogent question addresses the potential morbidity of regional lymphadenectomy in patients requiring surgery for renal cancer. The complications of an extended lymphadenectomy for renal cancer are similar to those of retroperitoneal lymphadenectomy for testis cancer. The major risks are bleeding, lymphocele formation, and prolonged operating time.

Some aspects of the biological behavior of renal cell carcinoma negate the role of regional lymphadenectomy. Renal cell cancer metastasizes equally via the bloodstream and lymphatics, and blood-borne metastases are common if lymph nodes are involved. A unique feature of renal cell carcinoma is the high rate of blood-borne metastases. Autopsy studies demonstrate that up to 30% of patients with distant (i.e., bone, lung) metastases do not have retroperitoneal node involvement. Metastases probably bypass the lymphatics and spread via hematogenous routes to distant sites. A regional lymph node dissection would therefore not benefit such patients. Furthermore, the variable lymphatic drainage and lymphatic crossover make it difficult to select the appropriate surgical margins for regional lymphadenectomy (Table 18.3). The therapeutic value of lymphadenectomy in renal cell cancers, at least regarding short-term survival and accurate staging, is generally accepted. A regional lymphadenectomy is usually performed as a standard part of a radical nephrectomy. However, the extent of the surgical dissection has not been clarified, and there is considerable variability among surgeons.

Unfortunately, the literature does not provide enough data to answer the question whether regional lymphadenectomy is of benefit in renal carcinoma. Recent data suggest that patients with T_3 disease and microscopic lymph node involvement, without evidence of distant metastases, are most likely to achieve cure with the addition of an extended regional lymphadenectomy. The therapeutic value of staging lymphadenectomy is uncertain, especially as nodal involvement is associated with a poor prognosis. However, the recent introduction of immunotherapy protocols (e.g., IL2-LAK cells, etc.) may lead to a reevaluation of the role of lymphadenectomy in renal cell carcinoma.

TESTIS CANCER

During fetal life the testes originate in the retroperitoneum near the kidneys and descend toward the scrotum. Because of these embryologic origins, testis cancer spreads via lymphatic channels to the retroperitoneal lymph nodes. Testicular germ cell tumors can be divided into four histologic types: seminoma, embryonal carcinoma, teratoma, and choriocarcinoma. Noninvasive radiologic staging of testis cancer has the same limitations as with other organs. CT scanning, MRI scanning, and lymphangiography cannot detect micrometastases in normal-sized nodes. It is therefore not surprising that retroperitoneal lymphadenectomy is the most accurate way of staging patients with testis cancer.

Most testicular cancers spread in a predictable fashion to the lymphatics (Figure 18.1). Vascular spread occurs early, particularly in non-

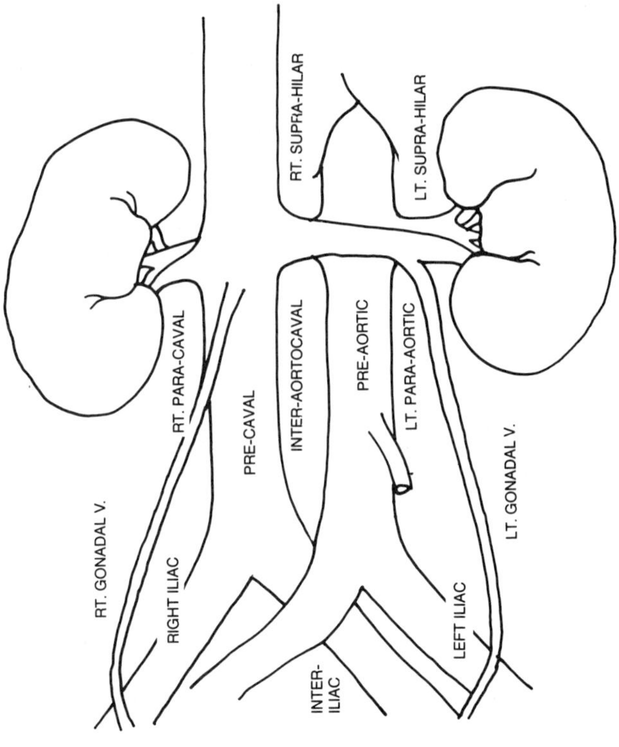

Figure 18.1: Landing sites of testicular cancer

seminomatous tumors (e.g., embryonal cell carcinoma) with microscopic vascular space (V positive) invasion. The primary drainage of the right testicle is the interaortocaval lymph nodes with subsequent spread to the precaval, preaortic, and paracaval nodes. Because of the right-to-left drain-age of the right testis, the left para-aortic nodes can be involved. The main drainage area of the left testis is the left para-aortic nodes just inferior to the left renal vein. Subsequent spread is to the preaortic nodes. Cross-metastases are more common with right-sided tumors. Iliac, inguinal, and suprahilar metastases are distinctly uncommon. Testis cancers are staged by the TNM or the Memorial Sloan Kettering Cancer Center System (Table 18.4).

Clinical and radiologic techniques frequently understage testicular cancer. The limit of detection of a retroperitoneal mass by CT scan is 1 to 1.5 cm, and this results in understaging of microscopic retroperitoneal disease. Lymphangiography can be used for staging, especially in seminomas, but this modality has not found widespread acceptance. The most accurate method for surgical/pathologic staging is retroperitoneal lymphadenectomy, especially in patients with low stage (A to B2) disease. Prior to the introduction of platinum-based multidrug chemotherapy, retroperitoneal lymphadenectomy was used not only for surgical staging but also as the primary mode of treatment.

Donohue has performed extensive analyses of the landing sites of testicular metastases in the retroperitoneum (Figure 18.2). On the basis of over 300 bilateral retroperitoneal lymph node dissections, he divided the retroperitoneal tissue into segments for zonal analysis: right paracaval,

Table 18.4: Staging of Testis Cancer

Memorial Sloan Kettering System	*TNM System*
Stage A: confined to testis	Tumor (T)
Stage B: retroperitoneal spread	T_1: tumor in testis
$B_1 < 5$ cm	T_2: tumor involves inguinal end of cord
$B_2 > 5$ cm	T_3: invasion through testis capsule;
$B_3 > 10$ cm	scrotal orchiectomy
Stage C: beyond retroperitoneum	Nodes (N)
	N_1: microscopic disease
	N_2: enlarged nodes
	N_3: extension into areolar tissue
	Metastases (M)
	M_0: no distant metastasis
	M_1: distant metastasis

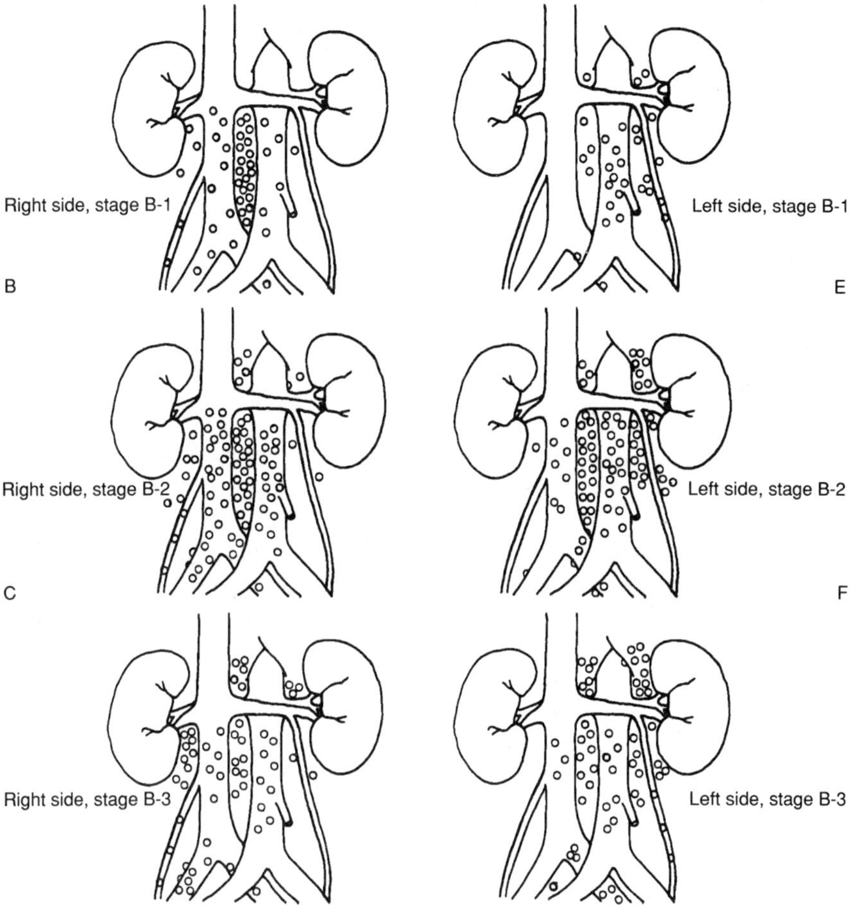

Figure 18.2: Nodal metastases in testis cancer. CD Donohue J Urol 1982;128:315

precaval, interaortocaval, preaortic, left para-aortic, right suprahilar, left suprahilar, right iliac, left iliac, interiliac, and gonadal zones. These tumor landing sites were analyzed with respect to the stage and the side of the primary tumor (Table 18.5). The interaortocaval zone just below the left renal vein is the most common site of tumor deposition from right-sided testis tumors. The preaortic and left para-aortic are the most common sites of tumor nodal metastases from the left testicle. There is a positive correlation between the extent of disease and involvement of suprahilar nodes. The suprahilar zones are rarely involved in low stage (B_1) disease. Suprahilar nodes are usually negative in stage B_1 disease if the primary tumor is on the right side. However, 20% are positive with

Table 18.5: Distribution of Nodal Metastases in Testis Cancer

Interaortocaval nodes for right-sided tumors
Para-aortic nodes for left-sided tumors
Suprahilar nodal disease
More common with left-sided tumors
Higher incidence with bulky retroperitoneal disease (B_2, B_3)
Ipsilateral iliac nodes rarely involved
Gonadal vein lymphatic involvement uncommon

left-sided B_1 disease. The suprahilar area is more often involved in stage B_2 disease: 13 to 33% if the primary is on the right, and 16 to 42% if it is on the left. Gonadal veins and their lymphatics are involved with tumor in 8 to 17% of patients. The ipsilateral iliac nodes are rarely involved in low stage disease. Thus, patients with minimal volume disease (stages A, B_1, B_2) undergoing retroperitoneal lymphadenectomy do not routinely require suprahilar dissection, especially for right-sided tumors. Occasionally, a left-sided tumor may have suprahilar spread due to the high insertion of the gonadal vein. For low-volume tumors, modified node dissections that spare the contralateral package (paracaval, para-aortic) are now recommended and result in better preservation of ejaculation and fertility and greater patient acceptability.

With this anatomic and pathologic foundation, the question of the role of retroperitoneal lymphadenectomy in the management of testis cancer can be addressed. It is wise to preface this discussion by stating that much controversy still exists over the optimal management of testis cancer. Because of the radiosensitivity of seminoma, the majority of patients with low stage disease (stage A, B_1) are treated with radiation therapy directed toward the periaortic and ipsilateral inguinopelvic lymph nodes. In bulky retroperitoneal disease (stage B_2, B_3) or in patients with distant metastases, initial treatment is usually with multi-drug chemotherapy. Chemotherapy protocols vary from institution to institution, but *cis*-platinum appears to be the most active chemotherapeutic agent.

Retroperitoneal lymph node dissection remains the cornerstone of treatment of nonseminomatous germ cell tumors (Table 18.6). Traditionally, clinical stage A nonseminomatous testis tumors have been treated with a retroperitoneal lymph node dissection. This treatment schema was based on survival rates of greater than 95% using surgical treatment for low stage disease. However, with the advent of more effective chemotherapy, as well as more accurate staging with CT scan and tumor markers, a case

Table 18.6: Rationale for Lymphadenectomy for Testis Cancer

Consistent pattern and progression of nodal metastases
Nodal disease greatly exceeds and predates hematogenous metastases
Suprahilar metastases uncommon with low-stage disease
Lymphadenectomy
Curative
Surgical margins defined
Limited, nerve-sparing operations
New approach by laparoscopic lymphadenectomy

can be made for observation alone in patients with clinical stage A disease. The rationale and attractiveness for this surveillance treatment approach are the avoidance of the morbidity of retroperitoneal lymph node dissection. Recent reports have demonstrated the utility of observation rather than retroperitoneal node dissection in carefully selected patients. Patients who elect to undergo surveillance for their testis tumors should have negative tumor markers, normal abdominal CT scans, and no evidence of vascular space invasion (lymphatic, vascular) by microscopic examination of the orchiectomy specimen.

Currently, 20 to 25% of patients with clinical stage I (stage A) disease are understaged using noninvasive radiologic imaging techniques. However, the recent impressive improvements in chemotherapy for metastatic disease have led to the emergence of surveillance protocols for patients with clinically localized disease (Table 18.7). Further impetus to the use of these protocols are the following: (1) approximately 70% of patients who undergo retroperitoneal lymphadenectomy will have nega-

Table 18.7: Surveillance Protocols for Stage I Nonseminomatous Testis Cancer

Advantages	*Disadvantages*
Attractive to patient	Requires compliant patient
No surgical/anesthesia risk	Careful, frequent clinic visits
No ejaculatory dysfunction	Long-term costs
Lower initial costs	Less favorable relapse model (lungs plus retroperitoneum)
Excellent cure rate in patients who relapse	Relapses require chemotherapy with increased toxicity
	Death rate higher than RPLND
	Patient anxiety

tive nodes (stage A disease) and derive no therapeutic benefit in spite of the risks of mortality and morbidity, (2) between 5 and 10% of patients relapse outside the field of the surgical dissection, and (3) the risks of postsurgical loss of ejaculation and fertility are eliminated. The overall relapse rate in surveillance protocols varies between 20 and 30%, and many relapses occur in more advanced stages. Although patients who relapse respond to four courses of platinum-based chemotherapy, the overall death rate is about 7%.

Patients who enter surveillance protocols should be carefully selected and actively monitored for compliance and tumor relapse. Frequent clinic visits are important (every month for 1 year, every 2 months for the second year, and every 3 to 6 months beyond the second year for at least 5 years). Several prognostic factors help to stratify the risk of relapse. High-risk groups include patients with embryonal carcinoma, the presence of vascular or lymphatic invasion, and tumor involvement of the epididymis or tunica albuginea.

As the treatment of testicular cancer has continued to evolve, efforts have been made to reduce the morbidity of retroperitoneal lymph node dissection. Based on the knowledge of the pattern and location of retroperitoneal lymph node metastases, a modified lymphadenectomy has been recommended for low stage nonseminomatous tumors so as to preserve ejaculatory function. This approach in low stage disease has resulted in preservation of ejaculation in approximately 80 to 90% of patients and a relapse rate of less than 10%. The anatomic dissection is complete above the level of the inferior mesenteric artery but limited to a unilateral, ipsilateral dissection below the inferior mesenteric artery in an attempt to preserve the sympathetic chain plexus around the terminal aorta and aortic bifurcation. The anatomical boundaries of the limited retroperitoneal node dissection are outlined in Figure 18.3.

The surgical limits of retroperitoneal lymphadenectomies performed before the modern era of multidrug chemotherapy included a complete bilateral dissection from above the renal arteries, bilaterally limited by the ureters down to the level where the ureters crossed the common iliac arteries. Complete removal of nodal tissue was essential to cure, especially before the advent of successful chemotherapy. The success of combination chemotherapy in curing testis cancer has led to greater attention being paid to such quality-of-life issues as fertility and ejaculation. Ejaculation depends on emission caused by contraction of the ampulla of the vas, seminal vesicle, and periurethral glands, and this coincides with closure of the bladder neck. The thoracolumbar sympathetic outflow (T-12 to L-3) is responsible for ejaculation. Nerve fibers arise from the sympathetic ganglia, converge and intermingle as a plexus anterior to the

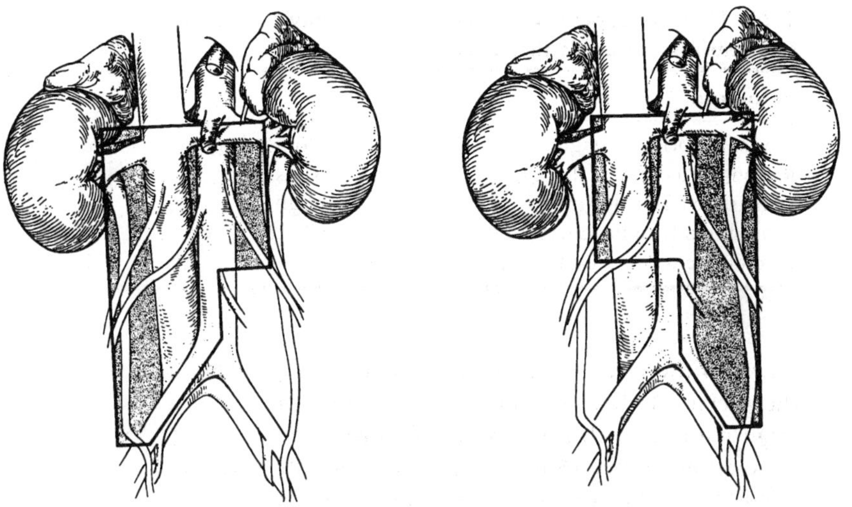

(a) Right (b) Left

Figure 18.3: Boundaries of modified retroperitoneal node dissection for testis cancer. Modified templates for retroperitoneal node dissection. Note complete bilateral dissection above the level of the inferior mesenteric artery and a unilateral dissection below this level. The tissues over the aortic bifurcation are spared. (After J.P. Richie.)

aorta and aortic bifurcation, and then course over the common iliac arteries into the pelvis as the hypogastric plexus and pelvic nerves. Surgical injury to these fibers, especially in the region of the aortic bifurcation, results in ejaculatory dysfunction.

Modification of the surgical boundaries of retroperitoneal lymphadenectomy results in preservation of ejaculatory function in most patients. The knowledge of the anatomy of the sympathetic preaortic plexus and the primary nodal drainage sites of low stage testicular cancer has resulted in a variety of modifications to the standard, complete retroperitoneal lymphadenectomy. In these modifications, the dissection is fully bilateral between the level of the renal veins and the inferior mesenteric artery. All lumbar vessels between these margins are divided to remove node-bearing tissue from behind the aorta and vena cava. Below the level of the inferior mesenteric artery, the dissection includes the ipsilateral great vessel including the common iliac artery and the ipsilateral side of the aorta. This modified dissection makes it possible to preserve the ipsilateral ganglia and postganglionic nerves, which are adjacent to the vertebral bodies. The ipsilateral spermatic vessels are excised

Table 18.8: Retroperitoneal Lymphadenectomy for Clinical Stage I Nonseminomatous Testicular Cancer

Advantages	*Disadvantages*
Precise pathologic staging	Nontherapeutic in majority (80%)
Rational selection of therapy	Risks of surgery, anesthesia
Antegrade ejaculation with modified lymphadenectomy	Higher initial cost
Predictable relapse model (lungs)	Chest relapses in 10%

down to the level of the internal inguinal ring, including the stump of the previously ligated spermatic cord. Modified dissections adequately stage patients with stage A and B_1 disease while preserving antegrade ejaculation (Table 18.8). In general, ejaculation is preserved more frequently in right-sided modified lymphadenectomies, especially when the Donohue template is used. Refinements in nerve-sparing techniques for retroperitoneal lymphadenectomy include identification of individual retroperitoneal sympathetic nerves during surgery in an attempt to preserve ejaculatory function. However, surgical lymphadenectomy presents certain risks and disadvantages (Table 18.8).

The success of nerve-sparing techniques in preserving ejaculation in patients with low-volume, early-stage retroperitoneal lymphatic metastases has been an important advance in surgical urologic oncology. Modified or limited retroperitoneal node dissections are an attractive alternative to observation protocols. They eliminate the risk of pathologic understaging, provide complete removal of nodal tissue from the primary drainage sites, and preserve ejaculation in the majority of patients. Staging lymphadenectomy in patients with persistent retroperitoneal masses following chemotherapy also provides information about the nature of such masses (fibrosis, mature teratoma, or residual carcinoma).

Until noninvasive staging techniques become more accurate, modified retroperitoneal lymphadenectomy will continue to play a critical role in the treatment of nonseminomatous testicular cancer.

BLADDER CARCINOMA

Invasive bladder cancer is an aggressive disease with the potential for metastatic spread. The pelvic lymph nodes constitute the first-echelon nodes for the spread of bladder cancer. Lymphatic metastases in bladder cancer, unlike renal cancer, occur early and are independent of blood-borne spread. The incidence of nodal metastases relates directly to the pathologic stage of the primary bladder tumor. Lymph nodes are involved in 75% of patients dying of bladder cancer. The obturator and external iliac nodes are the most commonly affected.

It remains controversial whether patients with positive lymph nodes can be cured with lymphadenectomy alone. A continuing dilemma in treating bladder cancer is that of clinical understaging. Transurethral tumor resection provides critical information about the depth of penetration of bladder cancer. However, the utility of preoperative staging by CT scans and other methods is limited by the sensitivity and specificity of the radiologic techniques. Lymphadenectomy is perhaps the most accurate method of evaluating the pelvic nodes in patients with bladder cancer. Lymphadenectomy provides accurate pathologic staging and may be of clinical benefit in patients with minimal nodal (i.e., microscopic) involvement (Table 18.9). Approximately 20 to 30% of patients undergoing radical cystectomy for clinically staged, organ-confined disease (by CT scan, etc.) have micrometastasis in their pelvic lymph nodes. This clinical understaging is a cogent argument to perform a regional pelvic lymphadenectomy in patients with bladder cancer undergoing radical cystectomy. Although it is rare for a bladder cancer patient with bulky nodal disease to survive for more than 18 to 24 months, a significant number of patients (up to 25 or 30%) with clinically undetectable nodal micrometastases survive beyond 5 years. The incidence of pelvic nodal metastases increases with tumor stage and grade, ranging from 10% in noninvasive tumors to 40% in high-grade, deeply infiltrating cancers. Interestingly, 35 to 65% of these nodal metastases are limited to 1 or 2 nodes below the iliac bifurcation and are microscopic.

The incidence of recurrence of local pelvic tumor is lower in patients who undergo an en-bloc pelvic lymphadenectomy at the time of radical cystectomy. The wide discrepancy between the clinical and pathologic staging of bladder cancer is a compelling rationale for regional lym-

Table 18.9: Nodal Disease in Bladder Cancer

Wide discrepancy between clinical and pathologic staging
Lymphatic metastases occur early and independent of blood-borne metastases
Micrometastases in 20–35% of patients with clinically staged, organ-confined disease
Lymphadenectomy
Useful in patients with micrometastases
En-bloc lymphadenectomy reduces chances of pelvic recurrence
Margins well defined

phadenectomy at the time of cystectomy. Despite the presence of positive nodes 2-, 3-, and 5-year survival rates of 46, 36, and 36%, respectively, have been reported. Thus, it appears reasonable to perform pelvic lymphadenectomy at the time of radical cystectomy. The limits of pelvic lymphadenectomy vary among surgeons. The standard lymphadenectomy includes the nodes from the iliac bifurcation to the femoral canal. A more cephalad dissection to the level of the aortic bifurcation is espoused by some urologists.

Over the past decade, with the advent of more effective chemotherapy, many urologists have modified their indications for pelvic lymphadenectomy in patients with invasive bladder carcinoma. Chemotherapy regimens such as M-VAC (methotrexate, vinblastine, doxorubicin, and cisplatin) have achieved partial and complete response rates in over 80% of patients with invasive bladder cancer, and complete remission was achieved in 37±10% of the patients. These data have caused most urologists to adopt new treatment approaches for the management of invasive bladder cancers.

Half of the patients with muscle invasive bladder cancer have occult/overt metastases elsewhere, and this limits the efficacy of locoregional forms of therapy such as lymphadenectomy. As advances in chemotherapy, radiation therapy, and combination therapy continue to evolve, surgery may play a less prominent role in the treatment of invasive bladder cancer. At present, pelvic lymphadenectomy provides accurate pathologic staging, and in selected patients it may contribute to surgical cure.

PROSTATE CANCER

Prostate cancer is the most common malignancy in American men, with approximately 132,000 new cases diagnosed annually. In general, regional nodal involvement in prostate cancer signifies a suboptimal outcome in patients undergoing radical prostatectomy. Such patients are believed to be better treated with radiation therapy or chemotherapy. Thus, the identification of nodal metastases is of paramount importance in the selection of therapy for patients with prostatic cancer. The obturator and iliac lymph nodes are the first-echelon nodes to be involved by metastatic prostate cancer. The distribution of nodal metastases in prostate cancer is outlined in Table 18.10.

The management of prostatic cancer is still controversial, and this makes the discussion of the role of lymphadenectomy problematic. Experience with bilateral pelvic lymphadenectomy and radical prostatectomy, with and without early hormonal therapy for stage D_1 disease, has

Table 18.10: Nodal Metastases in Prostate Cancer

Occur independently of hematogenous, bony, or local dissemination
Obturator nodes are primary drainage sites
Bilateral involvement 50%
Rare "skipping"
Low-volume metastases 20 to 30%
Lymphadenectomy
Most useful for pathologic staging
Modified, limited lymphadenectomy
Laparoscopic lymphadenectomy
Allows appropriate treatment selection
Node involvement by clinical stage
Stage A_1: 2%
A_2: 23%
Stage B_1: 18%
B_2: 35%
Stage C: 50–80%

been reported. Although early hormonal treatment is beneficial, particularly in patients with diploid tumors, all patients with D_1 disease who had bilateral pelvic lymphadenectomy and radical prostatectomy alone eventually had disease progression. The available data suggest that about 80% of men having microscopic pelvic lymph node metastases will develop distant metastases within 5 years. It is generally agreed that patients with stage D_1 cancer have systemic disease and that local therapy alone (surgery or radiation) is unlikely to be curative.

Therefore, it appears that the role of pelvic lymphadenectomy in prostate cancer is one of pathologic staging rather than therapy. The common sites of spread of prostate cancer are the pelvic lymph nodes, the periprostatic space, and the axial skeleton (i.e., pelvis, spine, thorax). Clinical data from patients undergoing radical prostatectomy indicate that capsular/periprostatic spread (e.g., perineural spaces, seminal vesicle involvement) is common and occurs in up to 30 to 40% of patients without nodal or bony metastases. Furthermore, unlike renal cell cancer, lymph node metastases occur independently of hematogenous and/or bone dissemination (Table 18.10). The main site of spread of prostate cancer is the pelvic lymph nodes, particularly the obturator nodes, nodes situated in the triangle bordered by the external iliac, obturator, and internal iliac vessels. Studies of involved nodes have shown the following: bilateral nodal involvement in over 50% of patients, near universal involvement of the obturator nodes, rare "skipping" of the obturator nodes to involve the external or common iliac nodes, and involvement (low-volume) of one to two nodes in up to one-third of patients (Table 18.10). This knowledge has led to the widespread use of a limited or modified bilateral pelvic lymphadenectomy for accurate pathologic staging of prostate cancer.

The obturator nodes not only are involved more frequently than other pelvic nodes but also are involved earlier. The occurrence of pelvic lymph node metastases is directly related to tumor volume and histologic grade. However, direct assessment and evaluation of the regional lymph nodes are essential to the process of selection of the appropriate treatment modality. The increasing use and sophistication of prostate specific antigen (PSA) levels as well as PSA density measurements may, in the future, lessen the need for accurate pretreatment assessment of nodal status.

A variety of techniques are available to determine the presence of nodal metastases. CT and MRI scanning have been somewhat disappointing for staging prostatic cancer. False-negative findings are not uncommon, especially in patients with low-volume nodal metastases. Pedal lymphangiography with visualization of pelvic nodes has also been used as a staging modality. However, this technique fails to visualize the obturator and hypogastric nodal chains consistently. Selective percutaneous nodal aspiration using CT or lymphangiographic guidance has been employed to assess the nodal status of patients with prostatic cancer.

Because of the limitations of PSA, CT, and MRI in predicting pelvic lymph node involvement, surgical staging remains the most accurate method of determining the pathologic status of the pelvic lymph nodes in patients with prostate cancer. Recently, a laparoscopic approach to pelvic lymphadenectomy has been introduced, and the initial experience suggests that laparoscopic pelvic lymphadenectomy offers the potential for accurate staging of pelvic nodes, with decreased morbidity.

Although Gleason score grading, lymphangiography, and CT/MRI scanning can be used, the definitive technique for identifying pelvic nodal metastases is pelvic lymphadenectomy: removal and pathologic analysis of the obturator nodes. The standard pelvic lymphadenectomy for prostatic cancer staging includes the external iliac, obturator, and internal iliac nodes. However, a modified dissection, preserving the lymphatics around the external iliac artery and those distal to the circumflex iliac vein, causes significantly less genital and lower-extremity lymphedema. The incidence of lymph node metastases with the modified dissection is similar (85 to 90%) to that of the standard pelvic lymphadenectomy. Lymphadenectomy has a potentially small survival therapeutic benefit in patients with well differentiated micrometastases in few lymph nodes. In general, however, patients with documented nodal disease may best be served by either radiation or chemotherapeutic treatment. The distribution of metastases in the pelvic lymph nodes is well known and has allowed the performance of limited or modified pelvic lymphadenectomy focused on the obturator and hypogastric nodes. If the pelvic nodes are not palpably enlarged, some surgeons eliminate the frozen-section analysis and proceed to definitive radical prostatectomy. Because most micrometastases occur in grossly normal nodes, routine frozen sections are still indicated despite the small but definite incidence of false-negative evaluations (5 to 10%). Patients in this category may well benefit therapeutically because of their low-volume disease status.

PENILE CANCER

In North America, penile cancer is the most infrequently encountered of the major urologic malignancies. Incidence rates for penile cancer have wide geographic variation, and penile cancer is the most common GU cancer in certain African and South American countries. The most commonly used classification system is outlined in Table 18.11. Clinical staging of patients with penile carcinoma is highly inaccurate. Up to 20% of patients with clinically negative nodes harbor occult nodal metastases, and as many as 50% with palpably enlarged nodes do not have nodal metastases on histologic examination.

The prognosis for patients with carcinoma of the penis correlates

Table 18.11: Penile Cancer

Jackson Staging System

Stage I: confined to glans/prepuce
Stage II: corporal invasion
Stage III: nodal metastases
Stage IV: distant metastases

Nodal Metastases

Much more common than blood-borne metastases
Micrometastases present in 20% of patients
Palpable inguinal nodes
 50% positive for cancer

Lymphadenectomy

Essential for disease cure
Deep pelvic nodal involvement associated with poor prognosis
Comparable survival with immediate versus delayed lymphadenectomy

with tumor stage. The 5-year survival rate for patients with stage I and II disease is 90 and 65% respectively. For patients with nodal metastases the 5-year survival rate is 30 to 40%. The presence or absence of lymph node metastases affects survival more than tumor grade. Penile cancers have a propensity for local spread to the corporal tissues or glans penis. Blood-borne metastases are rare, and lymphatic metastases are the common metastases. Death from penile cancer is usually from metastatic disease, and this makes the role of lymphadenectomy critical. Although the treatment of the local lesion is the main concern of the patients, survival depends on the status and management of the regional lymph nodes (inguinal, pelvic). Micrometastases are present in about 20% of patients with clinically negative (i.e., by palpation, CT scans, etc.) nodes.

The lymphatic drainage of the penis includes the superficial inguinal nodes and the pelvic nodes. The lymphatics of the penile skin and prepuce course to the superficial inguinal nodes primarily in the compartment of the femoral sheath medial to the femoral vein. The lymphatics from the glans penis and the corporal bodies drain into the superficial inguinal nodes as well as to the pelvic nodes. Pelvic lymph node involvement without inguinal node involvement is exceedingly rare. The presence of inguinal nodal metastases cannot be reliably assessed clinically. Approximately 50% of patients with palpable inguinal nodes do not have metastases on histological examination, and 20% of patients with clinically negative nodes have micrometastases present (Table 18.11).

Patients with palpable inguinal nodes should receive 4 to 6 weeks of antibiotics. If the nodes remain palpable after this course of antibiotics, the patient should undergo a bilateral ilioinguinal node dissection. A bilateral dissection is recommended on the basis of data reporting bilateral disease in about 60% of patients with metastatic penile cancer. Because of the morbidity associated with the superficial inguinal node dissection, the pelvic nodes should be examined first at the time of surgery. If extensive lymph node involvement is present above the external iliac vessels, surgical cure is unlikely, and the superficial inguinal node dissection should not be performed.

A more difficult question is what to do in the case of clinically and radiologically negative nodes. Three factors should be considered when deciding whether to operate on nonpalpable inguinal nodes in penile cancer. First, the extent of the primary lesion is of importance. Patients with stage I lesions have a reported 5 to 11% incidence of lymph node metastases, whereas patients with stage II lesions have a 66% incidence of positive nodes. Second, the inaccuracy of lymph node biopsies also impacts on the decision regarding surgery. Biopsy of the so-called "sentinel" node was initially advocated by Cabanas. This node is situated near the anteromedial aspect of the superficial epigastric vein near the junction with the greater saphenous vein. Cabanas reported that if the "sentinel" node biopsy was negative, patients were unlikely to have superficial inguinal node involvement with tumor. However subsequent investigators have failed to reproduce his findings, and it is now generally accepted that a lymph node biopsy is not a good predictor of metastases. Third, most reported clinical experiences suggest that cure rates are comparable for delayed versus immediate node dissections in patients with nonpalpable nodes at the time of initial presentation. For these reasons it would appear that close follow-up with surgical intervention if the inguinal nodes become palpable is the prudent therapy for patients with penile cancer who initially present with nonpalpable inguinal nodes.

The technique of ilioinguinal node dissection has undergone modification to try to minimize morbidity. The pelvic node dissection is performed first, and only if the pelvic nodes are negative is the superficial inguinal dissection performed. Various skin incisions for the inguinal node dissection have been described, but our preference is an incision that transverses the groin crease and affords better exposure. The use of the Scott ring retractor has proven valuable in minimizing handling of the skin edges and avoiding skin necrosis and wound breakdown. The saphenous vein, the first major landmark encountered, leads to the fossa ovalis. The limits of the superficial groin dissection are the inguinal ligament superiorly, the adductor longus muscle medially, the sartorius muscle laterally, and the apex of the femoral triangle inferiorly. At the conclusion of the dissection, the sartorius muscle is divided from the iliac crest and sutured to the inguinal ligament to cover and protect the femoral vessels in case a wound infection occurs. Hemovac drains are routinely left to minimize postoperative hematoma or lymphocele formation. The patients are asked to wear antiembolic stockings postoperatively and are given anticoagulation therapy until they leave the hospital.

CONCLUSIONS

The rationale for lymphadenectomy in genitourinary cancers is multifactorial. It frequently provides more accurate staging (i.e., pathologic) than the commonly used diagnostic radiologic imaging techniques such as CT scanning, MRI scanning, and lymphangiography. Furthermore, in some tumors, regional lymphadenectomy may confer added therapeutic benefit to patients with low-volume, microscopic nodal metastases.

The increasing use of immunotherapy protocols for renal cell cancer and the introduction of multidrug chemotherapy for bladder cancer further impact on the role of lymphadenectomy in these cancers. The current trend in surgical lymphadenectomy is toward more limited, selected dissection fields, and this results in significantly less morbidity in patients with nonseminomatous testis cancers. The indications and role of regional lymphadenectomy in the staging and treatment of urologic cancers may well undergo further evolution and change.

SUGGESTED READINGS

Marshall FF, Powell KC. Lymphadenectomy for renal cell carcinoma: anatomical and therapeutic considerations. J Urol 1982; 128:677.

Extensive review of the lymphatic drainage of the kidneys and its surgical implications with regard to lymphadenectomy.

Donohue JP, Zachary JM, Maynard BR. Distribution of nodal metastases in nonseminomatous testis cancer. J Urol 1982; 128:315.

Clearly written article on landing sites and nodal distribution of testis cancer. This is the basis of the modified, limited retroperitoneal lymphadenectomies.

Sogani P, Fair W. Surveillance alone in the treatment of clinical stage 1 nonseminomatous germ cell tumors of the testis. Semin Urol 1988; 6:53.

The case for nonoperative treatment of Stage I nonseminomatous germ cell tumors is presented.

Donohue JP, Foster RS, Rowland RG, Bihrle R, Jones J, Geier G. Nerve-sparing retroperitoneal lymphadenectomy with preservation of ejaculation. J Urol 1990; 144:287.

The description and rationale for modified retroperitoneal lymphadenectomy is presented with particular reference to the preservation of ejaculatory function.

Skinner DG. Management of invasive bladder cancer: a meticulous pelvic node dissection can make a difference. J Urol 1982; 128:34.

Presents the view that extensive lymphadenectomy can be curative in bladder cancer.

Herr HW, Whitmore WF Jr, Morse MJ, Sogani PC, Russo P, Fair WR. Neoadjuvant chemotherapy in invasive bladder cancer: the evolving role of surgery. J Urol 1990; 144:1083.

Current experience with multimodality treatment of bladder cancer is outlined and the changing role of surgery addressed.

Raghavan D, Shipley WU, Garnick MB, Russell PJ, Richie JP. Biology and management of bladder cancer. New Engl J Med 1990; 322: 1129.

Overview of current controversies regarding bladder cancer. Succinct discussion of the biologic determinants of bladder cancer and available treatment modalities.

McDougal WS, Kirchner FK Jr, Edwards RH. Treatment of carcinoma of the penis: the case for primary lymphadenectomy. J Urol 1986; 136:38.

Review of the controversial issues regarding the role of lymphadenectomy in penile cancer.

Wespes E, Simon J, Schulman CC. Cabanas' approach: is sentinel node biopsy reliable for staging of penile carcinoma? Urology 1986; 28:278.

Review of the "sentinel node" controversy.

Loughlin KR. Technique of ilioinguinal node dissection. Contemp Surg 1988; 33(2):33.

Outline of the surgical technique of the ilioinguinal node dissection.

Richie JP. Clinical stage I testicular cancer: the role of modified retroperitoneal lymphadenectomy. J Urol 1990; 144:1160.

Review of the indications and results of the modified retroperitoneal lymphadenectomy in low-stage testicular cancer.

Cabanas RM. An approach for the treatment of penile cancer. Cancer 1977; 39:456.

Classic paper describing the anatomy of the "sentinel node" and the role of the sentinel node biopsy in the management of penile cancer.

Index

D

O

Q

S